The Inseparable Nature of
Love and Aggression

··■··

Clinical and Theoretical Perspectives

The Inseparable Nature of
Love and Aggression

–■–

Clinical and Theoretical Perspectives

by

Otto F. Kernberg, M.D.

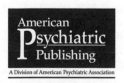

American Psychiatric Publishing

A Division of American Psychiatric Association

Washington, DC
London, England

Copyright © 2012 American Psychiatric Association
ALL RIGHTS RESERVED

Manufactured in the United States of America on acid-free paper
21   5 4 3 2
First Edition
Typeset in Centennial and Poppl-Laudatio.

American Psychiatric Publishing
A Division of American Psychiatric Association
1000 Wilson Boulevard
Arlington, VA 22209-3901
www.appi.org

Library of Congress Cataloging-in-Publication Data
Kernberg, Otto F., 1928-
The inseparable nature of love and aggression : clinical and theoretical perspectives / by Otto F. Kernberg. — 1st ed.
      p. ; cm.
  Includes bibliographical references and index.
  ISBN 978-1-58562-428-7 (pbk. : alk. paper) 1. Personality disorders—Treatment. 2. Psychotherapy. I. Title.
  [DNLM: 1. Personality Disorders—therapy. 2. Aggression—psychology. 3. Love. 4. Psychoanalytic Theory. 5. Psychotherapy. WM 190]
  RC554.K456 2012
  616.85′81—dc23
                                        2011022586

British Library Cataloguing in Publication Data
A CIP record is available from the British Library.

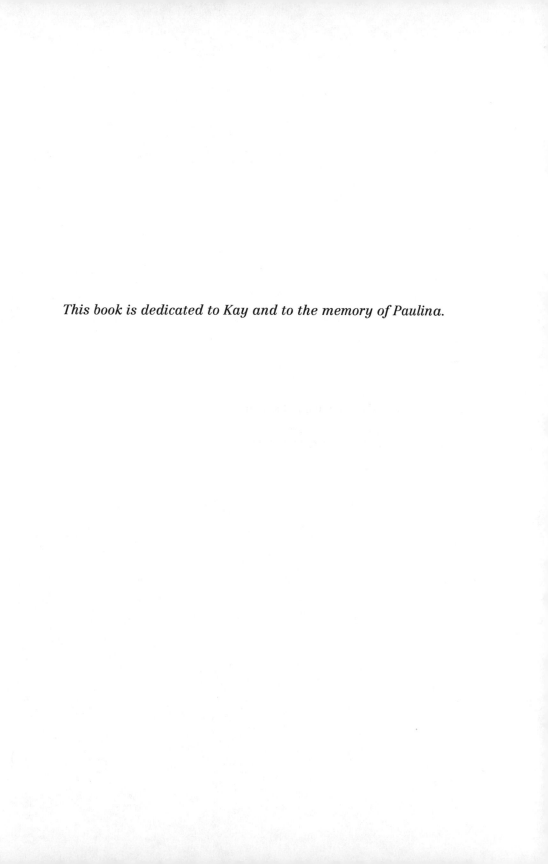

This book is dedicated to Kay and to the memory of Paulina.

Contents

PART I
Severe Personality Disorders

PART IV
Contemporary Challenges for Psychoanalysis

PART V
The Psychology of Religious Experience

About the Author

Otto F. Kernberg, M.D., is Director of the Personality Disorders Institute, Professor of Psychiatry, and DeWitt Wallace Senior Scholar at the Weill Cornell Medical College, New York, New York, as well as Training and Supervising Analyst of the Columbia University Center for Psychoanalytic Training and Research. Formerly, Dr. Kernberg served as Director of the C.F. Menninger Memorial Hospital, Supervising and Training Analyst of the Topeka Institute for Psychoanalysis, and Director of the Psychotherapy Research Project of the Menninger Foundation. The recipient of numerous awards for excellence in psychiatry and author or coauthor of more than twenty books in the field, Dr. Kernberg is also Past President of the International Psychoanalytical Association.

Introduction

This volume brings together my work in recent years with severe personality disorders, couples in conflict, and psychoanalytic research and education. This work has been strongly influenced by the collaborative research and clinical work of the Personality Disorders Institute at the Weill Cornell Medical College at the Westchester Division of the New York Presbyterian Hospital and reflects a major effort to carry out a boundary function between a psychoanalytic, a clinical psychiatric, and a neurobiological approach.

The title *The Inseparable Nature of Love and Aggression* refers to the corresponding major motivations of human psychology in Freud's classical drive theory of libido and the death drive. The confrontation with this theory in the light of contemporary knowledge, as well as the consistent encounter with this antinomy of disposition in clinical practice, has inspired this title.

This overall focus is reflected in the sections of this book: Part I explores new approaches to diagnosis and treatment of the most severe personality disorders, particularly the spectrum of severe narcissistic psychopathology. Our research findings have been published elsewhere, but here I am communicating our clinical experience and the development of new psychotherapeutic techniques.

Chapter 1 defines and updates the concept of identity and explains its central function in differentiating severe personality disorders from less severe ones, that is, the spectrum of "borderline personality organization" as differentiated from "neurotic personality organization." In the chapter, I analyze the developmental origins of normal identity and its relation to attachment and clarify the difference between identity and overall personality organization. In this context, a summary of contemporary psychoanalytic object relations theory places the concept of identity within a broader developmental frame. I then illustrate the clinical evaluation of identity with a detailed case explored with the technical approach of transference-focused psychotherapy (TFP)—a specific psychodynamic psychotherapy for borderline personality disorders and severe personality disorders in general developed in our Institute for Personality Disorders.

Chapter 2 provides an overall description of TFP, summarizing, in the process, the overall strategies, tactics, and techniques for the treatment of individual patients, followed by the application of this approach to group psychotherapy. TFP has been empirically studied, with randomized clinical trials demonstrating its efficacy and comparing it with alternative treatment methods carried out in our institute and replicated in a randomized controlled trial in Munich and Vienna. This chapter includes, in fact, a summary of the recently published updated version of the manual of TFP.

Chapter 3 focuses on essential mechanisms of change operating in psychodynamic psychotherapies in general, and in TFP in particular, namely, improvement in reflective function or "mentalization." In this chapter, I review critically the corresponding literature and relate it to the corresponding development, within cognitive-behavioral psychotherapies, of the concept of "mindfulness." This exploration leads to the role of interpretation as a central technique in TFP and its illustration with a detailed clinical case of a borderline patient where interpretation was carried out in an early treatment session.

Chapter 4 explores one other key element in the psychodynamic psychotherapy of severe personality disorders, namely, the therapist's management of the countertransference—that is, the activation of powerful affective reactions in the therapist as a consequence of his or her encounter with and efforts to understand the severely regressive emotional transference reactions of these patients. Here I review and update the management of countertransference under particularly difficult treatment situations, illustrating it with clinical case material.

The analysis of particularly challenging and difficult treatment situations, the almost "impossible" cases that often defy even experienced therapists' efforts, is explored in detail in Chapters 5 and 6. These two chapters focus on patients with severe narcissistic personality disorders, a frequent comorbidity of borderline personality disorders, that typically includes a significant group of treatment-resistant patients. In these two chapters, I describe difficult and challenging complications that may arise in the corresponding treatments and how to diagnose and deal with them. In particular, Chapter 6 points to a subtle but potentially highly destructive neglect of the passage of time in some severely ill patients and in the development of their corresponding treatments.

The treatment of severe personality disorders requires, on the part of the clinician at any level of expertise, the possibility of consulting with colleagues and, at times, obtaining supervision. In Chapter 7, I discuss the role of the consultant or supervisor of psychodynamic psychotherapies and his or her tasks and challenges, and, above all, I spell out realistic requirements for such delicate and responsible work.

Part II deals with new approaches within psychoanalytic theory and its relation to contemporary neurobiological findings. Here I try to illuminate the influences of neurobiological structures and intrapsychic conflicts on the development of the personality and argue against the temptations of reductionism on both sides. In Chapter 8, I examine contemporary affect theory, from the viewpoint of both developments in the understanding of the neurobiological structures and neurotransmitters involved in affect activation and the influence on affect development of early infant-caregiver interactions, and relate these findings to the psychoanalytic theory of drives. The relation between drive theory and affect theory becomes a complex, highly relevant field of psychodynamic and neurobiological interaction, and I propose an integrated view of this relation.

Chapter 9 examines the controversial psychoanalytic theory of the death drive, an inborn disposition to potentially severe, self-destructive motivation and behavior. In this chapter, I attempt to clarify, from a neurobiological viewpoint, the diagnosis and treatment of a group of severely ill patients who present a dominant motivation for self-destructiveness, not only in chronic suicidal or parasuicidal behavior but also in devastating self-destructive characterological features that may lead to death in many cases. Severely sadistic and masochistic pathology is explored in this connection, again with illustrative clinical material.

Chapter 10 explores another fundamental area of psychoanalytic theory in the light of contemporary clinical experience—namely, the process of mourning. This chapter is a counterpoint to the consideration of the death drive in Chapter 9, involving mourning over destruction and loss and the function of guilt feelings and concern as a reparative and potentially creative counterpart to death and loss.

The effort to relate psychoanalytic to neurobiological findings also influences Part III, the study of sexual love, ranging from neurobiological to psychodynamic understandings regarding the disposition and preconditions for the capacity of mature love relationships, the inhibition of this capacity, and the manifestations of sexual problems in patients and couples with severe personality disorders. Here I move from the organization of brain structures and neurotransmitters to the overall systems of erotic activation, attachment, and bonding to consider the nature of passionate love and the psychodynamic features of a couple's love relationship.

Chapter 11 represents the theoretical part of this exploration, the analysis of the development of the capacity for mature sexual love, starting from the neurobiology of sexual excitement and attachment, and exploring the transformation of the behavioral expression of these basic neurobiological systems, into the complex subjective experience of erotic desire and passionate love. I examine how the individual's potential to integrate erotic desire, passionate love, and idealization evolves to the conditions that permit the establishment of a mature love relationship and the threats to such a relationship by various psychopathological developments. In the process, the critique of the concept of the death drive is complemented here by a critique of the concept of the libidinal drive in psychoanalytic theory, thus completing a general critique of the psychoanalytic theory of motivation.

This developmental and structural analysis is followed, in Chapter 12, by the descriptions of the characteristics of the capacity for a mature love relationship. This chapter shifts radically from the theoretical integration of neurobiological and psychodynamic perspectives to a phenomenological, clinical description of that capability, which should help the clinician's orientation to conflicts in a couple's love relationship.

Chapter 13, finally, complements this section with the typical manifestations of pathology in the sexual realm prevalent in severe personality disorders, particularly in borderline patients.

Part IV explores serious problems facing psychoanalytic education, institutions, and the profession of psychoanalysis and proposes solutions to these difficulties geared to energize the contributions of psychoanalysis to scientific research and progress in the field of psychodynamic psychiatry and psychotherapy. In Chapter 14, I review critically present environmental and internal problems of psychoanalytic institutions, particularly of psychoanalytic institutes. I follow this critique with an exploration of the challenges that psychoanalysis faces at this point, the urgent need to strengthen and consolidate its integration with the academic environment, the university, and the corresponding changes required in the structure of psychoanalytic societies, institutes, and their educational methods. I review the important contributions of psychoanalysis to psychodynamic psychiatry, as well as to societal analysis and cultural life, but stress the need for radical innovation.

Chapter 14 deals with the social, political, and administrative problems facing psychoanalysis, whereas Chapter 15, under the heading of "dissidence" in the theoretical realm of psychoanalysis, considers the future of conceptual developments, the openness to new theoretical thinking and scientific testing of alternative hypotheses, while exploring the ideological interferences that such a development derived from the history of the psychoanalytic "movement." The implicit intention of this section is to contribute to the integration of psychodynamic, neurobiological, and psychosocial approaches, and that development demands a profound transformation of psychoanalytic institutions within the spirit of university research and teaching.

Part V, finally, addresses psychodynamic factors involved in the religious experience and the search for and functions of universal ethical values, examining the object relations fundamentals of a spiritual realm of experience. Chapter 16 explores the origins of the motivation for the consolidation of an integrated system of ethical values as an essential aspect of the personality and its relation to the religious experience. Here I take a critical view of Freud's negative attitude toward religion and point to the psychological function of religiosity as an expression of the development of the capacity for an internalized, integrated ethical guidance system. In the process, I summarize briefly the contemporary view of the development of the superego and the crucial function of the religious experience in dealing with the ideological challenges of social life.

Finally, in Chapter 17, I propose a general developmental model of internal object relations that, at a certain level of integration, facilitates the awareness and the development of a spiritual realm of experience that transcends the pragmatic aspects of mature object relations and opens the road to aspiration and commitment to universal ethical values.

Because, in my view, progress in psychodynamic understanding is so crucial for the psychology of normality and illness, the potential development of this field deserves to be examined critically and constructively. At the bottom, this volume is based on the conviction that neurobiology and psychoanalysis are two basic sciences that, in their collaboration, have the potential to significantly advance our understanding of the human mind in health and illness.

Acknowledgments

I am grateful to many colleagues and friends who, in our work together and in our discussion of all these issues, helped me to clarify my own thoughts and to gain new understanding regarding many subjects touched on in this book. They include, in the United States, Drs. Martin Bergmann, Harold Blum, Robert Michels, Robert Tyson, Robert Wallerstein, and the late William Grossman; in England, Drs. Anne Marie and the late Joseph Sandler; in France, Drs. André Green and Daniel Widlocher; in Germany, Drs. Peter Buchheim, Horst Kaechele, the late Irmhild Kohte-Meyer, Rainer Krause, Ernst Lürssen, Gerhard Roth, and Almuth Sellschopp; and in Austria, Drs. Stephan Doering and Peter Schuster. My views on psychoanalytic education have been profoundly influenced by Drs. Arnold Cooper, recently deceased, David Sachs, and Robert Tyson in the United States; André Lussier and Lina Normandin in Canada; Claudio Eizirik and Elias Mallet de Rocha Barros in Brazil; Sara Zac de Filc and Isidoro Berenstein in Argentina; and Cesar Garza Guerrero in Mexico.

I have already referred to the exciting stimulation I have received from colleagues at the Personality Disorders Institute at Cornell University, which I direct. I warmly thank the senior members of this institute—in particular, Drs. Eve Caligor, Diana Diamond, Eric Fertuck, Pamela Foelsch, Catherine Haran, James Hull, Kenneth Levy, Barry Stern, Michael Stone, and Frank Yeomans. Ms. Jill Delaney, another senior member of our group, deserves my special gratitude for her careful, critical editing of all the chapters in this volume.

Our research collaboration with Drs. Mark Lenzenweger, Michael Posner, and David Silbersweig in the United States and with Drs. Peter Buchheim, Stefan Doering, Melitta Fischer-Kern, Susanne Hoerz, Mathias Lomer, Phillip Martius, and Peter Schuster abroad has greatly influenced the entire clinical section of this volume. Above all, I express profound appreciation to Dr. John Clarkin, codirector of the Personality Disorders Institute and the mastermind in the transformation of our theoretical and clinical hypotheses into workable research designs.

I wish to thank Mr. Alvin Dworman and Mr. and Mrs. Michael Tusiani for their confidence and generous support in our work with severe personality disorders. Their interest and understanding have been crucial, stimulating factors in our research and educational functions. And I express my profound gratitude to Dr. Jack Barchas, professor and chairman of the Department of Psychiatry of the Weill Cornell Medical College, for his warm encouragement, concern, and support of our research enterprise and my personal work.

I thank Ms. Rosetta Davis, who diligently worked on the early versions of the manuscripts, and express my heartfelt gratitude to Ms. Louise Taitt, the administrative secretary of the Personality Disorders Institute, who, in fact, carried out the major work related to the transcription, organization, and final production of this volume. Her careful attention to the thousands of problems and details and her stoic efforts to protect my time were crucial in permitting the completion of this work.

Finally, I want to thank my wife, Dr. Catherine Haran, who, in her double function as a clinician and researcher at the institute as well as provider of unfailing emotional support under all conditions of professional and institutional weather, helped me to achieve this work. This book is dedicated to her and to the memory of my late first wife, Dr. Paulina Kernberg. Paulina's pioneering work on personality disorders in children and adolescents continues to inspire our present research endeavor.

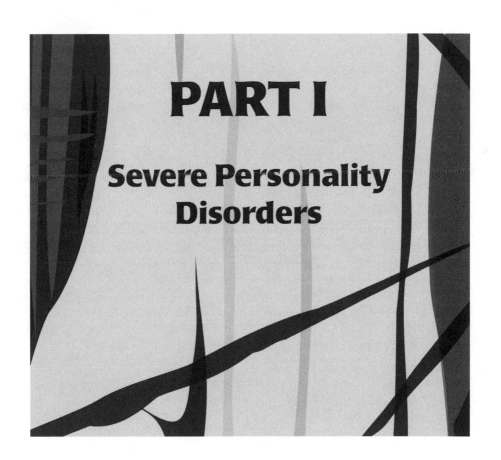

PART I

Severe Personality Disorders

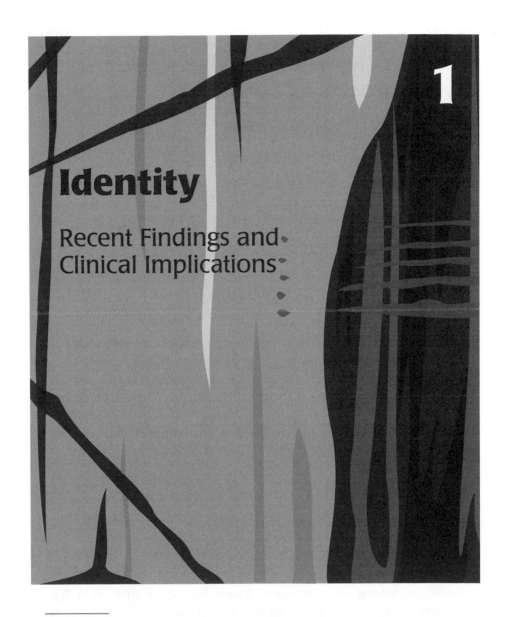

Identity

Recent Findings and Clinical Implications

This chapter was first published in © *The Psychoanalytic Quarterly,* 2006. Reprinted from Kernberg OF: "Identity: Recent Findings and Clinical Implications." *Psychoanalytic Quarterly* 75:969–1044, 2006. Used with permission.

This chapter represents work from the Cornell Psychotherapy Research Project supported by a grant from the Borderline Personality Disorder Research Foundation. The Foundation, and its founder, Dr. Marco Stoffel, are gratefully acknowledged.

In this chapter, I describe the psychological structures that dominate the clinical picture of severe personality disorders, what also has been called *borderline personality organization,* of which the borderline personality disorder represents a paradigmatic personality disorder. I focus on a central aspect of normal and pathological personality functions, the presence or absence of normal identity: *identity diffusion* is the most important, etiologically and symptomatically relevant, fundamental feature common to all severe personality disorders. I define the concept of *identity*, related to developmental features of the personality and clarified as part of the diagnostic evaluation of personality disorders. I describe a specific clinical interview, the *structural interview,* and apply it to the diagnostic evaluation of a patient, including a verbatim transcription of relevant parts of the interviewing process. In summary, the reader should be able to acquire the essential knowledge of this diagnostic method and its clinical relevance.

The subject matter of identity and pathology or breakdown of identity was barely touched by Freud, who referred, however, to the ego's ("Ich") tendency toward integration of its disparate instinctual dispositions and objectives (Bohleber 2000). It is only following the pathbreaking contributions by Erik Erikson (1950, 1956) that the concept of identity became a fundamental contribution to psychoanalytic theory and exploration of character pathology. The cultural and sociological concern with the vicissitudes of individual identity in a rapidly changing world may have contributed to the popularity of the concept following Erikson's theoretical and clinical formulations. More recently still, the concern with the development of the self has replaced the focus on the concept of identity in general psychoanalytic literature, although the study of normal and abnormal identity has become central in the research on the psychopathology of severe personality disorders.

What follows is a review of research findings of the Personality Disorders Institute of the Joan and Sanford I. Weill Medical College of Cornell University regarding the concepts of normal identity and identity diffusion as part of the psychopathology of personality disorders and their etiology, diagnosis, and treatment. The application of an object relations theory model to analyze the development of identity also clarifies the relation of individual identity with the social and cultural frame that influences identity formation and may amplify the effects of pathological identity development.

Review of Erikson's Contributions

The study of severe personality disorders has increasingly pointed to the importance of the differentiation of normal identity from the typical identity disturbances of severe personality disorders. In fact, the assumption that it is precisely the syndrome of identity diffusion that characterizes all severe personality disorders or borderline personality organization has made the clinical assessment of identity and identity disturbances most important diagnostically and in designing the strategies of treatment. The assessment of changes in identity disturbances has become for us an essential aspect of the evaluation of structural intrapsychic change.

Empirical evidence indicates that a temperamental disposition to negative affect, affective dyscontrol, and generalized impulsivity characterizes individuals prone to develop borderline personality disorder (deVagvar et al. 1994; Gurvits et al. 2000; Silk 2000; Steinberg et al. 1994; Stone 1992; van Reekum et al. 1994; Yehuda et al. 1994). But it is the presence of severe identity disturbances, added to these temperamental characteristics, that is directly related to the consolidation of this personality disorder (Kernberg 1984, 1992). This has made the study of identity and its origin, development, and psychopathology highly relevant for contemporary research on etiology, psychopathology, and treatment of severe personality disorders.

Erik Erikson (1950, 1956) first formulated in 1950 the concepts of *normal ego identity, identity crisis,* and *identity diffusion* as the crucial characteristics, respectively, of normal personality development, adolescence, and severe personality disorders. He returned to the definition of the concept of ego identity in 1956, stressing the importance of the conscious sense of individual identity, matched by the unconscious strivings for continuity of the individual's self-experience. He described identity as an overall synthesis of ego functions, on the one hand, and as the consolidation of a sense of solidarity with group ideals and group identity, on the other. Erikson stressed that ego identity has both conscious and unconscious aspects and that it develops gradually, until a final consolidation of its structure in adolescence.

Adolescence may present with an identity crisis—that is, a period of lack of correspondence between the view of the adolescent by his or her immediate environment derived from the past, in contrast to the adolescent's relatively rapid change of self-experience that, at least transitorily, no longer corresponds to others' view of him or her. Thus, identity crisis derives from a lack of confirmation by others of the adolescent's changing identity. This normal identity crisis, however, must be differentiated from identity diffusion, the pathology of identity characteristic for borderline patients.

Erikson (1956) described identity diffusion as an absence or loss of the normal capacity for self-definition, reflected in emotional breakdown at times of physical intimacy, occupational choice, and competition, and increased need for a psychosocial self-definition. He suggested that the avoidance of choices reflecting such identity diffusion led to isolation, a sense of inner vacuum, and regression to earlier identifications. Identity diffusion would be characterized by the incapacity for intimacy in relationships, because intimacy depends on self-definition, and its absence triggers the sense of danger of fusion or loss of identity that is feared as a major calamity. Identity diffusion, Erikson went on, is also characterized by diffusion of the time perspective, reflected either in a sense of urgency regarding decision making or in a loss of regard for time in an endless postponement of such decision making. Identity diffusion also shows in the incapacity to work creatively and in breakdown at work. Erikson described as one consequence of identity diffusion, the choice of a negative identity; that is, a rejection of normally assigned social roles, and the establishment of an identity on the basis of a socially unacceptable, rejected, oppositionally defined set of identifications, an abnormal identity found in a "totalistic" embrace of what society rejects.

Blos (1967, 1979), in his fundamental contributions to the analysis of developmental features of adolescence, has described a "second individuation," characterized by the adolescent's gradual detachment from the internalized infantile objects, through a process involving temporary regression to preoedipal conflicts and, particularly, the reactivation of the negative oedipal complex. Powerful regressive currents activating dependency needs, intense conflicts around homosexual and heterosexual urges, and defenses against these impulses evolve in the context of strengthening of a mature ego ideal and further development of ego identity. The restructuring of the adolescent's superego clarified by Jacobson (1964) represents an important aspect of this structural reorganization and overcoming of infantile oedipal prohibitions. It needs to be stressed that the normal symptomatic manifestations of these changes are represented by the identity crisis of adolescence. Cases of severe psychopathology—characterized, from early childhood on, by identity diffusion; pathological expressions of conflicts around dependency; "negative identity" (the rigid identification with a rebellious, antisocial, oppositional, alienated social subgroup); and chronic, chaotic dominance of polymorphous perverse infantile tendencies—illustrate the incapacity to resolve the challenges of adolescent psychic restructuring.

Westen (1985, 1992), in reviewing the empirical and theoretical literature on self and identity, summarized the major components of identity as "a sense of continuity over time; emotional commitment to a set of self-defining representations of self, role relationships, and core values and ideal self standards; development or acceptances of a world view that gives life meaning; and some recognition of one's place in the world by significant others."

Hauser (Allen et al. 1993; Hauser 1976; Hauser and Follansbee 1984) enlarged upon several types of identity problems and pathology originally mapped out by Erikson: identity achievement, moratorium, foreclosure, and identity diffusion. Identity achievement reflects normal identity; moratorium implies a postponement of the resolution of the integration processes leading to a normal identity; and foreclosure refers to a rigid role commitment to a group identity, or to a pathological parental identity, or to a combination of isolation and submission to the identity of a leader or a group: it refers to a particularly severe form of negative identity.

Marcia (1966, 1980) further studied the development of ego identity and its relevance for the evolution of adolescents.

Masterson (1967, 1972) and Rinsley (1982) had described the difference between the identity crisis of normal adolescence and identity diffusion in adolescents with severe personality disorders. Masterson, particularly, pointed to the permanence of the severe identity disturbances in adolescence, thus complementing Offer's (1973) research stressing the normal identity characteristic of adolescents without major psychopathology.

Wilkinson-Ryan and Westen (2000), in summarizing their research on identity disturbance in borderline personality disorder, concluded: "Identity disturbance in borderline personality disorders is characterized by a painful sense of incoherence, objective inconsistencies in beliefs and behaviors, over-identification with groups or roles, and, to a lesser extent, difficulties with commitment to jobs, values, and goals. These factors are all related to borderline personality disorder regardless of abuse history, although a history of trauma can contribute substantially to the sense of painful incoherence associated with dissociative tendencies."

At our Institute, we developed an Inventory of Personality Organization (IPO), which assesses reality testing, primitive psychological defenses, and identity diffusion, applying this instrument to both clinical and nonclinical samples. We found that the hypothesized combination of identity diffusion and primitive defenses, with maintenance of reality testing, was significantly correlated with a high level of negative affects and aggressive dyscontrol, the phenotypes characteristic of borderline personality disorder (Lenzenweger et al. 2001).

Identity and Object Relations Theory

At the Personality Disorders Institute, we have studied the psychopathology, clinical diagnosis, and psychotherapeutic treatment of identity diffusion on the basis of the application of contemporary psychoanalytic object relations theory. We have applied this theory to the understanding of the development of normal and pathological identity and, in the process, defined and explored further the characteristics of identity diffusion (Kernberg 1976, 1984, 1992).

In essence, our basic assumption in the application of contemporary object relations theory is that all internalizations of relationships with significant others, from the beginning of life on, have different characteristics under the conditions of peak affect interactions and low affect interactions. Under conditions of low affect activation, reality-oriented, perception-controlled cognitive learning takes place, influenced by temperamental dispositions—that is, the affective, cognitive, and motor reactivity of the infant—leading to differentiated, gradually evolving definitions of self and others. These definitions start out from the perception of bodily functions, the position of the self in space and time, and the permanent characteristics of others. As these perceptions are integrated and become more complex, interactions with others are cognitively registered and evaluated, and working models of them are established. Inborn capacities to differentiate self from nonself, and the capacity for cross-modal transfer of sensorial experience, play an important part in the construction of the model of self and the surrounding world.

In contrast, under conditions of peak affect activation—be they of an extremely positive, pleasurable or an extremely negative, painful mode—specific internalizations take place framed by the dyadic nature of the interaction between the baby and the caretaking

person, leading to the setting up of specific affective memory structures with powerful motivational implications. These structures are
constituted, essentially, by a representation of self interacting with a
representation of significant other under the dominance of a peak
affect state. The importance of these affective memory structures
lies in their constituting the basis of the primary psychic motivational system, in the direction of efforts to approach, maintain, or increase the conditions that generate peak positive affect states and to
decrease, avoid, and escape from conditions of peak negative affect
states.

Positive affect states involve the sensuous gratification of the
satisfied baby at the breast, erotic stimulation of the skin, and the
disposition to euphoric "in tune" interactions with mother; peak
negative affective states involve situations of intense physical pain,
hunger, or painful stimuli that trigger intense reactions of rage,
fear, or disgust and may motivate general irritability and hypersensitivity to frustration and pain. Object relations theory assumes that
these positive and negative affective memories are built up separately in the early internalization of these experiences and, later
on, are actively split or dissociated from each other in an effort to
maintain an ideal domain of experience of the relation between self
and others and to escape from the frightening experiences of negative affect states. Negative affect states tend to be projected,
to evolve into the fear of "bad" external objects, whereas positive
affect states evolve into the memory of a relationship with "ideal"
objects. This development evolves into two major, mutually split domains of early psychic experience, an idealized and a persecutory
or paranoid one, idealized in the sense of a segment of purely positive representations of self and other, and persecutory in the sense
of a segment of purely negative representations of other and
threatened representation of self. This early split experience protects the idealized experiences from "contamination" with bad
ones, until a higher degree of tolerance of pain and more realistic
assessment of external reality under painful conditions evolves.

This early stage of development of psychic representations of self
and other, with primary motivational implications—move toward
pleasure and away from pain—eventually evolves toward the integration of these two peak affect-determined segments, an integration facilitated by the development of cognitive capacities and ongoing
learning regarding realistic aspects of self and others interacting under circumstances of low affect activation. The normal predominance
of the idealized experiences leads to a tolerance of integrating the

paranoid ones, while neutralizing them in the process. In simple terms, the child recognizes that he or she has both "good" and "bad" aspects, and so does mother and the significant others of the immediate family circle, while the good aspects predominate sufficiently to tolerate an integrated view of self and others.

This state of development, referred to by Kleinian authors (Klein 1940; Segal 1964) as the shift from the paranoid-schizoid to the depressive position, and by ego psychological authors as the shift into object constancy, presumably takes place somewhere between the end of the first year of life and the end of the third year of life. Here Margaret Mahler's (1972a, 1972b) research on separation-individuation is relevant, pointing to the gradual nature of this integration over the first three years of life.

Peter Fonagy's (Fonagy and Target 2003) referral to the findings regarding mother's capacity to "mark" the infant's affect that she congruently reflects to the infant points to a related process: mother's contingent (accurate) mirroring the infant's affect, while marked (differentiated) signaling that she does not share it while still empathizing with it, contributes to the infant's assimilating his or her own affect while marking the boundary between self and other. Under normal conditions, then, an integrated sense of self ("good and bad"), surrounded by integrated representations of significant others ("good and bad") that are also differentiated among one another in terms of their gender characteristics as well as their status/role characteristics, jointly determine normal identity.

The concept of ego identity originally formulated by Erikson included in its definition the integration of the concept of the self; an object relations approach expands this definition with the corresponding integration of the concepts of significant others. In contrast, when this developmental stage of normal identity integration is not reached, the earlier developmental stage of dissociation or splitting between an idealized and a persecutory segment of experience persists. Under these conditions, multiple, nonintegrated representations of self split into an idealized and persecutory segment, and multiple representations of significant others split along similar lines, jointly constituting the syndrome of identity diffusion. One might argue that, insofar as Erikson considered the confirmation of the self by the representations of significant others as an aspect of normal identity, he already stressed the relevance of that relationship between the self-concept and the concept of significant others, but he did not as yet conceive of the intimate connection between the integration or lack of it on the part of the concepts of self and the parallel achievement or failure in the corresponding concepts of others. In other words, he was aware of the importance of integration or lack of integration of the concept of self but not of the equally important function of the corresponding integration or lack of integration of the representations of others. It was the work of Edith Jacobson (1964) in the United States, powerfully influencing Margaret Mahler's conceptualizations, and the work of Ronald Fairbairn (1954) in Great Britain, that pointed to the dyadic nature of the development of early internalizations and created the basis for the contemporary psychoanalytic object relations theory.

Etiology of Identity Diffusion

Regarding the etiology of identity diffusion, we may now formulate a proposal that integrates the findings regarding temperamental predisposition to the development of severe personality disorders or borderline personality organization, particularly regarding the development of the borderline personality disorder in a restricted sense as formulated in DSM-IV-TR (American Psychiatric Association 2000), with early developmental and later psychosocial etiological factors. To begin, the genetic disposition to affect activation related to the pathology of neurotransmitter systems, involving particularly the biogenic amines (such as the serotonergic, the noradrenergic, and the dopaminergic systems), may determine an organismic hyperreactivity to painful stimuli represented by an inborn excessive development of aggressive affect. Presumably the genetically determined hyperactivity of the areas of the brain that involve affect activation, particularly hyperactivity of the amygdala, contributed to negative affect activation (deVagvar et al. 1994; Gurvits et al. 2000; Silk 2000; Steinberg et al. 1994; Stone 1992, 1993; van Reekum et al. 1994; Yehuda et al. 1994). A genetic disposition also may be involved in a potential primary inhibition of areas of the brain involved in cognitive control, particularly the prefrontal and preorbital cortex and the anterior portion of the cingulum, the areas involved in determining the capacity for "effortful control" (Posner et al. 2002). In a collaborative neuroimaging study with our Personality Disorders Institute, Silbersweig and colleagues (D.A. Silbersweig, K. Levy, K. Thomas, et al., "Exploring the Mechanisms of Negative Affect and Self-Regulation in BPD Patients and Controls Prior to Therapy," unpublished manuscript, 2003) found that patients with borderline personality disorder presented decreased activity in dorsolateral prefrontal and orbitofrontal cortex in contrast to normal control subjects during presentation of inhibitory words and an inappropriate increased amygdalar activity in these patients in neutral word conditions. These genetic and constitutional dispositions to excessive aggressive affect activation and lack of cognitive control would result in an inborn, temperamentally given predominance of the negative domain of early experience, one predisposing factor to the development of identity diffusion.

Then, from the beginning of the postnatal life on, the relationship between infant and mother, particularly under conditions of peak affect activation, reflected in the development of normal or pathological attachment, would represent a further and crucial determinant of the predominance of the negative domain of affective experience. Wilfred Bion (1967, 1970) stressed the crucial function of mother in transforming the infant's sensorial impressions that are projected onto mother in the form of "beta elements" into "alpha elements," reflecting mother's integrative emotional capacity. The infant's introjection of these modified sensorial elements would determine the infant's tolerance of early negative affective experiences. Failure of this maternal function leads to continued predominance of pathological projective identification, bringing about a dominance of the paranoid segment of early experience by amplifying intolerable negative affective experience.

More recently, Peter Fonagy (Fonagy and Target 2003) has proposed that mother, activating her normal capacity to mirror congruently the infant's dominant affect (particularly under conditions of negative affect activation) while signaling to the infant by means of her "marking" of the affect that she can empathize with it without sharing it, permits the infant to internalize mother's contingent, accurate and marked, differentiated emotional experience. The infant thus becomes able to reflect on his or her own affective experience, developing in the process the function of normal "mentalization." When mother is unable to mark her congruent reactions to the infant, that is, when she reflects to the infant an intensity of negative affect that would seem to mirror the infant's incapacity to contain it, this experience amplifies the infant's dread of his or her own primitive negative affect, thus leading, I would add, once again to the predominance of the paranoid domain of experience. Or else, when mother is unable to congruently mirror the infant's affect, thus reflecting a deficient empathy with him or her, this also determines an intolerable intensity of negative affect in the infant that cannot be "contained," thus also increasing the dominance of the negative segment of experience. By these mechanisms, then, the predominance of negative affect is reinforced and may lead to a severe restriction in mentalization.

There are several patterns of mirroring that may be risk factors for various types of psychopathology. Mirroring that is both unmarked and noncongruent may be a risk factor for borderline personality organization or even psychosis. As mentioned before, mirroring that is unmarked but contingent may contribute to exacerbate the infant's and small child's lack of capacity to contain negative affects. Marked but noncontingent mirroring—when the parent differentiates his or her own feeling from that of the infant, but there is not an accurate reflection of the infant's or young child's feeling—may pose a risk factor for narcissistic personality disorder (Allen and Fonagy 2003).

All insecure attachment patterns involve contradictory, incompatible working models of attachment (Main 1995). The preoccupied person oscillates between good and bad evaluation of self and others; the unresolved person shows logically inconsistent simultaneous beliefs or sudden breaks in discourse, whereas the dismissing individual holds an "idealized" working model at the semantic level and a "negative," contradictory one at the episodic level. The disorganized or unresolved individual is at still greater risk for identity diffusion because of the dissociated systems that are operative in such individuals (Diana Diamond, personal communication, 2005). Levy (2005) proposes that the Cannot Classify (CC) category may be the most extreme example of contradictory, incompatible working models of attachment. The Cannot Classify classification is assigned if an adult displays a combination of contradictory and incompatible linguistic patternings.

In short, insecure attachment is likely a risk factor for identity diffusion just as it is for borderline personality organization, but these three domains need to be clearly differentiated from one another. Attachment is a developmental sequence of particular modes of relatedness that codetermine the formation of internal models of self and other ("object") representations. The organization of these self and object representations lead, in turn, to identity integration or identity diffusion. In my view, identity diffusion is a structural, pathological consolidation of the internalized world of object relations, reflected in a stable lack of integration of the concept of self and of significant others. Borderline personality organization is a specific psychopathological syndrome with common features characterizing all severe personality disorders that reflects the subjective and behavioral consequences of identity diffusion and presents secondary defensive operations and symptoms that maintain it. Insecure attachment is an important risk factor for identity diffusion, probably superimposed on the temperamental disposition referred to before, and reinforced by other psychosocial risk factors to be mentioned further on.

Fonagy's concept of mentalization includes the child's capacity for both reflecting on his or her own affect and appropriately reflecting on the mother's affect; mentalization thus includes the capacity for "secondary representation" of one's own affect, the capacity to empathize with the affective experience of the other, and the capacity to appropriately differentiate between the affective experiences of self and other. In my view, the multiple meanings of mentalization do not consider sufficiently the difference between the early capacity for differentiation between self and object representation and the later integration of contradictory representations of others as well as of self. Although I agree with Fonagy's idea that the function of abnormal attachment is an important contributor to identity diffusion, it does not do justice to the concept of integration or lack of integration of representations of significant others—in parallel to the integration (or lack of it) of the concept of self—implied in the concept of normal identity and identity diffusion as defined before. In other words, identity diffusion implies internal working models that reflect disorganized/disoriented representation of self and of others, derived from the splitting mechanisms that fragment the representatives of self and the representations of others in terms of polar opposite affect dispositions (Paulina Kernberg, personal communication, 2003).

There is ample evidence that a history of severe physical abuse and sexual abuse and of the chronic witnessing of severe sexual and physical abuse are highly prevalent in borderline personality disorder (Stone 1993). There is also evidence that chronic pain related to physical illness in the first year of life is related to an accentuation of aggressive behavior (Grossman 1991; Zanarini 2000). The effects of chronic abandonment and of severe chaos within the family structure, particularly the breakdown of ordinary intergenerational boundaries and chronic unpredictability of parental behavior, are further factors that increase the predominance of the negative domain of early experience, contributing to the development of severe personality disorders and, in the context of this analysis, of identity diffusion. A study carried out by Ken

Levy (K. N. Levy, "The Role of Identity Disturbance in the Development of Borderline Personality Disorder," unpublished data, 2002) indicates that within a segment of a normal population that shows exaggerated negative affect and impulsivity as temperamental phenotypes, those subjects within that subgroup who, at the same time, evince severe identity disturbances also present with personality disorder, whereas those who do not present such identity disturbances do not. He concludes that, whereas negative affect and impulsivity may be broadband risk factors for the development of borderline personality disorder, identity disturbance appears to be a specific risk factor. This finding is consistent with earlier work (Garnet et al. 1994), which found that identity disturbance was the best predictor of the continuance of borderline personality disorder from adolescence into young adulthood.

In short, the major proposed hypothesis regarding the etiological factors determining severe personality disorders or borderline personality organization is that, starting from a temperamental predisposition to the predominance of negative affect and impulsivity or lack of effortful control, the development of disorganized attachment, exposure to physical or sexual trauma, abandonment, or chronic family chaos predispose the individual to the abnormal fixation at the early stage of development that predates the integration of normal identity: a general split persists between idealized and persecutory internalized experiences under the dominance of corresponding negative and positive peak affect states. Clinically, this state of affairs is represented by the syndrome of identity diffusion, with its lack of integration of the concept of the self and the lack of integration of the concepts of significant others. The question still remains, what other temperamental, psychodynamic, or psychosocial factors may then influence the development of the specific constellations of pathological character traits that differentiate the various constellations of severe personality disorder from one another, a subject that remains to be explored. The fact that much of the relevant research involves borderline personality disorder points to the need to carry out such studies involving other severe personality disorders.

From a clinical standpoint, the syndrome of identity diffusion explains the dominant characteristics of borderline personality organization. The predominance of primitive dissociation or splitting of the idealized segment of experience from the paranoid one is naturally reinforced by primitive defensive operations intimately connected with splitting mechanisms, such as projective identification, denial, primitive idealization, devaluation, omnipotence, and omnipotent control. All these defensive mechanisms contribute to distorting interpersonal interactions and create chronic disturbances in interpersonal relationships, thus reinforcing the lack of self-reflectiveness and of "mentalization" in a broad sense, decreasing the capacity to assess other people's behavior and motivation in depth, particularly, of course, under the effect of intense affect activation. The lack of integration of the concept of the self interferes with a comprehensive integration of one's past and present into a capacity to predict one's future behavior and decreases the capacity for stable commitment to professional goals, personal interests, work and social functions, and intimate relationships.

The lack of integration of the concept of significant others interferes with the capacity of realistic assessment of others, with selecting partners harmonious with the individual's actual expectations, and with investment in others. All sexual excitement involves a discrete aggressive component (Kernberg 1995). The predominance of negative affect dispositions leads to an infiltration of the disposition for sexual intimacy with excessive aggressive components, determining, at best, an exaggerated and chaotic persistence of polymorphous perverse infantile features as part of the individual's sexual repertoire and, at worst, a primary inhibition of the capacity for sensual responsiveness and erotic enjoyment. Under these latter circumstances, severely negative affects eliminate the very capacity for erotic response, clinically reflected in the severe types of sexual inhibition that are to be found in the most severe personality disorders.

The lack of integration of the concept of self and of significant others also interferes with the internalization of the early layers of internalized value systems, leading particularly to an exaggerated quality of the idealization of positive values and the ego ideal and to a persecutory quality of the internalized, prohibitive aspects of the primitive superego. These developments lead, in turn, to a predominance of splitting mechanisms at the level of internalized value systems or superego functions, with excessive projection of internalized prohibitions, while the excessive, idealized demand for perfection further interferes with the integration of a normal superego. Under these conditions, antisocial behavior may emerge as an important aspect of severe personality disorders, particularly in the syndrome of malignant narcissism and in the most severe type of personality disorder—namely, the antisocial personality proper, which evinces most severe identity diffusion as well, underneath a pathological grandiose self (Kernberg 1984, 1992). In general, normal superego formation is a consequence of identity integration and, in turn, protects normal identity. Severe superego disorganization, in contrast, worsens the effects of identity diffusion (Jacobson 1964).

The treatment of personality disorders depends, in great part, on their severity, reflected in the syndrome of identity diffusion. The presence or absence of identity diffusion can be elicited clinically in initial diagnostic interviews focused on the structural characteristics of personality disorders. The dimensional aspects—greater or lesser degrees of identity diffusion—still require further research. From a clinical standpoint, the extent to which ordinary social tact is still maintained or lost is the dominant indicator of the severity of the syndrome. The diagnosis of identity diffusion or of normal identity, in short, acquires fundamental importance in the clinical assessment of patients with personality disorders.

Clinical Assessment of Identity

At the Personality Disorders Institute at Cornell, we have developed a particular mental status examination designated "structural interviewing," geared to the differential diagnosis of personality disorders. In essence, this interview, which ordinarily takes up to one and one-half hours of exploration, consists of various steps of inquiry into the patient's functioning. The first step evaluates all the patient's symptoms, including physical, emotional, interpersonal, and generally psychosocial aspects of malfunctioning; inappropriate affect experience and display; inappropriate behavior; and inordinate difficulties in assessing self and others in interactions and in negotiating ordinary psychosocial situations. This inquiry into symptoms is pursued until a full differential diagnosis of prominent symptoms and characterological difficulties has been achieved.

The second step of this interview explores the patient's present life situation, including his or her adaptation to work or a profession, love life and sexual experiences, family of origin, friendships, interests, creative pursuits, leisure activities, and social life in general. It also explores the patient's relations to society and culture, particularly ideological and religious interests, and his or her relation to sports, arts, and hobbies. In short, we attempt to obtain as full a picture as possible of the patient's present life situation and interactions, raising questions whenever any aspect of the patient's present life situation seems obscure, contradictory, or problematic. This inquiry complements the earlier step of exploration of symptoms and, at the same time, makes it possible to compare the patient's assessment of his or her life situation and potential challenges and problems with the patient's interaction with the diagnostician as this exploration proceeds.

A third step of this structural interview consists of raising the question of the personality assessment by the patient of the two or three most important persons in his or her present life, followed by the assessment of the description of himself or herself as a unique, differentiated individual. The leading questions here are: "Could you now describe to me the personality of the most important persons in your present life that you have mentioned, so that I can acquire a live picture of them?" "And now, could you also describe yourself, your own personality, as it is unique or different from anybody else, so that I can acquire a live picture of it?"

As the fourth step of this interview, and only in cases with significant disturbances in the manifestations of their behavior, affects, thought content, or formal aspects of verbal communication during the interview, the diagnostician raises tactful questions about that aspect of the patient's behavior, affect, thought content, or verbal communication that has appeared as particularly curious, strange, inappropriate, or out of the ordinary, warranting such attention. The diagnostician communicates to the patient that a certain aspect of his or her communication has appeared puzzling or strange to the diagnostician and questions whether the patient can see that and what his or her explanation would be for the behavior that puzzles the diagnostician.

Such a tactful confrontation will permit the patient with good reality testing to be aware of what it is in himself or herself that has created a particular reaction of the interviewer and provide him or her with an explanation that reduces the strangeness or puzzling aspect of that behavior. This response, in other words, indicates good reality testing. If, to the contrary, such inquiry leads to an increased confusion, disorganization, and abnormal behavior in the interaction with the diagnostician, reality testing is presumably lost. The maintenance of reality testing is an essential aspect of the personality disorders; patients may have lost the subtle aspects of tactfulness in social interactions but maintain good reality testing under ordinary social circumstances. Loss of reality testing presumably indicates an atypical psychotic disorder or an organic mental disorder: that finding would lead to further exploration of such behavior, affect, or thought in terms of a standard mental status examination. In any case, a clear loss of reality testing indicates that an active psychotic or organic mental disorder is present and that the primary diagnosis of a personality disorder cannot be established at this time.

Otherwise, with reality testing maintained, the interview would permit the diagnosis of a personality disorder, the predominant constellation of pathological character traits, and its severity in terms of the presence or absence of the syndrome of identity diffusion. The capacity to provide an integrated view of significant others and of self indicates normal identity. Good interpersonal functioning that does not even raise the question of any strange or puzzling aspect of the present interaction would not warrant the exploration of reality testing. Patients with borderline personality organization, who present identity diffusion, also typically evince behaviors reflecting primitive defensive operations in the interaction with the diagnostician. These findings are less crucial than the diagnosis of the identity diffusion, but they certainly reinforce that diagnostic conclusion.

Although this method of clinical interviewing has proven enormously useful in the clinical setting, it does not lend itself, unmodified, for empirical research. A group of researchers at our institute are presently transforming this structural interview into a semistructured interview, geared to permit the assessment of personality disorders by way of an instrument (Structured Interview for Personality Organization [STIPO]; J.F. Clarkin, E. Caligor, B. Stern, et al., "Structured Interview of Personality Organization (STIPO)," unpublished manuscript, 2003) geared to empirical research. The clinical usefulness of the structural interview, however, may be illustrated by typical findings in various characterological constellations.

To begin, in the case of adolescents, structural interviewing makes it possible to differentiate adolescent identity crises from identity diffusion. In the case of identity crises, the adolescent may present with a sense of confusion about the attitude of significant others toward himself or herself and puzzlement about their attitude that does not correspond to his or her self-assessment. Asked to describe the personality of significant others, however, particularly from his or her immediate family, the description is precise and in depth. By the same token, while describing a state of confusion about relationships with others, the adolescent's description of his or her own personality also conveys an appropriate, integrated view, even including such confusion about relationships that corresponds to the impression that the adolescent gives to the interviewer. In addition, adolescents with identity crisis but without identity diffusion usually show a normal set of internalized ethical values, interests, and ideals, commensurate with their social and cultural background. It is remarkable that even if such adolescents are involved in intense struggles around dependence and independence, autonomy, and rebelliousness with their environment, they have a clear sense of these issues and their conflictual nature, and their description of significant others with whom they enter in conflict continues to be realistic and cognizant of the complexity of the interactions.

To the contrary, in the case of identity diffusion, the descriptions of the most important persons in his or her life on the part of an adolescent with borderline personality organization are vague and chaotic, and so is their description of the self, in addition to the emergence of significant discrepancies in the description of the adolescent's present psychosocial interactions, on the one hand, and the interaction with the interviewer, on the other. It is also typical for severe identity diffusion in adolescence that there exists a breakdown in the normal development of ideals and aspirations. The adolescent with identity diffusion may display a severe lack of internalized value systems or a chaotic and contradictory attitude toward such value systems.

The most typical manifestations of the syndrome of identity diffusion—that is, a clear lack of integration of the concept of self and of the concept of significant others—can be found in patients with borderline personality disorder and, to a somewhat lesser degree, in patients with histrionic or infantile personality disorder. In contrast, in the case of the narcissistic personality disorder, what is most characteristic is the presence of an apparently integrated, but pathological, grandiose self, contrasting sharply with a severe incapacity to develop an integrated view of significant others: the lack of the capacity for grasping the personality of significant others is most dramatically illustrated in the narcissistic personality disorder. An opposite situation may emerge in patients with schizoid personality disorders, in which a lack of integration of the concept of the self may be matched by very subtle observations of significant others. In the case of schizotypal personality, in contrast, both the concept of self and the concept of significant others are severely fragmented, similarly to the case of the borderline personality disorders.

Diagnostic Structural Interview

What follows is the summary of an initial interview using the technique of structural interviewing to illustrate identity diffusion. Part of the interview has been summarized, but the crucial segments illustrating identity diffusion are reproduced verbatim with the exception of minor distortions involving names, professions, and places referred to in the interview in order to protect the confidentiality of this material.

> The patient was a 21-year-old postgraduate student, married to a 21-year-old university student, who consulted because of depression, significant marital conflict, and decreasing functioning leading to interruption of her present studies at this point. She presented a history of long-term depression since early adolescence, occasional self-cutting, and chaotic adolescent interpersonal relationships. She had had a number of sexual relationships during her college years. Although, in consultation with a college psychologist, the possibility of a bipolar illness had been considered, there was definitely no history of a bona fide hypomanic episode, nor did the depressions present features that would justify their classification as a major depression. Following her parents' divorce during the patient's early childhood, mother remarried, and the patient described a chaotic relationship with both her mother and her stepfather. The severe difficulties with stepfather in her adolescence led to bitter fights between the patient and mother, with mother kicking the patient out of the house. She then lived with an aunt for a time, until her marriage at the time of graduation from college. She has several younger siblings and always felt that her mother preferred all of them while she was the black sheep of the family. Her relationship with her husband has been highly ambivalent, the patient stating that she loves him, but she does not know whether she did the right thing in getting married to him. Their sexual life was initially active and satisfying, but she gradually began to feel that all he wanted her for was sex, and she pulled away from him sexually. When their conflicts become particularly intense, she leaves him, to go back to her mother for weeks, disrupting her attendance at school. In addition, her tendency to be late to class and to some provocative behavior has irritated her teachers and gotten her suspended from one class.

This was the information we had before the initial interview with her.

The interview itself began with the therapist asking her to describe her difficulties, to which she summarized, in a rather chaotic way, many of the issues mentioned above.

He then asked several questions to clarify the nature of her depression, in an effort to make the differential diagnosis between a chronic dysthymic reaction or characterological depression, on the one hand, and a major depression, on the other. Her information seemed clearly to confirm that it was the case of a chronic characterologically related depression. In order to clarify further her present problems, he then asked her about what the difficulties were at school. The patient said that she had only been failing in one class, but she was dropping out because her teacher told her she was no longer allowed to attend school(!) After several attempts of his to clarify what really happened, the patient provided the following information.

PATIENT: Yeah, because I was trying, you know. The teacher, he was completely unreasonable with me, being on medical leave, when I was obviously very ill. Um, you know, the first time that my cell phone went off in class and I left early was because my mom was coming to take me to the hospital because I had bronchitis. You know, and he was just, he didn't even talk to me about it. I just got this e-mail saying you're no longer allowed to attend. I had talked to my T.A., and even my T.A. was saying that my grades were pretty good, you know, even on the exam where I had only attended one of the lectures, I got an eighty—a B on the exam. So, my numerical grades were fine, but he just felt that I was a disruption in class.

THERAPIST: But why did he do that? Does he have a bias against you? Or is there something in your behavior that provoked that reaction in him?

PATIENT: I think that it's both. You know, he's very rigid, um, and he's very hard to be reasonable with when it comes to making, um, exceptions for persons who have difficulties. Um, like I said, with the medical leave, he wouldn't let me make up any of the work. He wasn't even trying to understand—.

THERAPIST: So it sounds as if it was his problem?

PATIENT: Yeah, but like, I mean, I did, I did come late, like, later than a few minutes a couple of times, like, twice, and I left early twice. Like I said, the first time was when my mom was coming to take me to the hospital....

The interview then shifted in the direction of his exploring the difficulties in her marriage. What follows are significant extracts from the transcript, again in sequential order.

PATIENT: I just feel like no matter how hard I try to work with John about things, like with problems we have between us, it just doesn't go anywhere. And you know, like communication, I try to communicate with him, but there are times when he, and he just closes up. He just shuts me out, and he also, like, when I try to talk to him about things that are upsetting me, he doesn't seem to get it. I just always, no matter how well things are going I feel like, you know, things are going well, something bad is going to happen. You know, like, things are too good. You know, what's going to happen to bring everything back down again. Even when we're getting along, I feel like something bad is going to happen, like it's too good to be true.

They then talked about the patient's sexual relationship with her husband.

PATIENT: Like, I'm, like a lot of times, I'm just not, you know, ready or just not in the mood, you know, and feel, and he'll be like, c'mon, and so I'll be like, sure, you know, and let's go ahead and, but, a lot, again, you know, it's me trying to do something for him, you know, and make him think he's doing something for me—

THERAPIST: You don't see it as something you're doing for yourself?

PATIENT: No.

THERAPIST: And you don't see it as him showing his interest in you as a woman?

PATIENT: Not really. Like yes and no. Like yes because he does say, you know, you're so beautiful, whatever, but not, because a lot of the times he's just like, you know, he's just a horny teenager, whatever, you know. I don't even know how to describe it.

To this point of the interview, the therapist had focused first on the evaluation of her present symptomatology, particularly her chronic depression, and then, on the main conflictual features of her personality as they might be influencing the conflicts linked to her depression. He now shifted to evaluate identity integration by asking her to describe the most important persons in her present life, first, and then herself as a person. What follows are relevant extracts, again, verbatim interchanges in sequential order.

THERAPIST: Now, can you describe John a little more to me? How he is as a person, what makes him different from anybody else. What's unique about him?

PATIENT: He's very academic, highly intelligent, you know. His studies mean a lot to him, in fact, they come first. Um, he's very smart. I mean, he's made Dean's List every semester that he's been full time. And he's very professional about his work, um, you know. He's in a Research Lab on campus as a work study, and he's just very professional about his work. And I feel that his work comes before I do. Um, he, he likes to, when he has time, he likes to sit back and relax and not have to worry about things. But, and he tells me this all the time, you know, he realizes how important it is for us to be able to communicate openly, but when he does get upset about things, he shuts himself off, and he crawls within himself, and he won't talk to me at all. Half, like, 95% of the time, I don't even know what's bothering him when he's upset. Um, he's, he gets very upset over things that I know that if I were to get upset over something and he doesn't understand why, it would upset me. He gets angry at me, you know, basically, the idea how can you let something so small bother you. He's very quiet, very shy. He's very antisocial almost. Um, at family gatherings he's okay if he knows everyone, but if you put him in a situation where he's meeting more than two or three people at a time—that maybe I know, but he doesn't—he gets very flustered, very introverted, very upset. Um, you know, he likes to observe rather than take part. If he goes to, like he went to one party before I was up here, with a friend he went, and while everyone else was interacting, he just kind of sat back and watched everyone else. He's very, very about physical health. Such as, you know, he sees, okay, heart disease is the number one cause of death in this age group, this gender, whatever, and so what can I do to prevent myself from being at risk for heart disease? And so his diet is very low sugar, low fat, low sodium, and he works out two or three times a week. And you know, he's very imposing of, you know, that's bad for you, don't do it. Whether it's something as minimal as tanning or something as big as a tattoo or my belly button pierced or whatever, you know, the little things I want to do for myself that I wanted for so long, long before he was even in the picture, and he's very imposing against them. Like, no, you can't go tanning; it's so bad for you.

THERAPIST: Now that you've described him, it seems that another person that is important in your life is your mother.

PATIENT: Yes, she is.

THERAPIST: Can you describe her to me? What kind of person she is, so that I get a picture of her. What makes her different from other people? What's unique about her?

PATIENT: Well, my mom is really young, she's 45. Um, I actually fought with my mom for the, about seven years out of the past eight. You know, we're just very alike, so we butt heads a lot. It was always the big joke that the only things I inherited from my mother were her stubbornness and her anger. Yeah, because if my mom is right she's going to argue to the end, you know. And I'm the same way. If I know that I'm right, I'm going to argue until you realize that I am, or whatever, you know. And when it comes to anger, I'm not an angry person generally, outwardly, at least, but more pent-up rage. But when I get angry, it's like lighting a cloth that's soaked in kerosene or something, you know. It's just, once I start, it's hard for me to stop. She is, she can be very open, very warm, but she can also be very harsh, very demanding, very, I don't know, just very self-centered. I've heard her talk about me and my two brothers, and I'm the "fucked-up child," Frank is the one with problems that can be worked with and Bob the little angel. And, you know, yeah, I had my problems, but you know, when your mom tells you that she wishes that you were someone else, it has a big impact. You know, she can—when we get along, we get along really well—but when we're, when we don't get along, we don't get along, you don't want us in the same room as each other. And, the funny thing, though, is that our fights are always her yelling at me. I never fight back.

THERAPIST: Why don't you tell me a little more about yourself. How would you describe yourself as a person, what is unique about you, what makes you different from other people, what you would tell me to get a picture of you as a person?

PATIENT: I'm a religious person. I try very hard to be accepting of everyone in my religion—a lot of people who are Christians will say, oh, you know, gays are going to hell, whereas I say, so what, we're still taught to love. Because it's not like, even if somebody isn't going to heaven when they die, you're still supposed to love them as you would have them, or somebody else, love you. I'm a very accepting person, very empathic, empathetic person. Who, even if a stranger came to me and said I need somebody to talk to, I would sit down with them and listen and talk to them, if they needed a hug, or whatever, a shoulder to lean on, a shoulder to cry on. And that's something that I think is very unique about me, people have told me that it's unique about me, that I have been the type of friend that you'd want a friend to be. You know, whereas everyone else, you know, somebody told me that like, all of their other friends, they thought they were friends, but when they needed them the most, they weren't there and, you know, how in all these different ways I was such a good friend. And I think that's something that's definitely the most unique thing about me. You know, I can just pour out love, no matter how upset I am on my own, if somebody else is going through a rough time, I'll push me aside, and I'll just, I'll say, you know, why don't you talk to me, you need to talk, what's going on—just try to be there for them. As I said, I'm not easy to get angry, but when I do, you know, I go off. And another thing is, I love kids, I love working with kids. I love playing with them, being around them, you know. Like I was down at the diner, and this woman and her husband were there with their four kids, and one of the kids was crying and was really upset, and I went over to him and started singing the "bumblebee song," you know, just to make him in a better mood. That's just how I am, I love kids, I love working with them, being there.

THERAPIST: You told me that you tried to be open and loving.

PATIENT: Yeah.

THERAPIST: Would it be fair to say that that works with most people, but not with your husband? Because from what you've told me, some of it is that you can get rather easily angry at him and resentful, or am I wrong?

PATIENT: I don't know, like, I get frustrated with my marriage because I don't feel like he hears me. If I need somebody to talk to, he should be the first person to be there for me, and often times he's not. You know, I do love him, and I try not to push him away, but he doesn't make it very easy for me. If I'm upset and turn to my friends instead of him, he'll get upset about that, but what he doesn't realize is that I've been trying to talk to him. To open up to him.

In the last part of the interview, the therapist tactfully attempted to confront her with contradictions in her descriptions of her husband and of herself and in regard to the situation that led to her suspension at school, to evaluate, first of all, reality testing and, in addition, the capacity for emotional introspection. Again, what follows are selected segments of that interaction.

THERAPIST: But what I'm asking is to what extent are you really trying to take initiative in a loving way towards him, or to what extent you're contributing to create an atmosphere by which he feels that most of the time you are sensitive, irritated, rejecting. I mean, I'm not saying that you may be doing the wrong thing by contributing to the problems, but the way you are talking to me about him gave me the sense of a kind of resentful attitude, as if you had a smoldering resentment; this is how you sound. Are you surprised that I should say that?

PATIENT: No.

THERAPIST: Am I the first person to say that?

PATIENT: To my face, I think.

THERAPIST: Well, let me remind you that you had told me that other people had told you that the only way that you are like your mother is in being stubborn. So, to what extent is it possible that this is going on with your attitude with your husband? Perhaps without you even knowing it? Second nature.

PATIENT: I guess it's possible.

THERAPIST: What do you think?

PATIENT: A lot of times, you know, I don't know why I, why I'm like that towards my husband.

THERAPIST: I'm exaggerating here a little, but in the relationship with your professor, one could raise the question, why was he so irritated with you? Why would he have bad feelings towards you? Without being aware of it, were you contributing to it?

PATIENT: I guess, I mean, again, I don't know, I guess it's possible, that I was without realizing it.

THERAPIST: And I was impressed by your saying that when everything goes well, that you feel it can't last. Because the implication is that if you're afraid of destiny not tolerating your being happy, that you may be tempted to mess up your life because at least then you know what's going on; nothing worse can happen.

PATIENT: A lot of times it doesn't get to that point—

THERAPIST: I beg your pardon?

PATIENT: A lot of times it doesn't get to that point, though, you know.

THERAPIST: Why not?

PATIENT: I tend to stay in my depression, I tend to stay at the point where I know, you know, like, well, everything else is messed up, so this is gonna happen too…whatever.

Toward the end of the interview, they talked about her plans to go back to her mother, once again, at least temporarily separating from her husband and abandoning her efforts to continue her studies. The therapist raised the question to what extent there might be self-defeating forces in her at play, reminding her of her fantasies that things couldn't go well for her and that they had already talked about how she might have contributed to the resentment of her professor as well as to the angry responses of her husband to her. He gained the impression that she was clearly able to understand what he was saying and able to think about it and present arguments in opposition to what he was saying as well as thoughts that implied a thoughtful acknowledgment of what he was saying. The contradictory nature of her description of her husband's personality and of that of her mother, and of herself—the latter perhaps the most striking aspect of the interview, in which completely contradictory self-representations of stubbornness and opposition, on the one hand, and loving openness, on the other, coexisted without touching each other—made him conclude that she presented significant identity diffusion. Reality testing, however, seemed intact.

The overall diagnostic conclusion was that this was a patient with a personality disorder and borderline personality organization, with predominantly infantile or histrionic and masochistic features, presenting with a chronic characterological depression intimately linked to the self-defeating patterns in her relationship with her husband, with her studies, and in her social life.

After the interview, the therapist commented to the treatment team on the impression he had of her interaction with him during the session. Her presentation had self-defeating features. She conveyed the impression of somebody fearful, submissive on the surface, but suspicious and resentful underneath. She clearly seemed depressed and had a history of not responding satisfactorily to several selective serotonin reuptake inhibitor antidepressants in the past.

The recommendation for treatment was transference-focused psychotherapy, an empirically tested, effective, modified psychodynamic psychotherapy for severe personality disorders (J.F. Clarkin, K.N. Levy, M.F. Lenzenweger, et al., "Evaluating Three Treatments for Borderline Personality Disorder: A Multiwave Study," unpublished manuscript, 2005; Clarkin et al. 2006).

References

Allen JP, Fonagy P: The Development of Mentalizing and Its Role in Psychopathology and Psychotherapy (Technical Report No 02–0048). Topeka, KS, The Menninger Clinic, Research Department, 2003

Allen JP, Hauser ST, Bell KL, et al: Longitudinal assessment of autonomy and relatedness in adolescent-family interaction as predictors of adolescent ego development and self-esteem. Child Dev 65:179–194, 1993

American Psychiatric Association: Diagnostic and Statistical Manual of Mental Disorders, 4th Edition, Text Revision. Washington, DC, American Psychiatric Association, 2000

Bion WR: Second Thoughts: Selected Papers on Psycho-Analysis. New York, Basic Books, 1967

Bion WR: Attention and Interpretation. New York, Basic Books, 1970

Blos P: The second individuation process of adolescence. Psychoanal Study Child 22:162–186, 1967

Blos P: Modifications in the classical psychoanalytic model of adolescence. Adolescent Psychiatry 7:6–25, 1979

Bohleber W: Indentität, in Handbuch psychoanalytischer Grundbegriffe. Edited by Mertens W, Waldvogel B. Stuttgart, Germany, Kohlhammer, 2000, pp 328–332

Clarkin JF, Yeomans FE, Kernberg OF: Psychotherapy for Borderline Personality: Focusing on Object Relations. Washington, DC, American Psychiatric Publishing, 2006

deVagvar ML, Siever LJ, Trestman RL, et al: Impulsivity and serotonin in borderline personality disorder, in Biological and Neurobehavioral Studies of Borderline Personality Disorder. Edited by Silk KR. Washington, DC, American Psychiatric Press, 1994, pp 23–40

Erikson EH: Growth and crises of the healthy personality, in Identity and the Life Cycle. New York, International Universities Press, 1950, pp 50–100

Erikson EH: The problem of ego identity. J Am Psychoanal Assoc 4:56–121, 1956

Fairbairn WRD: An Object Relations Theory of the Personality. New York, Basic Books, 1954

Fonagy P, Target M: Psychoanalytic Theories: Perspectives From Developmental Psychopathology. Philadelphia, PA, Whurr, 2003, pp 270–282

Garnet KE, Levy KN, Mattanah JJF, et al: Borderline personality disorder in adolescence: ubiquitous or specific? Am J Psychiatry 151:1380–1382, 1994

Grossman WI: Pain, aggression, fantasy, and concepts of sadomasochism. Psychoanal Q 60:22–52, 1991

Gurvits IG, Koenigsberg HW, Siever LJ: Neurotransmitter dysfunction in patients with borderline personality disorder. Psychiatr Clin North Am 23:27–40, 2000

Hauser ST: Self-image complexity and identity formation in adolescence: longitudinal studies. Journal of Youth and Adolescence 5:161–177, 1976

Hauser ST, Follansbee D: Developing identity: ego growth and change during adolescence, in Theory and Research in Behavioral Pediatrics. Edited by Fitzgerald H, Lester B, Yogman M. New York, Plenum, 1984

Jacobson E: The Self and the Object World. New York, International Universities Press, 1964

Kernberg OF: Object Relations Theory and Clinical Psychoanalysis. New York, Jason Aronson, 1976

Kernberg OF: Severe Personality Disorders: Psychotherapeutic Strategies. New Haven, CT, Yale University Press, 1984

Kernberg OF: Aggression in Personality Disorders and Perversions. New Haven, CT, Yale University Press, 1992

Kernberg OF: Love Relations: Normality and Pathology. New Haven, CT, Yale University Press, 1995

Klein M: Mourning and its relation to manic-depressive states, in Contributions to Psycho-Analysis, 1921–1945. London, Hogarth Press, 1940, pp 311–338

Lenzenweger MF, Clarkin JF, Kernberg OF, et al: The Inventory of Personality Organization: psychometric properties, factorial composition, and criterion relations with affect, aggressive dyscontrol, psychosis proneness, and self-domains in a nonclinical sample. Psychol Assess 13:577–591, 2001

Levy KN: The implications of attachment theory and research for understanding borderline personality disorder. Dev Psychopathol 17:959–985, 2005

Mahler MS: On the first three subphases of the separation-individuation process. Int J Psychoanal 53:333–338, 1972a

Mahler MS: Rapprochement subphases of separation-individuation process. Psychoanal Q 41:487–506, 1972b

Main M: Recent studies in attachment: overview with selected implications for clinical work, in Attachment Theory: Social, Developmental, and Clinical Perspectives. Edited by Goldberg S, Muir R, Kerr J. Hillsdale, NJ, Analytic Press, 1995, pp 407–474

Marcia JE: Development and validation of ego-identity status. J Pers Soc Psychol 3:551–558, 1966

Marcia JE: Identity in adolescence, in Handbook of Adolescent Psychology. Edited by Adelson J. New York, Wiley, 1980, pp 159–187

Masterson J: The Psychiatric Dilemma of Adolescence. Boston, MA, Little, Brown, 1967, pp 119–134

Masterson J: Treatment of the Borderline Adolescent: A Developmental Approach. New York, Wiley-Interscience, 1972

Offer D: Psychological World of the Teenager: A Study of Normal Adolescent Boys. New York, Harper & Row, 1973

Posner MI, Rothbart MK, Vizueta N, et al: Attentional mechanisms of borderline personality disorder. Proc Natl Acad Sci U S A 99:16366–16370, 2002

Rinsley BR: Borderline and Other Self Disorders. New York, Jason Aronson, 1982

Segal H: Introduction to the Work of Melanie Klein. New York, Basic Books, 1964

Silbersweig DA, Levy K, Thomas K, et al: Exploring the mechanisms of negative affect and self regulation in BPD patients and controls prior to therapy. (2003, manuscript in preparation)

Silk KR: Borderline personality disorder: overview of biologic factors. Psychiatr Clin North Am 23:61–75, 2000

Steinberg BJ, Trestman RL, Siever LJ, et al: The cholinergic and noradrenergic neurotransmitter systems and affective instability in borderline personality disorder, in Biological and Neurobehavioral Studies of Borderline Personality Disorder. Edited by Silk R. Washington, DC, American Psychiatric Press, 1994, pp 41–62

Stone M: Etiology of borderline personality disorder: psychobiological factors contributing to an underlying irritability, in Borderline Personality Disorder: Etiology and Treatment. Edited by Paris J. Washington, DC, American Psychiatric Press, 1992, pp 87–102

Stone M: Abnormalities of Personality. New York, WW Norton, 1993

van Reekum R, Links PS, Fedorov C: Impulsivity in borderline personality disorder, in Biological and Neurobehavioral Studies of Borderline Personality Disorder. Edited by Silk KR. Washington, DC, American Psychiatric Press, 1994, pp 11–22

Westen D: Self and Society: Narcissism, Collectivism, and the Development of Morals. New York, Cambridge University Press, 1985

Westen D: The cognitive self and psychoanalytic self: can we put ourselves together? Psychoanalytic Inquiry 3:1–13, 1992

Wilkinson-Ryan T, Westen D: Identity disturbance in borderline personality disorder: an empirical investigation. Am J Psychiatry 157:528–541, 2000

Yehuda R, Southwick SM, Perry BD, et al: Peripheral catecholamine alterations in borderline personality disorder, in Biological and Neurobehavioral Studies of Borderline Personality Disorder. Edited by Silk KR. Washington, DC, American Psychiatric Press, 1994, pp 63–90

Zanarini MC: Childhood experiences associated with the development of borderline personality disorder. Psychiatr Clin North Am 23:89–101, 2000

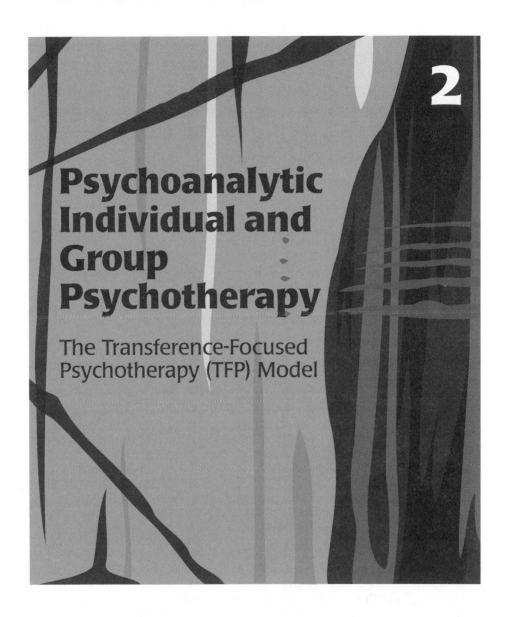

2

Psychoanalytic Individual and Group Psychotherapy

The Transference-Focused Psychotherapy (TFP) Model

This chapter was reprinted from Kernberg OF: "Psychoanalytic Individual and Group Psychotherapy: The Transference Focused Psychotherapy (TFP) Model." *Persönlichkeitsstörungen Theorie und Therapie* 13:79–93, 2009. Used with permission.

In this chapter, I present an overview of transference-focused psychotherapy (TFP), a psychoanalytically derived, specific psychodynamic psychotherapy for severe personality disorder. This method has been manualized and empirically tested, as summarized in this chapter. A synthetic description of the strategies, tactics, and techniques of TFP for individual patients as developed and tested at the Personality Disorders Institute at Cornell University is followed by the application of this method to dynamic group therapy. In this latter application, so far, we only count on our clinical experience, and this chapter is a first report of our effort to systematically explore this approach. Implicitly, this latter approach illustrates the application of an object relations theory model to small group psychology.

TFP was based upon the Menninger Foundation's psychotherapy research project (Kernberg et al. 1972), which indicated that the optimal treatment of patients with severe personality disorders or "low ego strength" was a psychoanalytic psychotherapy, with systematic interpretation of the transference in the hours and the provision of as much external support as the patient required outside the hours to permit the treatment to develop successfully. In contrast, neither the treatment with standard psychoanalysis nor with a purely supportive modality based on psychoanalytic principles was as effective. On this basis, at the Personality Disorders Institute of the Weill Cornell Medical College and The New York Hospital, we developed a psychoanalytic psychotherapy centered upon the principle of systematic interpretation of the transference and the setting up of a treatment structure, including limit-setting when needed, in order to protect the patient and the treatment from the severe acting out that is practically unavoidable in the treatment of these patients.

These efforts, over a period of approximately 15 years, culminated in the development of a manualized psychoanalytic psychotherapy, TFP, that fulfilled these general characteristics mentioned above. We tested the possibility of training psychotherapists in carrying out this manualized treatment, and after sufficient adherence and competence in carrying out that treatment was confirmed, we carried out a set of psychotherapy research projects; the first confirmed the efficacy of this treatment in comparison to treatment as usual for borderline patients, and then a randomized controlled trial compared TFP to dialectic behavior therapy (DBT) and to a supportive psychotherapy based on a psychoanalytic model. All three treatments were manualized, carried out by therapists who were convinced about the helpfulness of this model and proficient in carrying it out. The findings revealed the efficacy of all three forms of therapy and showed significant differences regarding the treatment of suicidal and parasuicidal symptoms, more effective with TFP and DBT than with supportive psychotherapy. TFP was more effective in reducing various aspects of aggressive affects and behavior of these patients in comparison to the other modalities (Kernberg et al. 2008).

At various points of our developing work, we studied the possibility of applying the principles of TFP to psychoanalytic group psychotherapy and developed a tentative model that seemed clinically satisfactory. We have applied this mostly to a day hospital setting and in sporadic attempts applied it to an inpatient setting as well. While clinicians involved in this effort have felt encouraged to pursue it further, we have not yet carried out empirical research on the efficacy of such a group psychotherapy, and the present chapter is a first effort to spell out the general model of this form of group psychotherapy and its relation to other related models. I shall first present an outline of the basic principles of TFP as applied to individual patients and then present an overview of how these principles apply to a corresponding TFP group psychotherapy.

Overview of Transference-Focused Psychotherapy for Individual Patients

We evolved a differentiation of overall, long-range treatment objectives and corresponding "treatment strategies," the systematization of interventions in each session that are conditions necessary for working with a borderline patient population, or "treatment tactics," adopting specific instruments of psychoanalytic treatment throughout its course, or "treatment techniques." In what follows, I shall outline these treatment strategies, tactics, and techniques.

Strategies

Our assumption was that patients with severe personality disorders or borderline personality organization have the syndrome of identity diffusion—that is, a chronic, stable lack of integration of the concept of self and of the concept of significant others—and that the ultimate cause of that syndrome was the failure of psychological integration resulting from the predominance of aggressive internalized object relations over idealized ones. In an effort to protect the idealized segment of the self and object representations, these patients' ego was fixated at a level of primitive dissociative or splitting mechanisms and their reinforcement by a variety of other primitive defensive operations predating the dominance of repression— namely, projective identification, omnipotence and omnipotent control, devaluation, denial, and primitive idealization. Identity diffusion is reflected clinically in the incapacity to accurately assess self and others in depth, to commit in depth to work or a profession, and to establish and maintain stable intimate relationships and in a lack of the normal subtlety of understanding and tact in interpersonal situations. Primitive defensive operations, which correspond to patients' split psychological structure and identity diffusion, are manifest in patient's behavior and are an important feature of their maladaptive dealing with negative affect and conflictual interpersonal situations, contributing fundamentally to chaos and breakdown in intimacy, in work, in creativity, and in social life. In the paper included as Chapter 1 of this volume, I have described in detail the etiology, psychopathology, empirical research, and clinical assessment of the syndrome of identity diffusion.

The main strategy in the TFP of borderline personality organization consists in the facilitation of the (re)activation in the treatment of split-off internalized object relations of contrasting persecutory and idealized natures that are then observed and interpreted in the transference. TFP is carried out in face-to-face sessions, a minimum of two and usually not more than three sessions a week. The patient is instructed to carry out free association (in a detailed, precise way), and the therapist restricts his or her role to careful observation of the activation of regressive, split-off relations in the transference and to help identify them and interpret their segregation in the light of these patients' enormous difficulty in reflecting on their own behavior and on the interactions they get involved in. The interpretation of these split-off object relations is based upon the assumption that each of them reflects a dyadic unit of a self-representation, an object representation, and a dominant affect linking them and that the activation of these dyadic relationships determines the patient's perception of the therapist and occurs with rapid role reversals in the transference, so that the patient may identify with a primitive self-representation while projecting a corresponding object representation onto the therapist, while ten minutes later, for example, the patient identifies with the object representation while projecting the self-representation onto the therapist. Engaging the patient's observing ego in this phenomenon paves the way for interpreting the conflicts that keep these dyads, and corresponding views of self and other, separate and exaggerated. Until these representations are integrated into more nuanced and modulated ones, the patient will continue to perceive himself or herself and others in exaggerated, distorted, and rapidly shifting terms.

The oscillation or alternative distribution of the roles of the dyad has to be differentiated from the split between opposite dyads carrying opposite (idealizing and persecutory) affective charges. The final step of interpretation consists in linking of the dissociated positive and negative transferences, leading to an integration of the mutually split-off idealized and persecutory segments of experience with the corresponding resolution of identity diffusion. The interpretation of these split-off relationships occurs in a characteristic sequence of three steps. Step one is the formulation of the total relationship that seems to be activated at that point, using metaphorical statements to present the situation as completely as possible in a way that can be understood by the patient, and the clarification of who enacts what role in that interaction. The therapist's comments are based on his or her observations, countertransference utilization, and clarifications that have been sought of the patient's experience of the relationship at each moment.

Step two consists in the observation of the interchange of the corresponding roles between patient and therapist, an extremely important step that permits the patient, throughout time, to understand his or her unconscious identification with the object representation as well as the self-representation, leading to a gradual awareness of the mutual complementarity of these two roles. Step two is carried out in the clarification and confrontation of both the oscillating poles of a given dyad. However, since the idealized and persecutory relationships that are activated remain typically split off from each other in different dyads, the patient becomes more able to recognize the extreme dyadic nature of each of them while still maintaining the split or dissociated nature that separates all good from all bad relationships. Understanding the motivation for keeping these dyads separate is one of the main objectives of the interpretive work, the focus of the next step.

Step three, finally, consists in an interpretive linking of the mutually dissociated positive and negative transferences, the transferences reflecting the idealized and persecutory relationships, thus leading to an integration of the mutually split-off idealized and persecutory segments of experience, the corresponding resolution of identity diffusion, and the modulation of intense affect dispositions as primitive euphoric or hypomanic affects are integrated with their corresponding fearful, persecutory, aggressive opposites. This third step brings about a significant integration of the patient's ego identity, as an integrated view of self—more complex, rich, and nuanced than the simplistic and extreme split-off representations—and a corresponding integrated view of significant others replaces their split-off previous nature, and an experience of appropriate depressive affects, reflecting the capacity for acknowledging one's own aggression that had previously been projected or experienced as dysphoric affect, with concern, guilt, and the wish to repair good relationships damaged in fantasy or reality becoming dominant.

Step one of this sequence begins in the first therapy session, and step two follows relatively quickly after the first few weeks and months of treatment. Step three characterizes the mid and advanced stages of the psychotherapy. At the same time, however, this three-step sequence is a highly repetitive process. Some step three interpretations may become possible relatively early, and step one, two, and three may recycle again and again, it first taking weeks to develop the entire sequence, then the course of a few sessions, and, in the advanced stages of the treatment, all three steps eventually may be elaborated in the course of the same session.

The overall strategy mentioned—namely, the resolution of identity diffusion and the integration of mutually split-off idealized and persecutory relationships—is facilitated by the fact that unconscious conflicts are activated in the transference mostly in the patient's behavior rather than in the emergence of preconscious subjective experiences reflecting unconscious fantasy. The intolerance of overwhelming emotional experiences is expressed in the tendency to replace such emotional experiences by acting out, in the case of most borderline patients, and somatization, in some other personality disorders (Green 1993). The fact that primitive conflicts manifest themselves in dissociated behavior rather than in the content of free association is a fundamental feature of these cases that facilitates transference analysis with a relatively low frequency of sessions, while the very intensity of those conflicts facilitates the full analysis of these transference developments. What is important in these cases is establishing very clear boundaries and conditions of the treatment situation, so that a "normal" relationship is defined in the therapy that immediately enters into contrast with the distortions in the therapeutic relationship derived from the activation of primitive transferences. This leads to the discussion of a second major aspect of the treatment: the tactics used by the therapist in each session that create the conditions necessary for the use of interpretation and the other techniques of treatment.

Tactics

The tactics are rules of engagement that allow for the application of psychoanalytic technique in a modified way that corresponds to the nature of the transference developments in these cases. The tactics are 1) setting the treatment contract; 2) choosing the priority theme to address in the material the patient is presenting; 3) maintaining an appropriate balance between, on the one hand, exploring the incompatible views of reality between the patient and therapist in preparation for interpretation and, on the other, establishing common elements of shared reality; and 4) regulating the intensity of affective involvement.

In the establishment of an initial treatment contract, in addition to the usual arrangements for psychoanalytic treatment and urgent difficulties in the borderline patient's life that may threaten the patient's physical integrity or survival, other people's physical integrity or survival, or the very continuation of the treatment, all are taken up and structured, in the sense of setting up conditions under which the treatment can be carried out that involve certain responsibilities for the patient and certain responsibilities for the therapist. What is important in these structuring arrangements at the beginning of the treatment is first, that the therapeutic structure eliminate the secondary gain of treatment and second, that in a situation where limits or restrictions need to be established in order to preserve the patient's life or the treatment, the transference implications of these restrictions or limit-settings need to be interpreted immediately. The combination of limit-setting and interpretation of the corresponding transference development is an essential, highly effective, and at times lifesaving tactic of the treatment. Yeomans et al. (1992) have described in detail the techniques and vicissitudes of initial contract setting; and the manual of the technical aspects of TFP (Clarkin et al. 2006) describes in detail the priorities to address in carrying out the therapy.

With regard to choosing which theme to address at any given moment in the material the patient brings to the session, the most important tactic is the general analytic rule that interpretation has to be carried out where the affect is most intense: affect dominance determines the focus of the interpretation. The most intense affect may be expressed in the patient's subjective experience, in the patient's nonverbal behavior, or, at times, in the countertransference—in the face of what on the surface seems a completely frozen or affectless situation (Kernberg 2004). The simultaneous attention, by the therapist, to the patient's verbal communication, nonverbal behavior, and the countertransference permits diagnosing what the dominant affect is at the moment—and the corresponding object relation activated in the treatment situation. Every affect is considered to be the manifestation of an underlying object relation.

The second most important consideration in determining the selection of what is interpreted is the nature of the transference. When major affect development coincides with transference development, that becomes easy to determine, but there are times when most affect occurs related to extratransferential conditions or the patient's external world. Such affective dominance in the patient's external world, of course, always has transference implications as well; the focus, however, has to start on the external affectively invested situation, only shifting into a transference interpretation when the corresponding transference development clearly occupies the center of the patient's present interaction with the analyst. This is an important tactic derived from Fenichel's (1939) technical recommendations and reflects a flexibility of this approach that focuses simultaneously on the transference and on developments in these patients' external life at any time.

Still another tactical approach relates to certain general priorities that need to be taken up immediately, whether they reflect affective dominance or not in the session, although they usually do so anyway. These priorities include, by order of importance: 1) suicidal or homicidal behavior, 2) threats to the disruption of the treatment, 3) severe acting out in the session or outside that threatens the patient's life or the treatment, 4) dishonesty, 5) trivialization of the content of the hour, and 6) pervasive narcissistic resistances that must be resolved by consistent analysis of the transference implications of the pathological grandiose self (Clarkin et al. 2006; Kernberg 1984). When none of these priorities seems dominant at the moment in the hour, the general tactic of affective dominance and transference analysis prevails.

An important tactical aspect of a treatment involves conditions of severe regression, including affect storms, micropsychotic episodes, negative therapeutic reactions, and "incompatible realities."

We have developed specific technical approaches to these situations, the description of all of which would exceed the limits of this chapter.

Techniques

While "strategies" refer to overall, long-range goals and their implementation in transference analysis and "tactics" to particular interventions in concrete hours of treatment, "techniques" refers to the general, consistent application of technical instruments derived from psychoanalytic technique. The main technical instruments of TFP are those referred to by Gill (1954) as the essential techniques of psychoanalysis—namely, interpretation, transference analysis, and technical neutrality. If psychoanalysis consists in the facilitation of a regressive transference neurosis and the resolution of this transference neurosis by interpretation alone carried out by the psychoanalyst from a position of technical neutrality, TFP may be defined, in terms of its technical utilization, by these same three instruments, somewhat modified, however, as I shall mention below, and the important contribution of countertransference analysis as an additional major technical instrument.

The use of interpretation focuses particularly on the early phases of the interpretive process—namely, clarification of the subjective experience of the patient (clarification of what is in the patient's mind rather than clarifying information to him or her) and confrontation, in the sense of a tactful drawing of attention to any inconsistencies or contradictions in the patient's communication—either between what the patient says at one point in contrast to another, between verbal and nonverbal communication, or between the patient's communication and what is evoked in the countertransference. Nonverbal aspects of behavior become extremely important in the psychoanalytic psychotherapy of severe personality disorders. Interpretation per se, that is, the establishment of hypotheses regarding the unconscious functions of what has been brought forth by clarification and confrontation, follows these two techniques. Interpretation as a hypothesis about unconscious meaning refers, first of all, to interpretation of unconscious meaning in the "here and now," the "present unconscious" (Sandler and Sandler 1987), in contrast to genetic interpretations that link the unconscious meaning in the "here and now" with assumed unconscious meanings in the "there and then" that become important only in advanced stages of the treatment of severe personality disorders. Interpretation, in short, is applied systematically, but with heavy emphasis on its preliminary phases, clarification and confrontation, and the interpretation of the "present unconscious."

Transference analysis differs from the analysis of the transference in standard psychoanalysis in that, as mentioned before, it is always closely linked with the analysis of the patient's problems in external reality, in order to avoid the dissociation of the psychotherapy sessions from the patient's external life. Transference analysis also includes an implied concern for the long-range treatment goals that, characteristically, are not focused upon in standard psychoanalysis, except if they emerge in the transference. In TFP, an ongoing concern regarding dominant problems in the patient's life is reflected in the occasional introduction of reference to major conflicts that brought the patient into treatment or that have been discovered in the course of the treatment, bringing such conflicts into the treatment situation even if they are not transference-dominant at that point. This introduction of "extratransference material" follows the therapist's assessment that a significant splitting operation is in process, shielding a certain important conflict in the patient's external life from exploration in the treatment. Here the therapist's overview of the total treatment situation and the total life situation of the patient may determine that he or she introduce a subject matter "arbitrarily" (at times, at least in the patient's mind) and then focus on the transference development that occurs as a consequence of introducing such a major life theme. While transference analysis starts from session one, and in this regard, the treatment has significant similarities with Kleinian technique (because of the dominant emphasis both on transference analysis and on primitive defenses and object relations), this bringing in of external reality is a fundamental difference from Kleinian and, to some extent, also from ego psychological psychoanalysis.

Technical neutrality, as has probably become evident from what has been said before, is an ideal point of departure within the treatment at large and within each session but at times needs to be disrupted because of the urgent requirement for limit-setting and even in connection with the introduction of a major life problem of the patient that, at such point, would seem a nonneutral intervention of the therapist. Such deviation from technical neutrality may be indispensable in order to protect the boundaries of the treatment situation and protect the patient from severe suicidal and other self-destructive behavior and requires a particular approach in order to restore technical neutrality once it has been abandoned.

What we do, following an intervention that clearly signifies a temporary deviation from technical neutrality (e.g., by taking measures to control a patient's accumulation of medication with suicidal intentions), is the analysis of the transferential consequences of our intervention, to a point where these transferential developments can be resolved and then be followed with the analysis of the transference implications of the reasons that forced the therapist to move away from technical neutrality. Technical neutrality, in short, fluctuates throughout the treatment but is constantly worked on and reinstated as a major process goal.

The utilization of countertransference as a major therapeutic tool has already been referred to as an important source of information about affectively dominant issues in the hour. The intensity of the countertransferences evoked by patients with severe character pathology and consequent severely regressive behavior and acting out in the transference require an ongoing alertness to countertransference developments that the therapist has to tolerate in himself or herself, even under conditions of significant regression in countertransference fantasies and impulses of an aggressive, dependent, or sexual kind. That internal tolerance of countertransference permits its analysis in terms of the nature of the self-representation or the object representation that is being projected onto the therapist at that point, facilitating full interpretation of the dyadic relationship in the transference, so that countertransference is utilized in the therapist's mind for transference clarification. It is important that countertransference not be communicated directly to the patient but worked into transference interpretations. In this regard, TFP follows strictly analytic criteria typical for the ego psychological, Kleinian, British Independent, and French approaches. At times, partial acting out of the countertransference is unavoidable, and the therapist has to be honest in acknowledging the reality of what his or her behavior shows to the patient, without exceeding this communication with guilt-determined "confessions" or denying the reality of a behavioral response on the therapist's part that has become obvious to the patient. This, in essence, is not different from what standard psychoanalytic technique would expect from the analyst, except that the very intensity and dominant nature of countertransference information is characteristic of the process of TFP with severe personality disorders.

These then are the essential elements of the techniques of TFP. It also needs to be said that the frequency of interpretive interventions, at whatever level of regression, is high in comparison with transference interpretation in psychoanalysis. As Green (2000) has pointed out, the avoidance of traumatogenic associations drives borderline patients to jump from one subject to the next, thus expressing their "central phobic position," and may seem bewildering to an analyst used to expect the gradual development of a specific theme in free association, thus leading to clarify the subject matter that is being explored. Here, waiting for such a gradual deepening of free association is useless because of this defensive jump from one subject to the next, also related to the splitting operations that affect the very language of the patient.

The corresponding technical approach in TFP consists of an effort to interpret rapidly the implication of each of the fragments that emerge in the hours, with the intention of establishing continuity by the very nature of the interpretive interventions that gradually establish a continuity of their own. This approach may be compared with the interpretive work with dreams, in which the interpretation of apparently isolated fragments of the manifest dream content leads gradually to the latent dream content that establishes the continuity between the apparently disparate elements of the manifest content. Chapter 3 offers a verbatim report of a segment of an early session of TFP.

Indications and Contraindications

The most general indication for TFP is for patients with borderline personality organization; that is, presenting severe identity diffusion, severe breakdown in work and intimate relationships and in their social life, and specific symptoms linked to their particular personality disorder. This indication includes most personality disorders functioning at a borderline level, such as the borderline personality disorder per se, the more severe cases of histrionic personality disorder, paranoid personality disorders, schizoid personality disorders, narcissistic personality disorders functioning on an overt borderline level (i.e., having all the symptoms of borderline personality disorder and narcissistic personality disorder at the same time), and patients functioning at a borderline level with severe complications typical for these cases, if and when such complications can be treated first and controlled. These include alcoholism; drug dependency; severe eating disorders, particularly severe anorexia nervosa; antisocial behavior but definitely not an antisocial personality proper (that has no indication for psychotherapeutic treatment at all); schizotypal disorders; and severe hypochondriasis. In all individual cases, we evaluate first whether, even for such severe personality disorders, psychoanalysis may be the treatment of choice, which is the case for many histrionic personality disorders. Patients with the broad spectrum of severe personality disorders, who, in addition, usually have severe, chronic anxiety; characterologically based depression; somatization; phobic symptoms; and dissociative reactions, are optimal candidates for TFP, which thus expands the total realm of patients that can be treated with a psychoanalytically based approach.

The main contraindications include, as mentioned before, the antisocial personality proper and some narcissistic patients with severe antisocial features, as well as patients with chronic dishonesty that affects their capacity for verbal communication, such as pervasively dominant pseudologia fantastica: in short, severe degrees of chronic dishonesty that limit the capacity for honest communication and make the resolution of these psychopathic transferences very difficult. In contrast, patients with aggressive, provocative, irresponsible social behavior who, however, still are able to experience some degree of loyalty and investment in friendship and work are optimal candidates for TFP.

Another major contraindication is overwhelming secondary gain of illness, provided by financial social support, supportive housing, and financial means provided to many patients with severe personality disorders, who, unfortunately, are treated as if they were chronic schizophrenic patients and whose capacity to lead a parasitic life depending on the state or on wealthy families becomes a major life-sustaining goal. Patients without any social life at all, reduced for many years to staying in their room, watching television, and drifting in some way through life, also have a reserved prognosis but in many cases can be treated if an adequate treatment contract is in place. Patients should optimally have a normal IQ in order to undergo TFP.

There are patients in whom an inordinate amount of self-directed aggression expresses self-destruction as a major life goal, and the wishes to destroy themselves may be more powerful than the wishes to live and be treated. Some of these patients can be recognized before the treatment starts, others only in the course of the treatment, although a long series of extremely severe suicidal attempts and a long history of what seems like almost willful destruction of life opportunities may signal this condition. The same is true for patients with the most severe degree of negative therapeutic reaction, reflecting a profound identification with a battering object, and patients with the syndrome of malignant narcissism, where self-destructiveness implies the only possible triumph over an otherwise envied external world not suffering from the same conditions that they do. Many of the patients with contraindications for TFP may have an indication for supportive psychotherapy, a subject that goes beyond the realm of this particular communication, but to which our Personality Disorders Institute has contributed significantly (Appelbaum 2006; Rockland 1992).

This completes the outline of TFP for individual patients. What follows is the outline of the application of the general theory of technique of TFP to a model of psychoanalytic group psychotherapy.

A Conceptual Model for Transference-Focused Group Psychotherapy

From the viewpoint of a therapeutic approach geared to the systematic analysis of the transference, one might divide the psychoanalytically derived group psychotherapies into two groups. In one type of group psychotherapy, the main focus is the analysis of the development and interactions of the individuals in the group setting. Here the utilization of group dynamics intensifies highlighting, confronting, and helping the individual members to resolve their intrapsychic and interpersonal conflicts activated in their transference in the group, with the combined help of the therapist's interpretation and the group's confrontative and supportive intervention. This approach may be called "supportive," in the sense of not focusing analytically primarily on group dynamics per se and in utilizing supportive approaches in dealing with individual conflicts in combination with interpretive efforts. The second approach is centered primarily in the analysis of group dynamics rather than the dynamics of individual patients. This latter approach is linked particularly to Bion (1961), Ezriel (1950), and Sutherland (1952), in contrast to the first approach, of which Slavson (1964), Scheidlinger (1982), and Foulkes and Anthony (1957) may be considered the principal exponents, although many other authors have been influenced by them (Kaplan and Sadock 1993).

From the viewpoint of the techniques employed in working with the group, the supportive type of group psychotherapy may be characterized by the following features: the stimulation of the group to share information and provide commonality of experiences to its members, fostering mutual identification of the members in the process; clarification, confrontation, and cognitive and emotional support provided by the group and further deepened by the therapist's interpretation and facilitated by "chain reactions" within the group, thus fostering individual patients' adaptive responses; helping patients to shift from damaging to effective defensive operations and compromise formations; direct supportive interventions by the therapist, by means of affective and cognitive support in patients' confrontation with their difficulties, and, under certain circumstances, extending such interventions outside the group situation itself; and selection by the therapist of general themes for the group discussion, determined by their practical importance, the possibility of their generalization throughout the group, the urgency of intervention regarding certain problems, and their focus on pathology-specific issues. Last but not least, the therapist in this general approach is acutely aware of transference developments, attempts to strengthen positive transferences, and attempts to dismantle the negative ones that might interfere with the work of the group.

There are important differences within this general spectrum of approaches. While Slavson (1964) focuses specifically on the psychotherapy of individuals in the group setting, and believes that the dilution of transferences within the group is helpful to work with it, Foulkes and Anthony (1957) used group themes actively to apply them to individual patients and, in the process, encourage mutual support of the group, while the leader would reinforce the expression of such group reactions.

Implicitly, in the analytic approach to the treatment of this analytically derived supportive spectrum of group psychotherapy, higher level of characterological defenses characteristic of patients with well-integrated identity predominates, and a corresponding dominance of oedipal conflicts emerges in the foreground, while primitive group defenses tend to recede. The direct focus on improved socialization of individual patients also contributes to reducing the regression of the group into primitive states of mind, while supporting a certain degree of intellectualized understanding of dynamic processes.

In contrast, the group analytic approach of Bion, Ezriel, and Sutherland depends strongly on Bion's (1961) contributions to the psychology of small groups and his analysis of unconscious group dynamics, particularly his description of the basic assumption groups of dependency, fight-flight, and pairing. The analysis of the dynamics of small unstructured groups by Bion focused on the regressive group processes activated when the group leader limits himself or herself to observing the group's reactions, helping to clarify the respective basic assumptions group, and systematically avoiding any directive intervention, other than stressing the group's task of free interventions by members and of observing the processes emerging in the group setting. In Bion's approach to groups, the dominant basic group assumption expresses a dominant valence, at that moment, of the corresponding conflicts within the psychology of the individual members.

In the dependency group, what may be described as predominantly oral dependency conflicts predominate, with the search for an omniscient and omnipotent leader, and a corresponding feeling of incompetent, deskilled, or needy on the part of the group members as dependent on such a leader. Intense longings to obtain knowledge and love from such a leader, with greedy mutual competition for a maximum share of his or her attention, permeate the group. The failure of the leader to fulfill the expectations of total gratification expected from him or her leads to the leader's devaluation and to efforts of replacing him or her with somebody else who may fulfill those expectations. This dependent group evinces a predominance of primitive defensive operations, particularly primitive idealization, projected omnipotence, denial of aggression, envy, and greed, and defenses against those emotions.

In the fight-flight group, a paranoid atmosphere predominates, a surge of what might be considered strongly anally influenced conflicts around power and control. The group is engaged in a search for a powerful leader against external enemies. There may be a development of ad hoc ideologies that differentiate the group from outsiders or, within the group, conflicts between an in-group and an out-group, a potential split of the group between those who submit to the admired leader—the in-group—and those who are in rebellion against the dominant, feared leader—the out-group. Here the main emerging defensive operations are splitting and projection of aggression, projective identification, general paranoid suspiciousness and efforts at omnipotent control, and dread of any attack on the idealization of the leader or the dominant ideology.

In the pairing group, finally, the atmosphere is much more "oedipal," in contrast to the condensed preoedipal and oedipal contents and primitive defensive operations prevalent in the dependency and fight-flight group. Typically, the group attempts to create within it an idealized couple, homosexual or heterosexual, with an implicit unconscious hope that that successful, happy couple will assure the meaningfulness and the future of the group. Here a sense of erotized intimacy and sexualized gratification emerges as a major defense against regressive dependency and aggression.

The approach of Ezriel and Sutherland constitutes a modification of Bion's approach. It needs to be kept in mind that Bion's approach to the analysis of small groups was originally geared to study the psychology of group processes and only secondarily applied to therapeutic efforts in a group setting. The experience at the Tavistock Clinic, where Bion's therapeutic work with groups was carried out, was that the application of a "pure Bion model" was difficult for patients to tolerate and was experienced as less helpful than the modifications of interpretation introduced by Ezriel that focused somewhat more on the individual members' reactions to rather than exclusively on the major group themes (John Sutherland, personal communication, 1971). Ezriel and Sutherland, in effect, combined the analysis of predominant group themes with the analysis of the position that individual patients adopted regarding the conflicts activated in the basic assumptions group. Thus, for example, if in a group with a predominant basic assumption of fight-flight, one individual appeared as consistently supporting of or submitting to the leader, while another member of the group became extremely critical of that behavior, the group leader would point out how the contradiction in the behavior of these two members reflected a general conflict between submissiveness and rebelliousness in the group and how different group members occupied a particular position within that conflict that resonated with the particular forms that this kind of conflict took in the psychopathology of each individual.

Ezriel systematized the analysis of the conflictual dynamics of dominant group themes by defining, at various times, "a common group tension." He analyzed this group tension in terms of a "required attitude" within the group that expressed a defensive function regarding an opposite, "avoided experience" of the group, because the activation of that avoided experience might produce a fantasied "calamitous situation" and corresponding relationships. The therapist's analysis of the general group tension would be followed by highlighting how various individuals in the group fit into this dynamic on the side of the required or on the side of the avoided reaction, and he or she formulated a hypothesis regarding the threatened situation that the group was in an unconscious collusion to avoid by all means. In both Bion's and Ezriel and Sutherland's approaches, the group therapist maintains a position of technical neutrality, attempting to diagnose the dominant themes in the development of the interactions in the group, interpreting those themes when the situation seemed ripe for it, and, generally speaking, avoiding the addressing of individual members rather than the group at large.

Bion as well as Ezriel and Sutherland paid an ongoing attention to the countertransference reactions evoked in them by the developments in the group, utilizing them systematically in the diagnosis of the prevalent group tension and basic assumption group. Psychoanalytic group psychotherapy, with the unstructured nature of the communications derived from the invitation to all members to speak freely about whatever is on their mind, generally tends to evoke powerful countertransference reactions that the therapist must attempt to understand without being controlled by them and then use in the formulation of his or her interpretive interventions. The almost obsessive punctuality of starting and ending group sessions, the ritualized utilization of the sitting arrangement in a circle, by which all members can see and directly interact with one another, provides a subtle but powerful "containing" structure that tends to reduce the fears of acting out in the group setting and facilitates the diagnosis of regressive group behavior.

In our work with TFP with borderline patients at the Weill Cornell Personality Disorders Institute, we have found strong similarities of the basic principles to the technical approach of Ezriel and Sutherland, on the one hand, and the TFP-based approach to the technique of psychoanalytic psychotherapy for borderline patients, on the other. What follows is an outline of our own proposed model for psychoanalytic group psychotherapy with borderline patients, clinically carried out in various settings of group psychotherapy as part of inpatient and day hospital settings, but, as mentioned before, our clinical experience reported below still needs to be tested in empirical research.

Strategies and Techniques

I shall outline, in what follows, strategies, tactics, and techniques of the TFP model of analytic group psychotherapy. The main strategy consists in facilitating the interpretation of basic assumption groups, in the context of a strict focus, on the part of the therapist, on the nature of the primitive object relations and corresponding defensive operations activated in the course of any basic assumption group. In practice, the defensive operations activated in the dependency and in the fight-flight group present the total repertoire of primitive defensive operations based upon splitting mechanisms characteristic for borderline patients. As such, they are eminently relevant for the exploration of the psychopathology of patients with severe personality disorders, who find their dominant emotional reactions powerfully activated in the group situation.

Rather than interpreting the sequential activation of individually determined dominant transferences activated in the course of the group sessions, the therapist's emphasis is on the sequence of group processes, the progressive and regressive fluctuations of the group tension that facilitate the activation of particular conflicts of individual patients—their "group valence"—at different times. The individual pathology of any particular patient comes into central focus at a point when he or she occupies one of the polarities of the conflictual dynamics of the group. The fact that the therapist's interpretations follow the dominant group dynamics, his or her pointing out how this dynamic is played out by different members of the group, practically facilitates interventions geared to individual patients at the time when their corresponding conflicts are affectively dominant. Thus, the TFP principle of interpreting affectively dominant conflicts holds for both the analysis of the group tension and the analysis of the position of key members of the group in the enactment of and reaction to this group tension.

In practice, therefore, after the therapist has interpreted the dominant unconscious dynamics of the prevalent group tension, he or she may address how this group conflict touches all the individual members' conflicts in terms of their position taken regarding that particular group conflict. Insofar as individual patients' transferences are directed to other members of the group, to the group as a whole, and to the group leader, moments when all these three vectors come together may provide a powerful source for emotional understanding for individual patients. For example, a patient who attempts to erotize the relation with another patient under conditions when the group seems to be involved in a struggle with the authority of the group leader may both reflect this patient's participation in rebellious opposition to the group as such by isolating himself and this couple from it and illustrate the upsurge of erotic strivings at points where they fulfill a defensive function against the threat of mutual aggression.

The therapist's interventions in the group are guided by the same principles as the interventions in individual TFP sessions:

first, by what is affectively dominant in the group; second, by the nature of dominant transferences operating within the group atmosphere; and third, by his or her countertransference. The therapist's interventions consist in clarifications—namely, efforts to clarify the dominant issues affecting the group at a certain point; confrontation—namely, pointing to the nonverbal behaviors that accompany and often overshadow the verbal communication among group members and of the entire group toward the leader; and interpretation per se—namely, of the unconscious conflict inherent in the activation of determined group tension and the corresponding basic assumption group. The interpretation consists in focusing on the dominant group theme, by first pointing to the predominant conscious and preconscious experience of the group; then, the opposite, avoided theme and the motives for this avoidance; and finally, the nature of the experienced threat connected with what is avoided.

The therapist maintains an attitude of technical neutrality regarding the developments in the group, limited by establishing clear rules about what is not tolerated: particularly, physical aggression against the therapist, other members, and property; gross sexual harassment, such as seductiveness in the form of stripping; or self-destructive behavior, such as self-cutting or burning. The techniques utilized, in short, are interpretation, transference analysis, technical neutrality, and countertransference utilization. *Countertransference utilization* refers to the analysis in the therapist's mind of both concordant and complementary identifications he or she experiences regarding the group as a whole and individual members, followed by the utilization of the understanding of these developments as part of the interpretive formulations.

For example, the attraction a male therapist may feel for a female member of the group, while subtle comments within the group refer to a "special relation" between the two, may correspond to an unconscious collusion of the group to seduce the therapist to abandon his therapeutic role in an unconscious effort to dethrone and corrupt him, while an oedipal temptation combined with an unconscious masochistic acting out of sexual fantasies toward the unavailable father-therapist may be dominant in the woman patient's momentary affect activation.

The technical approach, therefore, follows the same general principles and guidelines of the technical approach in TFP, while the overall strategy of highlighting and resolving the dominant split-off or dissociated primitive internalized object relations of these patients is systematically explored in the order in which these object relations are achieving dominance as part of the group regression. Dominant object relations may be enacted by the group as a whole in relation to the group leader or by individual members toward the group, the leader, and other individual members. By means of the activation of projective identification, the role of self- and object representations may be rapidly exchanged among the members of the group as well as between the group and the group leader. For example, a process of total, contemptuous devaluation of the group leader, while the group assumes a controlling and omnipotent attitude, may reflect conflicts around narcissistic pathology of individual members, activating depreciatory behaviors while projecting the inferior, devalued aspects of the self onto the leader and these patients identifying themselves or the group with a pathological grandiose self.

Tactics

So far, I have examined the strategic and technical applications of TFP to this modified Ezriel-Sutherland model. From the viewpoint of tactical interventions, they include general arrangements that are specific for a group therapy approach and particular ones corresponding to the specific application of a TFP model. Regarding general tactical interventions, they refer to the selection of members of the group, a complex decision-making process that, in general terms, corresponds to the same criteria for indications of TFP in individual patients mentioned before. Contraindications include patients with an intelligence level below an IQ of 85 or 90; severe, uncontrollable secondary gain of illness; significant antisocial behavior that would risk the confidentiality of group processes to which the participants have to commit themselves and objectively threaten other group members; and severity of acting out or comorbid conditions that could not be easily handled by an individual therapist taking care of those aspects of treatment outside the setting of the group psychotherapy. For example, some patients with an active, major depression may present a contraindication for participating in this type of group psychotherapy, while others may be treated in a group while being followed up by an individual psychopharmacologist outside the group setting. In this connection, a specific contraindication for group psychotherapy is the case of severely depressed patients with negative therapeutic reactions, who may get worse with the expression of sympathy or support to them, thus possibly triggering a serious suicidal attempt.

In general, there is a great advantage to psychoanalytic group psychotherapy if the group therapist limits interventions to the treatment within the group situation. We have found that an optimal frequency of the sessions is about an hour and a half meeting twice a week, and that after the group has reached a certain minimum number of patients, optimally not fewer than five and not more than twelve, the group should be closed and prepared for a long time of work together. Individual, specialized contract setting with some patients may be necessary as a precondition for accepting them in the group situation, such as, for example, responsibly taking care of other necessary medical treatment or responsibility under crisis conditions, suicidal threats, and self-mutilating tendencies: here the general principles of TFP contract tactics are relevant (Yeomans et al. 1992).

The development of particular complications and severe regression of individuals in the group usually can be managed when the overall group setting is clear and consistent. Chronic monopolizers can be managed easily by pointing to the group's tolerance or unconscious fostering of such behavior and its meanings under the concrete group circumstances. The chronically silent patient may be much more behaviorally active in the context of shifting group themes than what is revealed by language alone, and varying meanings of the defensive use of silence can be explored in the context of its function as part of the group process. The manifestation of group resistances in the form of shared, extended silences; trivialization of the contents of the group discussion; and demonstrative ignoring of the group leader and of his or her interventions all become part and parcel of potential transference interpretations.

It is essential for the group therapist to establish an individual contract with each patient before the start of psychoanalytic group psychotherapy, defining clearly what the responsibilities of the patients are and under what conditions his or her continuation in the group psychotherapy would become impossible if such essential responsibilities, which the patient has to carry out for himself or herself, were not fulfilled. In the treatment of patients with severe personality disorders, a question comes up naturally: whether the patient would not need an individual psychotherapist outside the group sessions and whether the group psychotherapist should be available to individual patients outside the sessions under certain circumstances. As mentioned before, it would be ideal if the group therapist would be able to limit himself or herself to be available to the group sessions, but there may be circumstances when an exception would seem reasonable: to save the patient's life or to protect him or her from serious consequences of destructive or self-destructive behavior. Under these circumstances, it is important to share such outside interventions as objective data with the group, because this may be an important precondition to understand the group dynamics implication and permit the interpretation of the group transference meanings of such developments.

In other words, the confidentiality of individual material that reaches the therapist has to extend to the group to avoid splitting processes and omnipotent control of the therapist by individual patients. By the same token, the therapist may flexibly use information provided by individuals outside the group sessions in pointing out that he or she is willing to receive such information with the understanding that, by common agreement reached with the patient, it may be used in the group setting or, if the patient were not willing to authorize the therapist to share such information with the group, with the rare possibility that the therapist might decide to discontinue the patient from that group. The implication is that there may be much information that is either irrelevant or would not impact on major group themes and that the therapist would not feel necessary to communicate to the group. At the same time, the therapist needs to maintain his or her freedom to use interpretively what is affecting an emotional relationship to the group, including information coming from outside the sessions. The therapist has to be prepared to intervene in cases when an acute psychotic regression severely disrupts the group session, as well as threatening the patient himself or herself. Such a situation may justify a shift in the technical neutrality of the therapist, at the service of protecting the boundaries of the group as such.

Group members themselves should feel free to interact with one another (or not) outside the group sessions: it is part of a technical neutral attitude that the therapist will refrain from intervening or influencing directly the patient's life outside the sessions. However, if the mutual relationships of members outside the group setting clearly affect the group situation itself, or seem obvious manifestations of transference acting out on the part of the group, this needs to be interpreted systematically. Antisocial behavior of one of the members of the group, aggressively affecting the life of another member of the group, obviously may become a reason for discontinuing that antisocially behaving member from the group. All group members need to be protected physically and psychologically from mutual attack.

As can be seen from the illustrations given before, the tactical interventions under certain circumstances may differ from those required in individual TFP, particularly under conditions of severe patient regression. Usually the group itself tends to maintain its structure and protects individual patients from excessive regression. There are relatively infrequent situations in which severe regressions occur, and these are a challenge to the group therapist that the general approach outlined should help him or her to master. It helps enormously if the group leader has a good grasp of strategies, tactics, and techniques of individual TFP, together with knowledge of group processes in depth, regarding both small and large unstructured groups. The fact that regression in small groups so clearly parallels the activation of primitive defenses and object relations observed in the individual psychotherapy of severe personality disorders provides a basic link between these two therapeutic approaches and definitely justifies, I believe, further research into this area.

References

Appelbaum AH: Supportive psychoanalytic psychotherapy for borderline patients: an empirical approach. Am J Psychoanal 66:317–332, 2006

Bion WR: Experiences in Groups. New York, Basic Books, 1961

Clarkin JF, Yeomans FE, Kernberg OF: Psychotherapy for Borderline Personality: Focusing on Object Relations. Washington, DC, American Psychiatric Publishing, 2006

Ezriel H: A psychoanalytic approach to the treatment of patients in groups. Journal of Mental Science 96:774–779, 1950

Fenichel O: Problems of psychoanalytic technique. Psychoanal Q 8:438–470, 1939

Foulkes SH, Anthony EJ: Group Psychotherapy: The Psychoanalytic Approach. Baltimore, MD, Penguin Books, 1957

Gill M: Psychoanalysis and exploratory psychotherapy. J Am Psychoanal Assoc 2:771–797, 1954

Green A: On Private Madness. Madison, CT, International Universities Press, 1993

Green A: La position phobique centrale, in La pensée clinique. Paris, Editions Odile Jacob, 2000

Kaplan HI, Sadock BJ (eds): Comprehensive Group Psychotherapy, 3rd Edition. Baltimore, MD, Williams & Wilkins, 1993

Kernberg OF: Severe Personality Disorders: Psychotherapeutic Strategies. New Haven, CT, Yale University Press, 1984

Kernberg OF: Aggressivity, Narcissism, and Self-Destructiveness in the Psychotherapeutic Relationship: New Developments in the Psychopathology and Psychotherapy of Severe Personality Disorders. New Haven, CT, Yale University Press, 2004

Kernberg OF, Burnstein ED, Coyne L, et al: Psychotherapy and psychoanalysis: final report of the Menninger Foundation's Psychotherapy Research Project. Bull Menninger Clin 36:1–275, 1972

Kernberg OF, Yeomans FE, Clarkin JF, et al: Transference focused psychotherapy: overview and update. Int J Psychoanal 89:601–620, 2008

Rockland LH: Supportive Therapy for Borderline Patients: A Psychodynamic Approach. New York, Guilford, 1992

Sandler J, Sandler AM: The past unconscious, the present unconscious, and the vicissitudes of guilt. Int J Psychoanal 8:331–341, 1987

Scheidlinger S: Focus on Group Psychotherapy: Clinical Essays. New York, International Universities Press, 1982

Slavson SR: A Textbook in Analytic Group Psychotherapy. New York, International Universities Press, 1964

Sutherland JD: Notes on psychoanalytic group therapy, I: therapy and training. Psychiatry 15:111–117, 1952

Yeomans FE, Selzer MA, Clarkin JF: Treating the Borderline Patient: A Contract-Based Approach. New York, Basic Books, 1992

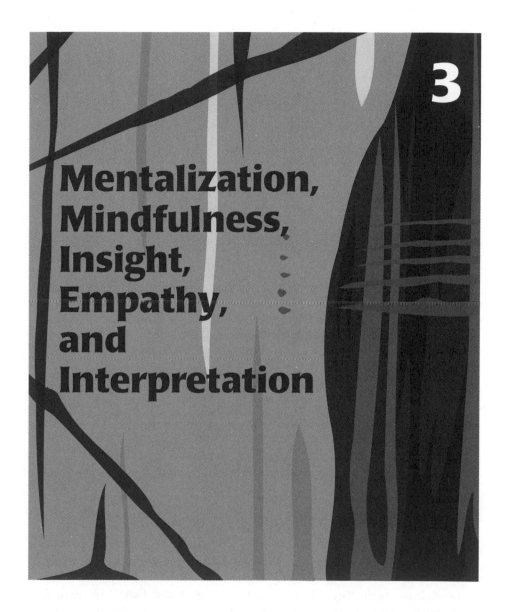

3

Mentalization, Mindfulness, Insight, Empathy, and Interpretation

To be published as a chapter in *Handbuch der Borderline Störungen,* 2nd Edition. Edited by Dulz B, Herpertz S, Kernberg OF, Sachsse U. Stuttgart, Germany, Schattauer, 2011. Used with permission.

In this chapter, I define the related concepts of *mentalization, mindfulness, insight,* and *empathy* and discuss their mutual relation and their relevance in the practice of behavioral and psychodynamic psychotherapy. Mentalization-based therapy (MBT) represents an alternative psychodynamic psychotherapy to transference-focused psychotherapy (TFP), and I attempt to clarify the relations between these two therapies that have been applied particularly to borderline personality disorder. Mindfulness is a key concept presently being utilized in cognitive-behavioral approaches, and the comparison of this concept with mentalization is relevant in the comparative analysis of different contemporary psychotherapies.

Another major issue explored in this chapter is the role of interpretation as a central psychodynamic technique in the treatment of severe personality disorders. It represents the viewpoint that early interpretive interventions—as defined in this context— are a helpful, essential component of psychodynamic approaches to severe personality disorders and illustrates this interpretive approach with a verbatim segment of an early session of TFP with a borderline patient.

The recent emphasis on mentalization as a particular focus and mechanism of change in the treatment of severe personality disorders within a psychodynamic approach has highlighted the confusingly broad spectrum of conceptualization of this term. Sugarman (2006), for example, in a comprehensive view, defines *mentalization* in the broadest sense. He equates mentalization with what he calls insightfulness, referring to the general developmental processes that foster self-reflectiveness, development of the capacity for symbolization, and acquisition of knowledge regarding the internal world: in psychoanalysis, insightfulness is fostered by interpretation and transference analysis. This broad conceptualization, I believe, loses the specificity of the corresponding technical approach to borderline conditions. In what follows, I shall propose a narrow, circumscribed definition of mentalization as a *specific* mechanism of change in the psychodynamic psychotherapy and psychoanalytic treatment of severe personality disorders, relate it to the technical interpretive approach to these conditions, and compare it with parallel developments in the cognitive-behavioral psychotherapeutic approaches.

I begin with some basic assumptions to frame the analysis that follows. A major goal of psychoanalysis is the patient's acquisition of insight into the unconscious mental processes (not only "content") that are the unconscious motivation and determinants of conscious behavior that overshadow conscious purposes. Insight involves self-reflective awareness of unconscious mental operations and of the interplay of past and present fantasy and reality in the context of which psychic processes evolve. Interpretation, I believe, is the fundamental psychoanalytic technique fostering insight, and I have discussed elsewhere the relation between transference analysis and the "real relationship" with the analyst as a therapeutic factor (Kernberg 2007b, 2009). Psychodynamic psychotherapies also have maintained this emphasis on acquiring insight on unconscious mental processes, stressing self-reflection facilitated by interpretive psychodynamic techniques to achieve such knowledge (Caligor et al. 2009; Kernberg 1999). In recent times, cognitive and behavioral psychotherapeutic approaches have started to pay attention to self-reflective awareness of intrapsychic processes under the heading of "mindfulness," an approach influenced by Buddhist philosophy, the efficacy of which is currently being investigated through empirical studies of psychotherapy outcome (Siegel 2007).

The recent emphasis on "mentalization," with its focus on increased awareness of mental processes of the self and of significant others, as a major aspect of psychoanalytic psychotherapies of severe personality disorders constitutes a special development within the search for increased insight (Bateman and Fonagy 2004; Levy et al. 2006a). MBT, a special form of psychodynamic psychotherapy for severe personality disorders, proposes that early interpretation may actually be contraindicated in the early stages of MBT, or any therapy, for severe personality disorders. Fonagy and his coworkers, the authors of MBT, have pointed to the risks of early interpretation of the transference in borderline patients, raising the question whether, indeed, interpretation, under certain circumstances, may actually hinder or inhibit a patient's ability to mentalize (Bateman and Fonagy 2004). A related question, frequently raised in recent times, is the relative importance of interpretation-derived insight as contrasted to the effects of the therapeutic relationship per se as a major mechanism of change (Kernberg 2007b). In addition, the prevalent broadening of the concept of insight to signify a general increase of knowledge of oneself, decoupling the concept from specific technical implications, may be occurring to the concept of mentalization as well. The latter, originally focused on therapeutic approaches to borderline patients, now tends at times to be applied to all psychotherapeutic processes focused on increased self-reflectiveness rather than related to a specific psychodynamic approach to severe personality disorders. This conceptual broadening blurs the concepts of insight and mentalization.

Mindfulness

In this context, the parallel development of the concept of mindfulness as a major technical concern of cognitive-behavioral therapies adds a related dimension regarding the importance of self-reflection in all psychotherapies. All of this, I believe, warrants an effort to define these related concepts and circumscribe their indications for general or specific technical employment, particularly from the viewpoint of a psychoanalytic approach. The comparison of the concept of mindfulness within cognitive psychotherapeutic approaches and mentalization within psychoanalytic psychotherapeutic approaches may provide a basic frame for clarifying the issues raised above. This task was first engaged in the original paper by Choi-Kain and Gunderson (2008), with a particular focus on the overlapping areas of these and related concepts. In what follows, I shall explore these concepts from the viewpoint of psychoanalytic object relations theory, attempting to circumscribe them and to sharpen their differential implications and utilization.

Mindfulness has been a central task of meditation, derived from Buddhist philosophical principles, and incorporated in cognitive-behavioral therapies, stimulating empirical research and attempts to sharpen the concept (Linehan 1993; Linehan et al. 2007). *Mindfulness* may be defined as a conscious effort to evaluate the subjective experience of the present moment by means of voluntary attentiveness, without exerting any judgment of this experience. It is a benign attention—active, focused, but without critical restriction—to the present experience of the self. It includes an emotional, empathic, open attentiveness regarding one's momentary thinking, feeling, and observing (Siegel 2007). Within dialectic behavior therapy (DBT), for example, this definition is further specified into various aspects—namely, observing and describing the conscious experience of the self in the moment and the effort to observe this experience while accepting it in a noncritical way (Carson et al. 2004; Germer et al. 2005; Hays et al. 2004; Shapiro et al. 2006). Mindfulness implies the focus on the experience of one's feelings without reacting to them or acting on their basis (which is closely allied with what within psychoanalytic terminology one would think of as the process of containing thoughts and feelings, in contrast to acting them out). The attention to and perception of one's feelings without reacting to them should include both pleasurable and painful feelings, sensations and perceptions, and an effort to verbalize them within a frame of tolerance rather than a critical disposition. Mindfulness, in essence, is a reflection about the nature of one's own psychic processes and subjective state in the moment, and it implies an attitude of curiosity, openness, acceptance, and love toward self. It is a form of relationship with one's self, an internal form of "attunement" to oneself, that has become an important technical approach of cognitive-behavioral therapies focused on stress reduction. The content of such self-observation includes sensations, images, feelings, and thoughts; the attention is on everything perceived in this moment by the self, including the experience of inanimate objects in the surrounding environment. From a psychoanalytic viewpoint, one might speculate that such an attitude of an accepting self-orientation as implied by mindfulness may reflect an unconscious identification with a loving maternal introject but also carries with it the temptation for narcissistic self-enhancement.

The therapeutic objectives of mindfulness within cognitive-behavioral therapies include the regulation of attention and attentiveness and of affect and self-esteem through the acceptance and openness regarding one's own experiences. It also has become an objective instrument for research on psychological integration. From the viewpoint of a psychoanalytic approach, this focus on mindfulness within the field of cognitive-behavioral therapies represents a significant progress in several ways: it is a recognition that even within cognitive approaches, the focus on affectivity and emotionality has become quite central. It is a new focus on patients' internal experiences in addition to their objective behavior and intellectual structures.

There is clearly some overlap between mindfulness and mentalization in regard to self-observation and the emphasis on reduction of impulsivity and reactivity in approaching one's affective experience (Choi-Kain and Gunderson 2008). An important difference, however, is that mindfulness is restricted to self-observation. In spite of efforts to expand the realm of self-observation, its very focus is on "the moment," and not on the self in relationship to the other, and on "conscious" factors, while mentalization also includes the consideration of unconscious phenomena and, importantly, the consideration of the patient's experience of the therapist. Perhaps the most important difference, from the viewpoint of contemporary object relations theory, is that the concept of mindfulness does not include the unconscious determinants of self-observation derived from dyadic and triadic internalized object relationships, such as the unconscious identification with parental figures, whose loving, accepting, indifferent, or critical and rejecting attitude toward the self is incorporated in the form of the internal relationship to the self as a perceived entity (Kernberg 2004b). Insofar as mindfulness also includes the present experience of perceived objects surrounding the individual, these include inanimate objects and not the perception of others as mindful objects relating to the self of the individual. And the concept of mindfulness does not consider the problems raised by normal and pathological narcissistic tendencies, experiences of grandiosity, humiliation, and inferiority. Indeed, there is the danger that mindfulness may actually reinforce omnipotent narcissistic object relations in certain cases, promoting self-idealization or the illusion that everything that is valuable emanates and resides in the experience of self in the moment.

Mentalization

Mentalization, in contrast, implies the understanding of the behavior of self and of others as meaningful, based on intentional, purposeful mental states that include personal wishes, needs, feelings, and convictions of both parties. These states of mind change constantly in the course of interaction as a reflection of the mutual influences in the relationships between self and other. In other words, it is a process of realistic understanding of one's own mental processes and one's own affective and cognitive experiences and also the realistic understanding of the corresponding processes of the other ("the object"), with the implication of a realistic, deep capability for object relations. The concept of mentalization also includes explicit conscious and implicit unconscious aspects. It has been operationalized through the development of the Reflective Function Scale, an instrument designed to assess mentalization within the context of attachment relationships and which has been studied extensively through research with the Adult Attachment Interview (Fonagy et al. 1997; Levy et al. 2006b).

Fonagy has described the origin of the development of mentalization in the early attachment processes and has demonstrated the important relationship of borderline personality disorder with insecure attachment and thus highlighted the importance of the earliest mother-infant relationship as a key etiological feature of that personality disorder. Disorganization, or lack of development, of the symbolic function under the influence of strong, dominant negative affects emerges as the expression of insecure attachment. Fonagy has proposed that in borderline patients under conditions of stress, there is an activation of the attachment system with regression in cognitive function, a surge of insecurity with disregard of rational considerations, and the activation of an "alien self." This alien self, Fonagy has proposed, is an alien, anxiety-evoking, dissociated representation of self, linked to experiences with a traumatizing other who has failed to mirror the individual in ways that are marked and contingent, that must be continuously projected onto the other, distorting the realistic relationship with the object (Bateman and Fonagy 2004).

In MBT, the therapist tries to help the regressed borderline patient to clarify his or her own mental state to correct the incapacity to assess the patient's own affective experience fully and appropriately, by providing (and thus helping the patient achieve) an empathic cognitive framing of the patient's experience and by communicating to the patient how the therapist perceives the patient's experience of the therapist at that point. This facilitates the cognitive framing of the patient's own affective experience; contributes to transforming the primitive, diffuse, overwhelming primary affective representations into secondary affective representations, more appropriately framed cognitively; and permits the therapist to raise the question with the patient regarding the possibility that the therapist's view of his or her own emotional experience might differ from that which the patient holds of him or her. This fosters further increase in the patient's capability to mentalize his or her experience of the therapist's experience.

Gradually, the effect of sequential clarification of the patient's mental states of self and of the other in each concrete experience of powerful affective activation, including the reason for the cognitive regression and loss of symbolization at points of perceived stress, increases the patient's realistic awareness of self and the therapist and significantly decreases the projection of the alien self, thus normalizing the therapeutic relationship. This development, in turn, gradually permits the therapist to introduce interpretive efforts regarding unconscious motivations for the patient's states of intense, regressive affect activation. Bateman and Fonagy (2011) have stated succinctly the goal of MBT: "The aims of MBT are modest:

this is not a therapy aiming to achieve major structural/personality change or alter cognitions and schemas; its aim is to enhance embryonic capacities of mentalization so that the individual is more able to solve problems and to manage emotional states particularly within interpersonal relationships or at least feel more confident about their ability to do so."

The concept of mentalization and its expression in reflective function has significantly enhanced the description of an essential mechanism of change in the treatment of borderline patients, namely, the increasingly realistic understanding of the concept of self and the concept of significant others, a crucial step in the resolution of pathological internalized object relations characteristic of severe personality disorders. Also, Fonagy's clarification of the functions of congruent and marked affective response of mother to the infant's affect activation as an essential etiological factor in determining secure or insecure attachment has related a crucial etiological feature of severe personality disorders to a specific therapeutic approach.

Theoretical Considerations Regarding Mentalization

There are, however, in my view, two major problems regarding the formulation of MBT: first, at a theoretical level, the relationship of mentalization to contemporary psychoanalytic object relations theory, and second, at a clinical level, the nature of the therapeutic interventions with borderline patients in psychoanalytic psychotherapy and psychoanalysis.

Regarding the theoretical issue, involving psychoanalytic object relations theory, MBT describes the presence within the mind of the borderline patient of an "alien self," a dissociated self-representation dominated by negative affect that "colonizes" the self and influences the patient's experience of self and other, especially in moments of severe affective regression, by projection onto the object. This formulation does not adequately address the fact that, under conditions of severe regression, a pathological, "all bad" object relation is enacted, with the development of both a distorted, aggressively infiltrated, frightful representation of self and a corresponding aggressively dominated representation of the significant object, in relation to which the self is a victim (Kernberg 2004a). Thus, under conditions of reactivation of the "alien self," there is a parallel activation of an "alien object." In other words, while the patient projects one of these representations (of self or object) onto the therapist, he or she simultaneously identifies himself or herself with the corresponding reciprocal representation (of victim or perpetrator of self or object). Typically, under conditions of such regression in the case of severe personality disorders, the respective identification with an aggressive self or object representation or a victimized self is rapidly exchanged, alternatively enacted, and, respectively, projected by the patient onto the therapist. By the mechanism of projective identification, the corresponding representation of self or object projected by the patient onto the therapist may induce a corresponding complementary identification in the countertransference (the role responsiveness of the therapist). The clinical example presented further on illustrates this process. The restricted concept of the "alien self," in short, misses the total nature of the reactivated, unconscious, internalized object relation in the transference.

From that viewpoint, also, it becomes clearer that in the course of normal mentalization, not only is a "theory of mind" developed normally in the infant or child, that is, the capacity to construct a realistic assessment of intentional mental states in self and others, but also the capacity to empathize with the emotional experience of the other develops. The cognitive implications of a theory of mind that incorporates the ability to comprehend intentional mental processes in the object are not automatically equivalent to the capacity to empathize with the emotional state of the other. This complex fact is well illustrated in cases of the antisocial personality disorder. These patients definitely have the capacity for a theory of mind. In fact, they often have a keen understanding of the intentions and mental states of the other but are incapable of empathy with the emotional reality of other human beings. From a neurobiological standpoint, different complex mechanisms seem to be involved in the realistic cognitive assessment of another's cognitive processes and in the capacity to "feel with" the other. This latter capacity may depend not only on the nature of internalized, dyadic self- and object representation units but also, importantly, on the developmental processes of the integration of internalized object relations, the shift—in Kleinian terms—from the paranoid-schizoid to the depressive position or, in ego psychological terminology, from part object to whole object internalized object relations, leading to the establishment and consolidation of ego identity. This shift consolidates the capacity for experiencing feelings of guilt over one's own aggression, the development of concern for self and others, and the deepening of the capacity for gratitude and higher levels of idealization.

Mentalization and Transference-Focused Psychotherapy

This brings us to the second clinical issue regarding mentalization, referred to before: the nature of therapeutic interventions based on a concept such as MBT and their relation with other psychoanalytically based approaches to treatment of borderline conditions, particularly TFP. TFP is a psychoanalytic psychotherapy for borderline and other severe personality disorders, centered on the objective of integrating self-representations and their corresponding internalized object representations, in an effort to establish and consolidate normal identity (Clarkin et al. 2006). This clearly coincides with the objective of mentalization as a realistic assessment of intentional cognitive-affective states in self and significant others. Research on TFP at the Personality Disorders Institute at Weill Medical College of Cornell University empirically confirmed that TFP significantly increases mentalization (Levy et al. 2006a, 2006b). Now, our approach is essentially interpretive from practically the first session of the treatment and, in this regard, is quite similar, in some ways, to the Kleinian psychoanalytic approach, although also significant differences with that approach need to be stressed (Kernberg et al. 2008).

The process of interpretation in TFP is a stepwise process tailored to the patient. The overall process of interpretation begins with the therapist's effort to clarify the patient's experience of self and of object (the therapist) under the condition of any particular, idealized or persecutory, split-off affect state, in the context of the activation of primitive transferences of these patients. Clarification is intended to make explicit what is in the patient's mind with respect to the present mental state and in this regard may be thought of as a bid to promote mentalization. Clarification of how the patient perceives himself or herself and the therapist may be followed, often enough in the same session, by further clarification of an opposite mental state, in which the roles of patient and therapist have been reversed. This first stage of interpretation involves analyst-centered interpretations in which the patient's immediate experience of the therapist in the moment is amplified and explored without any attempts to link it to previously divergent experiences or the patient's conflicts or history.

For example, in a session [described further on (session five of the treatment)], the patient first felt humiliated by her experience of a grandiose and dominating therapist, only to, shortly later in the session, then enjoy feeling superior to an incompetent and ignorant therapist. This permitted the therapist to point out to the patient that the patient alternatively felt herself threatened by a dominant man and then enjoyed making the therapist feel inferior while she identified herself with that dominant position. No motivation for the patient's oscillating identification was hypothesized at this stage of the treatment. The therapist was guided by what appears to be affectively dominant in the transference from moment to moment, session to session, merely pointing out to the patient what appears to be happening between them.

Usually, after a period of weeks or months in which this interpretive approach to the alternation of split-off idealized and persecutory relationships has taken place, the patient becomes better able to tolerate split-off identifications with self and object both under idealized and under persecutory conditions. The interpretive linkage between these two opposite positions can now be proposed by the therapist for the patient's consideration. At this point in the treatment, the typical interpretation would attempt to clarify the patient's need to maintain an absolute dissociation between idealized and persecutory experiences, to avoid the contamination and feared destruction of the relation with an idealized object by a threatening world of negative, hostile, catastrophic object relations.

This process of interpreting the defensive nature of maintaining internal splits is titrated to the patient's ability to tolerate and work with the hypothesis. If the patient does not appear to be ready to consider attributions of underlying unconscious motivations, the therapist would continue to clarify the patient's transient identification and pointing to contradictions within the patient's cognitive and affective states. Gradually, the patient comes to recognize his or her own repertoire of internalized self and object dyads (victim/persecutor; helpless child/scary adult; the one with no power/the one with all power) and can see the reversal of these identifications as played out in the transference.

Interpretation of the underlying motivations for dissociated, sequestered aspects of themselves allows patients to make sense of the chaotic internal experience. They become less self-condemnatory and begin to develop compassion toward their own internal states, leading to a more complex, nuanced experience of themselves and others.

Once that integration has taken place, and the patient's self has become integrated to an extent that permits him or her to tolerate the development of interpretive interventions centering no longer on splitting and related primitive defensive operations but on repression and the related defensive operations, interpretation will take the form of standard psychoanalytic interpretation as one would with the better-functioning patients who had an indication for standard psychoanalysis from the very beginning.

There are several implications of TFP for the relation between mentalization and ego identity, on the one hand, and between mentalization and the nature of interpretation, on the other. Regarding mentalization and identity, the implication is that mentalization as a technical approach has crucial relevance in the psychoanalytic treatment of severe personality disorders, in which generalized splitting operations are reflected in the activation of extreme affective states completely dissociated from other affectively extreme self-experiences, in which the patient "simply is what he or she now feels." Here no self-reflection can take place, because there does not exist an integrated self able to maintain a consistent cognitive frame sufficient to "weather the storm" of a momentary, discrepant self-state. And the same, naturally, corresponds to the borderline patient's difficulty of relating any momentarily perceived mental experience of another in the context of an integrated view of the other with which the momentary affective experience of the other may be compared.

Therefore, the activity of the TFP therapist in the early stages of treatment is primarily focused on clarifying the patient's mental experience in the present interaction with the therapist and helping the patient to establish a tolerable affective memory of the presently dominant perception of self and other. That affective memory, in turn, gradually will become available and tolerable when the same relationship occurs with reversed roles, because the patient is able to recognize aspects of his or her "former" self in what he or she now perceives in the therapist, as well as to recognize aspects of the previous experience of the therapist in what is now perceived as an aspect of self. This is the first step in the capacity to compare a present self-state with an alternative one, even under the influence of an intense or "peak" affect state and, thus, signals the beginning of mentalization.

Under the influence of the systematic repetition of the clarification of activated dyadic object relations with role reversals, the therapist's interventions represent the participation of an "excluded third party." The first step, as described before, is to help the patient understand and tolerate his or her identification with both self- and object representations of an idealized or a persecutory internal dyad. The second step is to help the patient tolerate and understand that the alternation between idealized and persecutory relations to the transference object serves a protective function for the "good" relation from the "bad" one, the defensive operation of splitting. This "excluded third party," outside observing function of the therapist contributes to the integration of the patient's concept of self as well as his or her integrating the concept of the significant other, leading to the advance from the paranoid-schizoid position into the depressive position and the establishment of ego identity. At that point, the patient begins to be able to mentalize, that is, to carry out a normal self-reflection even under conditions of intense negative mental states induced by stressful experiences. (Of course, all of us have limits to the extent to which we can maintain our rationality under conditions of extreme affect activation. It has been said that under conditions of extreme affects, we all become idiots....)

Interpretation in Transference-Focused Psychotherapy

What follows illustrates the application of interpretation in the early stage of treatment with TFP. It is a verbatim segment of session number five of the treatment of a patient with borderline personality disorder, severe suicidal attempts, severe chaos of social and intimate relationships, and breakdown in work functions of a woman in the middle twenties.

PATIENT: Well, I was talking about my father.
THERAPIST: Yes.
PATIENT: Because I have to listen to him, and I don't like to.
    (patient sounds suspicious)
THERAPIST: Okay.
PATIENT: I don't like to feel submissive. I don't like to feel—listening feels submissive sometimes. Cause he goes on and on, you know. So...*(long pause)* I'll probably put up some distance

between he and I so I wouldn't have to listen. Or either I'd listen, but I didn't really have to be there. I'm not sure...but... it's hard for me to listen *(chuckles)* when uhm, a male starts talking. *(subtly ironic)*

THERAPIST: Why? Because males are particularly prone to have you become submissive?

PATIENT: Yes. Yes. Yes, yes, yes. Sure, I grew up as my father's wife. You know.

THERAPIST: What do you mean?

PATIENT: My mother died when I was 7. I was daddy's little helper. Even now, he tells me things that if she were okay, he would tell her. You know, that kind of stuff. So I grew up, you know, wanting to please him, wanting to help him. So it's there, it's just there in the—and it does cause a lot of problems. And a lot of pain.

THERAPIST: What problems? Why is it painful?

PATIENT: Because I shot myself down. I don't talk about things and do things that make me happy, you know. I'm just conditioned this way. Makes me want to be like whatever boyfriends I have, makes me want to be like them, if I'm gonna have to listen to them anyway, I mean that's not the reason, but, it's just like, that's just how I grew up. *(sounds angry)*

THERAPIST: So are you saying that because of that, with all your boyfriends you tend to be very submissive; is that what you're saying? Or resentful because you felt tempted to be submissive or they were trying to—

PATIENT *(interrupts)*: Certainly, yes. Yes.

THERAPIST: Yeah, which?

PATIENT: All of it! I mean I felt—

THERAPIST *(interrupts)*: You were tempted to be submissive, they were trying to exploit that, and before you knew it, you were in a mess being exploited by your boyfriends; is that what you're saying?

PATIENT: Well, it feels like a mess. It may not appear to be a mess because most of my boyfriends have been quite faithful and loyal, they haven't been *(clears throat)*...otherwise....But the mess I find myself in is I feel lost. I don't like it that I can't talk well today.

THERAPIST: Well, I'm aware that you are divided in your view of me; I, I have a sense that in part of you, you trust that I'm being straight with you and that I mean what I say. But in part of you, you see me as one more of that series of males who are trying to take over the brainwashing. And as I become important and you feel like trying to please me, it would be very humiliating to think that you try to please somebody who is controlling you, criticizing you, manipulating you, putting you down, not a very nice perspective.

PATIENT: So what am I gonna do? It's always been that way. I mean that's why I'm here. *(Again, she sounds somewhat suspicious and annoyed.)*

THERAPIST: That's right, so this is an opportunity for exploring that reaction, what it's all about.

PATIENT: I'm trying to. Don't you agree? Do you agree with me that it has something to do with my father?

THERAPIST *(interjects)*: Yes.

PATIENT *(continues)*: and how I was raised?

THERAPIST: Yes, I would be surprised if it wasn't—

PATIENT *(interjects)*: Okay.

THERAPIST *(continues)*: It makes sense. What I'm trying to stress here is how powerful that part of you is that sees apparently all relationships with men as a replica of the relationship with your father. And makes you try to get away, when you feel again threatened with being taken over and humiliated.

PATIENT: You know...I, uhm, I think I'm experiencing some of that in my relationship with Jacob. Uhm...he has moved to England, you know— *(appears thoughtful)*

THERAPIST: He has left already?

PATIENT: Oh yeah, he left on Monday. I didn't care if he stayed or not; it didn't matter, really. I talked to him about it. He was willing to stay, or to consider staying, but...his response about you know whether this is going somewhere or not was, yeah, I don't want you to waste your time with me. And then I told him that I might leave, that I may have to not see him or talk to him that much. And then of course he is all the more coming towards me and not wanting to not talk, and will stay in touch, and has called me every night since he left. Except for one or two. And, you know, I took his picture down off the wall after two days cause I was so frustrated with how to stop thinking about him, how to let it go, how to think about going out with someone else, those kinds of things.

PATIENT: *(silence)* So my best judgment about the whole thing is the sounds of marriage and children scare him, certainly, but he seems to warm up to that whole idea and starts talking about the future in some sort of plan-type way, even had a dream, and I called right when he was having the dream or something the other night, about going ahead, and telling me that yes, he would give me a kid. And he felt good about it.

THERAPIST: That's the dream?

(Pause)

THERAPIST: That's a dream? *(therapist sounds confused)*

PATIENT *(laughing)*: Yup, that's the dream.

THERAPIST: So are you saying that because you dreamt that, it makes it more likely to happen?

PATIENT: You tell me what it means! *(clearly ironic)*

THERAPIST: I beg your pardon.

PATIENT: Well you tell me what it means.

THERAPIST: What the dream means? Well, it sounds to me from your attitude that at least the content of the dream reflects a wish of yours.

PATIENT: Yup, and maybe his.

THERAPIST: That's not clear to me.

PATIENT: He had the dream. *(with a triumphant smile)*

THERAPIST: Oh, I'm sorry, I misunderstood that. I thought you had the dream.

PATIENT: Ahhhhhhh!!! *(claps; she enjoys this development)*

THERAPIST: I misunderstood.

PATIENT: Good, so I'll stay suspicious of you cause you still didn't understand. *(chuckling)* I'm just kidding. I'm teasing. You misunderstood me, see! Why should I trust you? Why should I? You don't understand me anyway; I can spell it out, and you still don't get it. That's the way men are. That's the way my dad is. I can spell it out, write it in French, German, English, or Spanish—does he get it, does he understand me, the nature of me? No. Why should I? How many diffe—I could go to 20 years of therapy and learn how to express myself 20 different ways. I could wear 20 different outfits; would he still understand me? No. Why not? Cause he has his thing about women. So what am I to do?

THERAPIST: Because he has what?

PATIENT: A thing about women.

THERAPIST: What thing?

PATIENT: Women are either this or this. Who knows what his thing is. This is my father you know, not Jacob.

THERAPIST: I understand. You looked very happy when I said I had misunderstood.

PATIENT: Cause I'm right.

THERAPIST: Yes.

PATIENT *(laughing)*: Cause I was right. Is it me? Is it me because I don't explain it well? Is it normal just because people don't understand each other the first time sometimes? Yes. I will let it slide, you know; I'll get over this and get back to my point, but...I do get upset about it. I have intense reactions about not being understood. I get mad like that *(snaps fingers)*. *(sighs)* Jacob had the dream. Two nights ago. I picked up the phone to call him, uhm, because he had tried to call a couple of nights before, and while I called, he was having this dream, and he wouldn't tell me about it. He asked me how I was doing. Then he got to it. Anyway, I just sensed that, uhm, I can't, I'm having a hard time how I feel. I'm having a hard time feeling how I feel about it. And it's—what do you want to say?

(Therapist's expression indicates he wants to comment.)

THERAPIST: I'm still mulling over your feeling happy because you were right and I was wrong. Uhm, it puts you in a position of superiority—

PATIENT: Ahh, yes!

THERAPIST: Right?

PATIENT: Yes.

THERAPIST: Well, I wonder whether you feel that if I'm right in what

I'm saying, I may feel happy about it and feel superior to you, and one more reason to feel the danger here of being humiliated. So—

PATIENT *(interjects)*: I can't follow you.

THERAPIST *(continues)*: Do you follow me?

PATIENT: No, I have a hard time—

THERAPIST: Have a hard time following me?

PATIENT: I know what you're saying but I can't quite—

THERAPIST: Well, it creates a problem for you. If I'm right in what I'm telling you, you may perceive me as reacting the same way you do, feeling superior because I'm right, so I'm on top, you are down, and that's humiliating for you. If I'm wrong, you feel fine; you are on top, but by the same token, there's nothing to be expected from me. So you can't win.

PATIENT: I can't win?

THERAPIST: That's right.

PATIENT: Why can't I win cause I can't expect anything?

THERAPIST: You can't win because if I'm right, you feel humiliated. And if I'm wrong, you feel disappointed. Do you follow me?

PATIENT: If you're wrong, I feel disappointed because you're my therapist, and you're no good.

THERAPIST: Right. And if I'm right, you feel humiliated because I know better than you, and you feel put down.

PATIENT: Yeah, that one's very vague. The other one is the one that's more active.

THERAPIST: Yes.

PATIENT: I mean, I know what you're saying—

(Silence)

THERAPIST: Okay, well, let's stop here.

I trust this material illustrates one main point made in this chapter—namely, the activation of a dominant persecutory object relation between a superior, controlling, sadistic object (an image of father) and a humiliated, controlled, subjugated self (of the patient) and the rapid interchange of these two roles between patient and therapist in the context of this session. It also illustrates the therapist's effort to have the patient acquire awareness of the nature of this interaction and of the exchange of roles in it: This is the early step in the interpretive process referred to before. Other implicit object relations already present in this session were not yet touched, because they did not seem affectively dominant, such as the strong oedipal implication of the patient's "having replaced mother" in the relationship with her father and a subtly seductive aspect of her nonverbal behavior, silently expressed simultaneously with the verbal interchange in this hour. The therapist took note of these nonverbal processes but felt that they were not yet affectively dominant and that it would have been premature to explore them at this point.

Regarding the relationship of mentalization to interpretation, what I have described is the nature of interpretation under conditions of predominance of splitting operations and primitive mental organization of patients with borderline personality organization. Here, the concept of the dynamic unconscious is not represented by the structural characteristics of the mature, tripartite psychic structure (of superego, ego, and id), with repressive mechanisms maintaining dynamic conflicts out of conscious awareness. Under conditions of higher level or neurotic personality organization, in contrast to borderline personality organization, interpretation typically involves the establishment of hypotheses regarding unconscious meanings that have to be confirmed or disconfirmed by the patient's processes of free association and the related activation of corresponding transference developments (Caligor et al. 2007). In contrast, in the case of patients with a predominance of splitting mechanisms and identity diffusion, the dynamic unconscious is expressed in mutually dissociated dynamic structures; that is, idealized and persecutory internalized object relations reflecting both archaic oedipal conflicts strongly dominated by oral and anal aggression and more advanced oedipal conflicts synchronically integrated with them. In cases of borderline personality organization, interpretation refers, first, to the interpretive linkage of contradictory ego or self-states under the same "peak" affect state, reflecting alternating activation of self- and object representations of a determined internalized object relationship, as well as the alternative, mutually split-off activation of idealized and persecutory relations. A contemporary concept of interpretation has to include bringing into consciousness both repressed and split-off and dissociated conflicts and, therefore, cannot be limited to interpretation as cognitively framed for patients with an integrated identity and the corresponding integrated concept of self and significant others (i.e., neurotic personality organization) (Caligor et al. 2009). From this viewpoint, the critique Bateman and Fonagy formulate regarding the problematic effects of interpretation in the cases of patients with severe personality disorders refers to the type of interpretations that would be indicated in the case of patients with much better integrated psychic structures—based on repressive mechanisms—but would not be a good reason for assuming that interpretation in general is contraindicated in the early stages of the treatment of borderline patients. To the contrary, as we have found in our research at Cornell, interpretation corresponding to the structural conditions of borderline patients may be a powerful application of psychoanalytic theory and technique to cases in which the severity of the pathology may contraindicate standard psychoanalytic treatment.

Mentalization, Insight, Empathy, and Mindfulness

We are now in a good position to sharpen and compare the concepts of mentalization, insight, and empathy with each other and with mindfulness. *Insight* is a broad term, referring to the combination of cognitive awareness, emotional awareness, and concern over what has been discovered by interpretation throughout the entire spectrum of psychoanalytic treatment. As mentioned before, a major goal of psychoanalysis is the patient's acquisition of insight into his or her unconscious motivation and its influence on conscious behavior. Insight involves self-reflective awareness of the mental operations that shape present experience and behavior in terms of unconscious desires and fears that derive from the past but constitute an everlasting presence. It is the result of interpretation and the patient's gradually internalizing the interpretive function of the analyst.

It seems reasonable to assume that the capacity to mentalize is fundamental to the acquisition of insight. Under conditions of identity diffusion, severe dissociation, or splitting of contradictory, peak affect states, the capacity to mentalize is compromised. Mentalization refers to a specific form of acquisition of insight into the intentional mental states of self and others under those conditions. It requires technical interventions that foster the development of a realistic assessment and self-reflection regarding the experience of self and of a significant other. It is a process that leads to the integration of the concept of self and significant others and, therefore, to a development of normal ego identity. At this point, any particular state of self may be explored from the perspective of a background of an integrated, overall self, "surrounded" by or related to an integrated view of significant others.

Interpretation, under conditions of mentalization, has specific characteristics: it consists in the cognitive and affective bringing together of originally conscious, but alternatively activated, mutually

split-off self-states. Through repeated clarification and interpretation of the dual but oscillating identification with idealized and persecutory object relations, the patient becomes able to integrate his
or her internalized object relations and becomes better able to tolerate ambivalence. Once consolidation of the self and a clear differentiation of the tripartite structure of ego, superego, and id have
taken place, with a consistent repressive barrier separating consciousness from the dynamic unconscious, interpretation may take
the form of the establishment of hypotheses regarding assumed
unconscious meaning of the patient's material, the standard analysis of transference/countertransference developments. Here, the
achievement of insight can no longer be attributed to mentalization
in its specific meaning. Mentalization, in short, is a highly specialized method and process of achieving insight with a particular
interpretive approach, indicated particularly with patients presenting severe character pathology: the borderline level of ego
functioning.

Insight, in turn, has to be differentiated from psychological
mindedness as a general motivation and effort to learn about oneself, to increase one's self-awareness, that is not limited to psychoanalysis and does not necessarily imply learning about one's own
unconscious processes. Obviously, insight as a consequence of psychoanalytic exploration—including its specialized process of mentalization in the case of predominance of primitive mental operations—powerfully increases psychological mindedness.

Mindfulness also increases psychological mindedness but differs from psychoanalytic insight in its exclusive concentration on
the present state of self and its lack of focus on unconscious processes. In contrast to insight, and particularly to mentalization, it
does not focus on the basic dyadic object relations that, from a psychoanalytic viewpoint, constitute the building blocks of the psychic
apparatus and evolve into the tripartite structure of the mind.

By the same token, authentic emotional insight, as mentioned
before, implies concern not only for oneself but for others as well
and a related capacity for empathy; that is, a capacity of concerned
identification with the mental experience of others without losing
one's own boundaries in the process or without a sense of being
overwhelmed by such an experience. In effect, as a consequence of
normal identity, a sharp differentiation between representations of
self and representations of significant others is a prerequisite for
the capacity for intimate relatedness as well as affective empathy.
And the concept of empathy, in turn, in a general sense a crucial

aspect of psychological mindedness, as well as of insight in a more specific way, needs to be differentiated further from the function of therapeutic empathy.

Empathy refers to the capacity to feel with another person's feelings, not only to understand him or her cognitively but also to be able to identify emotionally with the other's feelings. As mentioned before, I believe it is an inborn capacity that is powerfully reinforced and extended as a consequence of the achievement of the depressive position. It is a combination of feeling with and concern for the other. Therapeutic empathy refers to the capacity of the psychoanalyst and the psychoanalytic psychotherapist to maintain empathy not only with patients' central subjective experience (concordant identification) but also with patients' dissociated and projected experiences (complementary identification); in short, therapeutic empathy includes the tolerance of both concordant identification and complementary identification in the countertransference, although counteridentifications (loss of distance in complementary countertransference identification) may be unavoidable at times (Kernberg 2007a).

This concept of therapeutic empathy within the psychoanalytic realm runs the danger of dilution, by means of its confusion with the ordinary capacity to feel with another person's feelings. The technical implications of therapeutic empathy specifically include the capacity of the therapist to be able to identify with the patient's subjective experience, to diagnose the object relationship activated in transference and countertransference, and still to maintain a position as "excluded third party." As mentioned before, the therapist's very attention to the patient's identification with the self and object of basic dyads facilitates the patient's identification with the significant other, the development of his or her capacity of empathy.

The risks of overgeneralization of our terminology need to be stressed. The overuse of the term *insight* in the past, neglecting its specific implication of the combination of cognitive awareness, emotional awareness, and concern, has contributed to an apparent flattening and loss of practical relevance of the term within the psychoanalytic literature; the overextension of the concept of mentalization, a fundamental contribution to our technical armamentarium, may lead to the same danger. There is, of course, still the important challenge to evaluate to what extent the mechanism of mentalization is, in effect, specifically correlated with psychoanalytic modalities of treatment, in contrast to the mechanisms of action of other forms of psychotherapy. This is an important task for present-day psychotherapy research. The fact that significant advances in this regard have been achieved both in the pioneering work of Fonagy and his group and in the empirical contribution of the Cornell group (Clarkin et al. 2007) should stimulate further research efforts in this area.

This concludes the effort to clarify the relationship between the concepts of mindfulness, mentalization, insight, and empathy and their relevance regarding the process of interpretation both in severely regressed and in healthier patients. Just as there is a new emphasis on patients' subjective experience in the cognitive-behavioral psychotherapeutic field, so also within the psychoanalytic realm, through the concept of mentalization, has there been a new emphasis on the clarification of intentional mental states of self and other as a precursor to more advanced or complex forms of interpretation. Significant differences between the respective concepts of mentalization and mindfulness have been highlighted.

References

Bateman A, Fonagy P: Psychotherapy for Borderline Personality Disorder: Mentalization-Based Treatment. New York, Oxford University Press, 2004

Bateman A, Fonagy P: Mentalization-based treatment and borderline personality disorder, in Handbuch der Borderline-Störungen, 2. Auflage. Edited by Dulz B, Herpertz S, Kernberg O, et al. Stuttgart, Germany, Schattauer, 2011, pp 566–575

Caligor E, Kernberg OF, Clarkin JF: Handbook of Dynamic Psychotherapy for Higher Level Personality Pathology. Washington, DC, American Psychiatric Publishing, 2007

Caligor E, Diamond D, Yeomans FE, et al: The interpretive process in the psychoanalytic psychotherapy of borderline personality pathology. J Am Psychoanal Assoc 57:271–301, 2009

Carson JW, Carson KM, Gil KM, et al: Mindfulness-based relationship enhancement. Behav Ther 35:471–494, 2004

Choi-Kain LW, Gunderson JG: A review of the concept of mentalization: its ontogeny, assessment, and application in the treatment of borderline personality disorder. Am J Psychiatry 165:2–4, 2008

Clarkin JF, Yeomans FE, Kernberg OF: Psychotherapy for Borderline Personality: Focusing on Object Relations. Washington, DC, American Psychiatric Publishing, 2006

Clarkin JF, Levy KN, Lenzenweger ML, et al: Evaluating three treatments for borderline personality disorder: a multiwave study. Am J Psychiatry 164:922–928, 2007

Fonagy P, Target M, Steele H, et al: Reflective Functioning Manual: Version 5. For Application to Adult Attachment Interviews. London, University College, 1997

Germer CK, Siegel RD, Fulton PR (eds): Mindfulness and Psychotherapy. New York, Guilford, 2005

Hayes SC, Follette VM, Linehan MM (eds): Mindfulness and Acceptance: Expanding the Cognitive-Behavior Tradition. New York, Guilford, 2004

Kernberg OF: A severe sexual inhibition in the course of the psychoanalytic treatment of a patient with narcissistic personality disorder. Int J Psychoanal 80:899–908, 1999

Kernberg OF: Aggressivity, Narcissism, and Self-Destructiveness in the Psychotherapeutic Relationship: New Developments in the Psychopathology and Psychotherapy of Severe Personality Disorders. New Haven, CT, Yale University Press, 2004a

Kernberg OF: Contemporary Controversies in Psychoanalytic Theory, Technique, and Their Applications. New Haven, CT, Yale University Press, 2004b

Kernberg OF: Countertransference: recent developments and technical implications for the treatment of patients with severe personality disorders, in Severe Personality Disorders: Everyday Issues in Clinical Practice. Edited by van Luyn B, Akhtar S, Livesley J. London, Cambridge University Press, 2007a, pp 42–58

Kernberg OF: The therapeutic action of psychoanalysis: controversies and challenges. Psychoanal Q 76(suppl):1689–1723, 2007b

Kernberg OF: Psychoanalysis: Freud's theories and their contemporary development, in New Oxford Textbook of Psychiatry, 2nd Edition. Edited by Gelder MG, Andreasen NC, López-Ibor JJ Jr, et al. London, Oxford University Press, 2009, pp 293–305

Kernberg OF, Yeomans FE, Clarkin JF, et al: Transference focused psychotherapy: overview and update. Int J Psychoanal 89:601–620, 2008

Levy KN, Clarkin JF, Yeomans FE, et al: Mechanisms of change in the treatment of borderline personality disorder with transference focused psychotherapy. J Clin Psychol 62:481–502, 2006a

Levy KN, Meehan KB, Kelly KM, et al: Change in attachment and reflective function in the treatment of borderline personality disorder with transference focused psychotherapy. J Consult Clin Psychol 74:1027–1040, 2006b

Linehan MM: Cognitive-Behavioral Treatment of Borderline Personality Disorder. New York, Guilford, 1993

Linehan MM, Bohus M, Lynch TR: Dialectical behavior therapy for pervasive emotion dysregulation: theoretical and practical underpinnings, in Handbook of Emotion Regulation. Edited by Gross JJ. New York, Guilford, 2007, pp 581–605

Shapiro SL, Carlson LE, Astin JA, et al: Mechanisms of mindfulness. J Clin Psychol 62:373–386, 2006

Siegel DJ: The Mindful Brain. New York, WW Norton, 2007

Sugarman A: Mentalization, insightfulness, and therapeutic action: the importance of mental organization. Int J Psychoanal 87:965–987, 2006

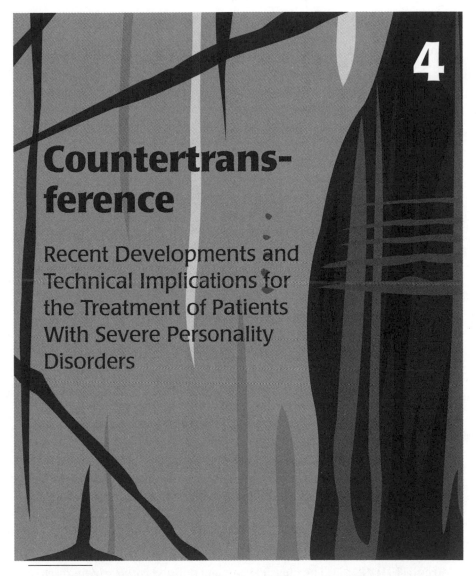

Countertrans-ference

Recent Developments and Technical Implications for the Treatment of Patients With Severe Personality Disorders

4

This chapter was reprinted from Kernberg OF: "Countertransference: Recent Developments and Technical Implications for the Treatment of Patients With Severe Personality Disorders," in *Severe Personality Disorders*. Edited by Bert van Luyn, Salman Akhtar, and W. John Livesley. New York, Cambridge University Press, 2007, pp. 42–58. Copyright © 2007 Cambridge University Press. Used with permission.

This chapter represents work from the Cornell Psychotherapy Research Project supported by a grant from the Borderline Personality Disorder Research Foundation. The foundation and its founder, Dr. Marco Stoffel, are gratefully acknowledged.

The concept, the diagnostic evaluation, and the therapeutic utilization of the therapist's countertransference reactions are a major, controversial area of intensive psychodynamic psychotherapy. In this chapter, I explore questions regarding the assessment of concordant and complementary identifications in the countertransference; whether countertransference reactions should or should not be communicated to the patient; and the relation between technical neutrality, communication of empathy, the "real relationship," and countertransference acting out, with a particular focus on countertransference developments in the intensive, long-term psychotherapy of severe personality disorders. A general, updated review of the corresponding literature is followed by my position regarding all (or most) of these issues. In this context, the particular approach of transference-focused psychotherapy (TFP) is further elaborated in this chapter.

What follows is an overview of the clinical experiences regarding countertransference that we have gathered over 25 years in the treatment of severe personality disorders at the Personality Disorders Institute of the Weill Cornell Medical College and the Westchester Division of the New York Hospital. My earlier experiences in work with the psychotherapy research project of the Menninger Foundation provided a conceptual and clinical background that influenced the development of new technical approaches and the reshaping of the relevant concepts.

The Contemporary Concept of Countertransference

At this time, the "totalistic" or "global" concept of countertransference clearly has replaced the classical concept as originally defined by Freud (1910/1957). The classical concept defined *countertransference* as the analyst's transferences toward the patient or the analyst's unconscious reactions to the patient's transference; the accent was on the unconscious aspect of the analyst's reaction, with the implication that only further analytic work by the analyst on himself or herself would help him or her to "overcome" the countertransference, as Freud recommended. The contemporary "totalistic" or "global" concept, in contrast, defines *countertransference* as the therapist's total emotional reaction to the patient at any particular point in time (Kernberg 1975). The implication of this modern, contemporary concept is that the therapist needs to monitor his or her countertransference consistently to deepen the understanding of the patient by relating it to the developments in the transference. For practical purposes, in fact, often, nowadays, the process of psychoanalysis and psychoanalytic psychotherapy is described as the gradual development of transference/countertransference binds in the context of a boundary-controlled psychotherapeutic interaction within which the therapist attempts to maintain a position of technical neutrality.

In this connection, it needs to be stressed that the concept of technical neutrality often is misinterpreted as implying a "studied indifference," suggesting a lack of appropriate investment and concern on the part of the therapist. In reality, technical neutrality refers to the therapist's interventions as remaining neutral regarding the intrapsychic conflicts of the patient or, more concretely, neutral in relation to the patient's superego, id, acting ego, and external reality. Technical neutrality implies a concerned objectivity characterized by interpretive interventions from the position of an alliance with the observing part of the patient's ego. This classical definition of technical neutrality, first formulated in this form by Anna Freud (1936/1966), still holds, I believe, as a necessary precondition for the analysis of countertransference reactions rather than simply acting them out. The therapist is not "neutral" in terms of not having emotional reactions to the patient but in his or her effort and capacity to contain them and use them for better understanding of the therapeutic situation rather than discharging these emotions in the relationship with the patient.

It is well known that in the psychoanalytic psychotherapy of patients with severe regression in the transference, countertransference acting out may, at times, be unavoidable and constitute a special complication in the management of the treatment of these patients, to which I shall return. As DeLeón and Bernardi (B. De-León and R. Bernardi, "Countertransference and Vulnerability of the Analyst," unpublished manuscript, 2005) have pointed out, the contemporary concern with countertransference should not be overly broadened to include the analyst's general disposition toward self-analysis and his or her reflective ability to understand what goes on in his or her mind as well as in that of the patient. These authors also caution us against the tendency to expand the utilization of countertransference to the extent of favoring narcissistic self-involvement of the therapist.

Returning to the classical concept of countertransference, it should be kept in mind that Freud's introduction of the term *counter-*

transference, together with his stress on the need to "overcome" it, reflected his reaction to the frequency of boundary violations by his early male disciples, leading to their sexual involvement with female patients. That early threatening experience determined a counter-phobic attitude toward this concept, lasting from the 1910s to the 1950s, reflecting, I believe, the hidden concern over those past boundary violations within the psychoanalytic community. As is well known, it was only in the 1950s that new, significant contributions opened the field of countertransference to its contemporary enrich-ment of psychoanalytic and psychotherapeutic theory and tech-nique. Here the contribution of Paula Heimann (1950), pointing to the projection of patient's unconscious experiences as part of the countertransference reaction of the psychoanalyst and to the anal-ysis of countertransference as a significant contribution to clarifying transference developments, was an important landmark. The con-tributions of the Argentinean school, particularly by Racker (1957) and Madeleine and Willie Baranger (1961–1962, 1969) and Baran-ger et al. (1983), further expanded the field of countertransference analysis and utilization in the treatment.

It was particularly Racker's clarification of concordant and complementary identification in the countertransference that pro-vided the most important, practical clinical applications of the new understanding of countertransference as a composite structure, constituted by aspects of both the patient's and the analyst's con-scious and unconscious contributions. In effect, the contemporary concept of countertransference implies that the therapist's mo-ment-to-moment emotional reaction to the patient is codetermined by 1) the patient's transference, 2) reality aspects of the patient's life, 3) reality aspects of the therapist's life that may be influenced directly or indirectly by the patient, and 4) the therapist's counter-transference disposition in a restricted sense, as defined by the classical concept.

What I have stressed in earlier work, based on these contributions to our understanding of the countertransference stemming from the 1950s on, is the fact that the more severe the patient's psychopathol-ogy, the more the countertransference is determined by the patient's transference; so that, in practice, countertransference analysis has become a fundamental instrument for the understanding in depth of transference developments of borderline pathology (Kernberg 1976). As we described it in our manual *Psychotherapy for Borderline Per-sonality: Focusing on Object Relations* (Clarkin et al. 2006), TFP was developed at the Cornell Personality Disorders Institute as a modified psychodynamic psychotherapy for severe personality disorders, in which the material that constitutes the raw data for the analysis of the patient's moment-to-moment transference developments is expressed by means of the patient's verbal communication, his or her nonverbal communication, and the countertransference.

In summary, when dealing with borderline or severely regressed patients, in contrast to those presenting less severe personality disorders, the therapist tends to experience, rather soon in the treatment, intense emotional reactions, having more to do with the patient's premature, intense, and chaotic transferences and with the therapist's capacity to withstand psychological stress and anxiety than with any specific problem of the therapist's past. Thus, countertransference becomes an important diagnostic tool that provides information as to the degree of regression in the patient, his or her predominant emotional position in relation to the therapist, and the changes occurring in this position. The more intense and premature the therapist's emotional reaction to the patient, the more threatening it becomes to the therapist's neutrality, and the more it has a quickly changing, fluctuating, and chaotic nature, the more we can think the therapist is in the presence of a severe personality disorder or a severe regression in the patient.

Classification of Countertransference, With Particular Implications for the Treatment of Severe Personality Disorders

The previously mentioned classification of countertransference into concordant and complementary identifications by Racker is of fundamental importance. Concordant identification, in which the therapist emotionally identifies with the patient's central subjective experience, "self with self," corresponds particularly to ordinary empathy and reflects the therapist's capacity to share the patient's experience in the transference. It leads to deepening of emotional understanding on the part of the therapist and to the patient's sense of being understood; its risk is an excessive identification with a patient that may correspond to conscious or unconscious seductive efforts by the patient or to a resonance with the patient's experience of a reactivated conflict from the therapist's past. Such an "overidentification" of the therapist with the patient may lead to countertransference acting out and, insofar as the therapist is tempted to share with the patient a common denial of a particular aspect of the patient's psychic reality, to "bastions" in the therapeutic situation. *Bastions* are areas of unconscious collusion between patient and therapist, determining a "blind spot" in the therapist's understanding (Baranger and Baranger 1969). Such unconscious collusions between patient and therapist, as DeLeón and Bernardi (B. DeLeón and R. Bernardi, "Countertransference and Vulnerability of the Analyst," unpublished manuscript, 2005) have pointed out, may constitute problems particularly with traumatized patients; for example, victims of political persecution and torture. One related problem is the patient's and the therapist's sharing a socially or culturally determined bias or prejudice that may restrict the analytic work. For example, if a patient has been persecuted politically, subjected to torture or other highly traumatic experiences, and both patient and therapist share the same political ideology, a "bastion" may evolve that may significantly hamper the deeper aspects of the psychotherapeutic work.

Complementary identification in the countertransference is, as a practical matter, the most important form that countertransference dispositions take in the treatment of patients with severe personality disorders. The mechanism of projective identification is the principal defensive operation by means of which patients induce complementary identification in the countertransference. Here the therapist identifies with what the patient cannot tolerate in himself or herself and is projecting onto the therapist, while the patient complements this projection with an unconscious role induction of the therapist to facilitate his or her identification with that projected aspect. Simultaneously, the patient attempts to control the therapist in order to neutralize the dangerousness of that which is projected, most frequently related to intense, primitive aggressive impulses. It needs to be stressed, however, that projective identification does not always elicit complementary identification in the countertransference and that, at times, complementary identification may evolve in sessions with a patient who is not utilizing the mechanism of projective identification at that point. In other words, it is important to avoid an excessive extension of the concept of projective identification, including the complementary countertransference response as part of it.

Joseph Sandler's (1976) concept of the "role responsiveness" of the analyst refers to how certain projections by the patient may resonate with particular dispositions in the psychoanalyst and become part of countertransference responses. With patients presenting severe personality disorders and the corresponding severe regression in the transference—particularly intense, primitive aggression directed at the therapist over an extended period of time, the therapist's habitual defenses against aggression, from both external and intrapsychic sources, may become activated, so that he or she may appear as having "reactivated" his or her most conflictual characterological traits in the treatment of a particular patient. Such developments are also part of chronic countertransference reactions, to which I shall return, and require careful and sometimes painful self-analysis by the therapist outside the sessions with a patient or, of course, consultation. In this connection, I do not believe that any therapist is free from such developments and from the need occasionally to consult with a trusted colleague in the course of the treatment of very sick patients.

Although intense projective identification and the resulting complementary identification in the countertransference may be disturbing, anxiety-producing developments in the sessions, they are potentially of great value in identifying the nature of the dominant object relationship activated in the transference. While in the case of concordant identification in the countertransference, the therapist's self is identified with the patient's self-experience at that moment, under conditions of complementary countertransference, the therapist may be identified with the patient's object representation while the patient identifies with his or her self-representation, or, to the contrary, the therapist may be identified with the patient's projected self-representation while the patient is enacting his or her identification with the object representation of the corresponding dyadic unit. In this regard, then, the analysis of complementary countertransference is a powerful tool to clarify the nature of the activation of specific object relations in the transference.

A young man who was failing in his studies at college because of an attitude of contempt toward teachers and books, with attendant fantasies of not having to study to understand and know everything, came to a session seriously disturbed because he had just learned that he had failed a major test. He was quite dejected, felt like a failure, and thought that he was going to be depreciated by teachers and his colleagues. I, on the other hand, struggled with an internal reaction of "I told you so," the sense that this failure served him well after my unsuccessful efforts to confront him with the dangerous, self-destructive nature of neglecting his studies. On further reflection, it seemed to me that he was now enacting, in his experience of despair and the fear of being depreciated and devalued by others, his worthless, inferior, depreciated self, while now projecting the grandiose, derogatory aspects of his self onto his classmates and, I wondered, presumably also onto me. I thought that I was in the position of a projected aspect of his grandiose self, condensed with a primitive, sadistic superego image.

I wondered with him whether his disturbance in this session also might be related to his attributing to me both an attitude of devaluation of him and a highly critical, sadistic, triumphant sense of superiority because I had forewarned him regarding the neglect of his studies. The patient immediately was able to recognize these aspects of his internal world projected onto me. As we explored his experience of me, it also became apparent that he could not conceive, at this point, that there was an authentic concern for him in my confronting him with the neglect of his studies. The defensive nature of his grandiose self against a profound conviction of not being loved by mother could only be explored much later.

On the negative side, an excessive intensity of complementary identification in the therapist may evolve into "projective counteridentification," a concept coined by Leon Grinberg (1956, 1979) to refer to the analyst's "getting stuck" in an unconscious identification with the patient's projective identification—being unable, therefore, to carry out the internal division between the emotional enactment in the countertransference and the secondary self-reflection that is part of the analytic task. This situation relates to one other aspect of countertransference that deserves further exploration, namely, the difference between acute countertransferences—countertransferences that vary from moment to moment in the therapeutic situation—and chronic countertransferences, which distort the experience of the patient in the therapist's mind over an extended period of time (Kernberg 2004a). The latter represent a chronic "blind spot," of which the therapist may gradually become aware, without, at first, being able to resolve it. It is particularly with patients presenting severe personality disorders that such development of chronic countertransference reactions are frequent and, as I pointed out in earlier work (Kernberg 1999), require self-exploration by the therapist outside the sessions or consultation. I believe this situation needs to be differentiated from moment-to-moment projective counteridentification and potential acting out of the countertransference under conditions of severe, regressive acting out of the transference in the sessions: here projective counteridentification is a transitory phenomenon that can be analyzed and resolved in the course of the same or a few sessions.

In short, the analysis of countertransference in terms of its concordant or complementary nature, and in terms of its moment-to-moment fluctuating nature in contrast to chronic transference developments, reflects two major, clinically useful classifications of countertransference reactions. These distinctions, at times, may not be so easy to establish quickly and not only require reflection regarding the countertransference in an ongoing process of the therapist analyzing his or her sources of information (the patient's verbal communication, the patient's nonverbal communication, and the therapist's countertransference) but also require the analysis of what happens with the patient's material in the therapist's mind outside the sessions. As Tower (1956) observed many years ago, chronic countertransference reactions may emerge so discreetly and so gradually that, at times, the analyst only becomes aware of them retrospectively, as the successful resolution of a transference stalemate reveals a chronic countertransference disposition.

Analysis and Management of Countertransference

Whatever the psychotherapeutic approach of the therapist, it cannot but help that one be attentive to the countertransference reactions triggered by any particular patient in any particular session. Psychoanalysis and psychoanalytic psychotherapy intensify transference regression by systematic analysis of the defenses against such a development, and, by the same token, countertransference reactions are magnified by the sharp analytic focus on the nature of the patient/therapist relationship enacted at conscious and unconscious levels. Even in supportive and cognitive-behavioral treatments, which attempt to utilize the positive aspects of the relationship and to reduce whatever negative aspects evolve, the awareness of one's changing emotional dispositions to the patient cannot but help the therapist apply his or her technical approach more appropriately and effectively.

In psychoanalytic psychotherapy and psychoanalysis, systematic countertransference analysis is part of the technical approach. It plays a less crucial role in the standard psychoanalysis of patients

with neurotic personality organization and the less severe personality disorders than in sicker patients when countertransference,
as mentioned before, is activated rapidly and intensively and dominates the treatment throughout. With less severely regressed patients, the projection of complex, elaborated superego features
or attribution of broad attitudinal characteristics to the therapist
may keep the countertransference, at least initially, at a relatively
low affective level, but the typical countertransference with more
primitive patients presents more specific, highly individualized,
primitive regressive features that correspond to reactivated primitive infantile object relations of the patient and hence can be very
useful.

Under these circumstances, the therapist may become temporarily enmeshed in a fantastic, primitive emotional experience, reflecting sadistic or masochistic, sexually excited or puritanical,
punishing or abandoning, unconscious parental images of the patient or a condensation of various parental representations activated under the impact of a certain emotional attitude. At other
moments, the therapist may experience emotions similar to those
experienced by the patient but momentarily disavowed and now
projected onto the therapist, such as intensely dependent, aggressive, sexualized feelings and fantasies that invade the therapist's
mind in the process of attempting to understand what is going on in
the relationship with the patient. In these moments, the therapist's
task is to diagnose the nature of the self- and/or object representations activated in himself or herself, in order to include that diagnostic understanding in the forthcoming transference interpretation.

A patient with a severe paranoid personality disorder and a history of extreme prohibitions against any sexual behavior stemming
from his fundamentalist religious parents talked in a session about
the good understanding he now had with his girlfriend and how
happy he felt about the relationship. For many years he had not
been able to be involved in an intimate relationship because of his
fears that women with whom he would become sexually engaged
would become extremely controlling and manipulative. Because,
in the past, he had told me about his fears and reservations about
getting involved with his girlfriend sexually, I asked the patient
whether there had been any change in their sexual intimacy. The
patient looked at me as if astonished by my question. When I tried
to find out what brought about this reaction, I became the object of
an intense barrage of indignant protests: given the fact that his

relationship with this new girlfriend had only lasted a few months, it was absurd, he said, that I should suggest that they should get involved sexually at this point. I had not, of course, suggested that they get involved sexually and had limited myself to ask about whether there had been any change regarding their relationship. The patient, however, was adamant in insisting that I was trying to push him into a premature sexual relationship, which, in his mind, reflected the immorality of the liberal establishment, characteristic of psychotherapists, of which I was a member.

It is difficult to convey in a few words the intensity of his attack, but my reaction was one of total impotence in the face of the problematic nature of his reasoning, which he saw as obvious, incontrovertible facts. I had a sense, at this point, that I was forced to identify with the patient's attacked sexual self, while he was identifying with his puritanical and prohibitive parents. This reflection then permitted me to point out to the patient that what was happening in the session reminded me of his painful feelings of being "brainwashed" by his parents, who in his adolescence had been severely disapproving of any manifestation of sexual interests or behavior on his part. What I missed at that point, however, was the fact that the patient responded with a tirade against sexuality in general when I had asked him whether there had been any change in his "sexual intimacy" with his girlfriend, indicating an inhibition in telling me what his concrete wishes, fears, and prohibitions involved. I thus remained caught up in a deeper level of his defensive operations against sexual fantasies of which I was not aware at that point.

Interpretive interventions that include utilization of countertransference understanding require several fundamental preconditions: first, a clear, stable, firm boundary of the therapeutic frame to prevent acting out on the part of the patient and, worst case scenario, acting out on the part of the therapist with violation of the therapeutic boundaries. The first precondition, therefore, for transference and countertransference analysis is the consistent assurance of the safety of the therapeutic relationship by maintaining a reliably stable frame of the therapeutic situation.

A second aspect of the task of countertransference analysis is for the therapist to tolerate the full development of the emotional regression that may occur in his or her mind, the primitive fantasies that may suddenly emerge in his or her mind and sometimes be of a frightening primitivity or crudeness, be it of a passive dependent, masochistic, sadistic, sexually excited, or punishing quality.

Full tolerance of dependent, aggressive, and sexual fantasies that may emerge in the therapist's mind is a precondition for raising the question: "Why am I reacting at this point in this way?" or "What is it in the patient's material or in my own disposition that has triggered my reaction to be stimulated in this way?" In other words, the therapist has to tolerate the full experience of his or her emotional reaction in the countertransference without acting on it and then using it for understanding its origin and meaning.

Third, to carry out this task, the therapist has to remain in role. This does not mean that the therapist has to be an indifferent robot or an emotionally nonresponsive human being but that he or she maintains the therapeutic stance throughout, regardless of the developments at any particular point, even under conditions of violent affect storms that not infrequently puncture the treatment of borderline patients. To be in role requires a combination of natural, honest behavior and a controlled, discreet maintenance of strict therapeutic boundaries, which guard against personal disclosure or gratification of personal needs out of countertransference acting out. Fourth, and finally, the introspective analysis of the countertransference, its meaning in terms of the transference situation of the patient, and its elaboration within the interpretation of the total object relationship activated in the transference at this point is the culminating task of countertransference analysis.

In short, maintenance of a therapeutic frame, tolerance of full development of countertransference fantasies and emotions, consistently staying in role, and finally the internal analysis of the meaning of the countertransference to utilize it in the building up of transference interpretations constitute an optimal management of the countertransference.

Borderline patients will test the therapeutic limits and, under the impact of severe regressive conditions, attempt to provoke the therapist, again and again, to cross the boundaries of the therapeutic relationship. In our various research projects, we have had experiences of patients who attempted to assault the therapist physically or sexually or destroy objects in his or her office; one patient even divined a therapist's password and was reading all his e-mail. Under such extreme conditions, the therapist, of course, first has to assure his or her own safety and the safety of the objects in his or her office. This safety, and the establishment of conditions for treatment that realistically assure its feasibility, are part of the frame of the treatment, set up in the therapeutic contract at the beginning of the treatment: to maintain this frame becomes the highest priority under the threatening conditions just described. Concern for the safety of the therapist comes before concern for the safety of the patient! In our teaching seminars, we use the metaphor of the airline policy by which adults have to put on the oxygen mask before they put it on the face of small children.

Even under less extreme conditions, there may be moments in which partial acting out of the countertransference is unavoidable: for example, when a patient, by means of an aggressive act, provokes the therapist to an outburst of anger, or another patient, in an impulsive "strip-tease behavior," manages to elicit a sexually interested demeanor of the therapist. It is important that the therapist not deny any momentary loss of appropriate behavior but rather acknowledge it as calmly as he or she can and then invite the patient to explore what this reaction on the therapist's part means to him or her. This approach, which combines the therapist's honest admission of error with a return to the focus on the transference, will prevent further acting out of guilt feelings by self-revelation, acting out a "guilt trip," or, to the contrary, vehemently denying a behavior that the patient has clearly observed. The general principle involved implies the need to preserve honesty and, as much as possible, technical neutrality.

Particular Countertransference Complications

There are certain treatment situations with patients presenting severe personality disorders that may generate emotional reactions in the therapist that, if not resolved, may end up paralyzing his or her therapeutic efforts. A typical example of such a situation is the case of some severely masochistic patients, involved with a sadistic partner who actually threatens their lives or threatens to blackmail them in a way that would threaten their marriage or social or economic survival. The therapist's efforts to analyze this masochistic behavior does not seem to lead anywhere; it is as if the patient, unconsciously, were triumphantly asserting his or her self-destructiveness, projecting his or her frightened self onto the therapist while professing a blind, fascinated submission to the persecutor in the outside world. At times, the therapist may fear for the patient's life and feel uncertain about whether to intervene by establishing preconditions for the treatment to continue or else, under even worse circumstances, suspecting the patient of communicating the content of the therapeutic hours to the persecutor, thus redirecting the hatred and the aggression of that object onto the therapist. Under these latter conditions, the therapist may fear becoming the victim of a revengeful attack of an antisocial third party.

Retrospectively, many of these situations seem a clear case of violation of the therapeutic contract and, possibly, of the boundaries of the therapeutic situation: but they may develop in surreptitious, gradual fashion that, first, induces an intended countertransference paralysis before the therapist recovers his or her objective stance, only then concerned over the therapeutic frame and for his or her own safety, and recovers his or her freedom to establish firm preconditions for the continuation of the treatment. There are other patients who, without being involved in such extremely dangerous circumstances, develop such an intense hatred in the transference that the therapist becomes afraid of that hatred being transmitted into action—fearing, for example, that the patient might spread false, damaging information about the therapist to third parties; initiate legal action against the therapist; or even commit a dangerous, aggressive assault on the therapist. Here, the chronic development of fear and distrust toward the patient leads to the therapist's secret desire to end the treatment, and intense guilt feelings over such a wished-for abandonment of the patient may paralyze the therapist over time. In these cases, consultation with a trusted senior colleague may be helpful and, eventually, facilitate making decisions regarding the continuation of the treatment, once the safety of the therapist and the boundaries of the therapeutic relationship are assured. With these preconditions in place, testing the patient's capacity to tolerate the interpretation of the severely aggressive sadomasochistic transference may proceed.

Another less extreme but more frequent complication is the development of the syndrome of arrogance described by Bion (1967), characterized by the patient's extremely arrogant behavior in the hours and apparent loss of all capacity for ordinary reasoning or accepting such ordinary reasoning on the part of the therapist, coupled with inordinate curiosity about the therapist and his or her life that may escalate into spying on the therapist or attempting to obtain information about him or her from third parties, invading his or her e-mail communications, etc. Here, the therapist's realistic hatred in the countertransference may threaten to evolve into projective counteridentification. The key to resolving this development, in addition to maintenance of the therapist's safety and the frame of the treatment, is the interpretation of the defensive elimination of rational thinking on the part of the patient to avoid the awareness of his or her own hatred. The acting out of the hatred protects against the emotional awareness of it in the transference, particularly against the tolerance of the pleasure that such hatred would give the patient. The interpretation of the defensive function of the acting out of an impulse that could not be tolerated as an emotional experience may gradually transform this acting out into a meaningful resumption of the work in the therapy hours.

Another type of complication is the complete apparent absence of any emotional relationship with the therapist, typical for some patients with severely narcissistic personality disorders who develop predominantly narcissistic defenses in the transference. Under these circumstances, the patient seems to be talking only to himself or herself, with the therapist tolerated as a shadowy witness, or he or she talks to the therapist in an effort to control the therapist, without really communicating anything about an internal experience. In either case, in spite of an apparent "animation" in the hours, the lack of an emotional relationship may induce a countertransference marked by emptiness and boredom. Boredom, the most typical affect reflecting the absence of a presently significant object relationship, may be an early warning signal before the therapist has even captured the extent of the narcissistic transference. The therapist's boredom may evolve into distractibility, sleepiness or actually falling asleep, or having to struggle with that impulse in every hour with that particular patient. Here the solution is obviously a systematic analysis of narcissistic defenses: this is one situation where the therapist's knowledge about the psychopathology and the technical requirements in the psychoanalytic therapy with narcissistic patients may help dramatically and rapidly to resolve this impasse (Kernberg 1984). In Chapter 5, I explore further the technical difficulties presented by narcissistic patients.

Perhaps the most difficult situation to tolerate is that presented by patients who are remarkably "unemotional," presenting a facade of polite indifference and, while apparently willing to talk openly about themselves and their difficulties, convey not only a sense of complete hopelessness over their situation but also what may impress the therapist as a cynical rejection of any effort on the therapist's part to understand the patient and to help by means of understanding. In contrast to patients with a major depression, whose tendency toward negative therapeutic reaction derives from an unconscious sense of not deserving help and who, in effect, may get worse as a reaction to the concerned, helpful attitude of the therapist, the patients I am referring to here are not depressed at all but present a life trajectory of chronically self-destructive, self-defeating behavior, with a combination of narcissistic grandiosity and superiority and yet pessimistic self-devaluation. It is as if the main objective in their lives were to destroy any hope and loving attitude presented to them by others.

Perhaps the most typical example of this type is a patient who presents what André Green (1993) described as the syndrome of the "dead mother." These are patients with an intense unconscious tendency to destroy all object relations, as if, by renouncing any human contacts, they could find the happiness of nonexpectations, nonfrustration, a kind of psychic death that, unconsciously, signifies their attachment to and identification with the symbolically dead mother. With some frequency, these are also the characteristics of some patients with chronic, severe self-damaging and self-mutilating tendencies, taken to the extreme of loss of limbs and/or carefully prepared, calmly desired suicide. These patients may induce a gradually intensifying unconscious and, eventually, conscious giving up on the part of the therapist, who becomes both victim and unconscious perpetrator of psychic death in the countertransference. Some of these patients can be helped by recovering the traumatic early experiences that are buried underneath their efforts to destroy all significant object relations and, particularly, the therapeutic one. In other cases, the countertransference reaction of internal abandonment may be a realistic indication that, at that point and with that therapist, the treatment has no future.

Contemporary Controversies Regarding Countertransference

One major issue that divides the psychoanalytic community in their view of the transference/countertransference bind, at this time, is the controversy between a "two-person psychology" and the assumed "one-person psychology" of Freud. In my view, the real issue here is insufficient attention to the fact that, in reality, we are always dealing with a "three-person psychology," as has been stressed particularly in the French psychoanalytic literature (De Mijolla and De Mijolla 1996). Those who have proposed a "two-person psychology" criticize Freud for his having focused exclusively on what was going on inside the patient's mind rather than on the interaction between patient and analyst, to which the analyst also contributes with countertransference. Analytic treatment, from that perspective, is the analysis of the bipersonal or intersubjective field, contributed to by both patient and analyst. The relational analytic school, self psychology, and the intersubjective approach all stress this "two-person psychology" (Kernberg 2004b). Within this approach, the patient's experience in the therapeutic situation is considered almost symmetrical to that of the analyst's experience of the situation, in terms of the construction of the meaning of transference and countertransference. Transference, from this viewpoint, is considered in part as a reaction to the countertransference, in parallel to countertransference being a reaction to the transference. This approach highlights the importance of the analysis of the countertransference and also is linked, in the view of some of the proponents of this approach, to the tendency to communicate the countertransference to the patient under certain circumstances.

The alternative position, reflected in what may be considered the psychoanalytic mainstream, constituted by the growing confluence of the British schools (the Kleinian as well as the Independent British approaches) and American ego psychology, and also sustained by the French psychoanalytic school, is that we must assume a "three-person psychology." The implication is that the analyst, in making the analysis of countertransference part of the technical task, is split between one part of him or her that, under the effect of countertransference, contributes to the transference/countertransference bind of the analytic situation, and another part of his or her mind, an "excluded third party," that would analyze this total situation as an aspect of the analyst's interpretive clarification and resolution of the transference. This view corresponds to my own approach and is consistent with the analysis of countertransference presented in this chapter.

I believe that the communication of the countertransference, a derivative of the relationist or interpersonal approaches, undoubtedly helps at times to reassure the patient against feared fantasies, strengthens the reality aspects of the therapeutic situation, and, particularly, reduces the impact of negative transference developments. At the same time, however, communication of the countertransference may drive deeper aspects of the negative transference underground and maintain the dissociative or splitting processes that are so typical for patients with severe personality disorders. In

these cases, communication of the countertransference may correspond to a strong pull toward action in the therapist, reflecting intense countertransference activation, and move the treatment into
a more reality-oriented, supportive approach. This may improve
behavioral aspects of the patient's psychopathology in the short
term but, in the long run, militates against the understanding
of deeper aspects of the patient's unconscious mind. This reduces,
I believe, the possibility of obtaining significant characterologic
change and resolution of the underlying personality disorder.

I have already mentioned that if a partial acting out of the countertransference occurs, in the sense that there is an actual behavior by
the therapist that implies that he or she has abandoned the position of
technical neutrality (i.e., of the concerned objectivity toward the patient), and the patient is aware of that inappropriate or changed behavior of the therapist, the therapist should acknowledge that
observation and not deny it. However, I reiterate that the therapist
should not go any further in stating what the nature of his or her countertransference problems are. The therapist may acknowledge that
he or she has been concerned with personal issues, that he or she may
temporarily not have fully done justice to the patient's needs and is
aware of the responsibility, either to be able to resolve these internal
issues to an extent that would not influence the relationship with the
patient or, should that not be possible, to interrupt, for this session or
for the time necessary, the treatment of this patient.

Again, I believe that such an honest statement is important yet
protects the patient from being overloaded with the therapist's
problems and preserves the possibility of a full analysis of the
transference that, in my view, would be lost under conditions of
communication of the countertransference. There may be extremely difficult life situations on the therapist's part that may interfere with his or her work, but insofar as our work uses our own
psychic responsivity to our patients, we owe it to them to treat them
only when our analytic instrument permits us to do so.

Searles (1979) has stressed that it is unavoidable that unresolved issues of the analyst's personality be activated as part of his
or her countertransference reaction. For example, the analyst's
conflicts over sadism and fragmentation, over guilt and concern,
may be triggered under circumstances when the patient's fears in
the transference activate his or her sense of not being able to help
the fragmented parent to deal with the patient's guilt over the patient's sadism in punishing the parent with the illness and with the
patient's grief over not being able to establish a bond of love with

his or her parent. Under such conditions, the tolerance of the analyst's own unresolved conflicts in the countertransference is a precondition for the therapeutic symbiosis, in which mutual humanization, tolerance, and the acceptance of the identity of the other and of a new bond with the other may take place. The fact that, even under ordinary circumstances, such developments may occur in the countertransference makes the need for the analyst's capacity to split himself or herself into an experiencing and an observing part so important.

Adler (1985) refers to the countertransference to the devaluing borderline patient, from what may be considered a Kohutian perspective, in the sense of an indication for the therapist to explore the patient's enactment of the relationship with a selfobject by whom the patient is not sufficiently "mirrored." The patient is unable to accept the competence of the analyst, whose behavior profoundly threatens the patient's self-assurance. There are serious risks, Adler states, of countertransference acting out under such conditions, and the analyst has to explore to what extent he or she may have contributed to fail the patient as a selfobject, carrying out insufficient mirroring in response to excessive demands or to the frustration of the analyst's own needs. Adler proposes that the analyst explore his or her countertransference from that viewpoint but not to communicate it to the patient.

Another controversial countertransference issue, less frequently debated but implicitly present, particularly with patients who, as part their psychopathology, show profound deviation from habitual social behavior, antisocial tendencies, or esoteric and strange lifestyles, involves the extent to which the therapist should and may be able to maintain a position of concerned objectivity, that is, of technical neutrality, rather than attempting to influence the patients with his or her own value systems. It has been said that the therapist should be moral without being moralistic (Ticho 1972) and that he or she should make a concerted and consistent effort to let the patient evolve his or her own ideological choices and commitments. I think we have to accept the limits of the position of technical neutrality insofar as it may be more dependent on cultural norms jointly adhered to by patient and therapist than what we are usually aware of. The changing view within the psychiatric and psychoanalytic community on homosexuality, for example, illustrates how socially prevalent beliefs may influence assumedly scientific thinking and attitudes toward patients: with this word of caution, I conclude this review of countertransference.

References

Adler G: Devaluation and countertransference, in Borderline Psychopathology and Its Treatment. New York, Jason Aronson, 1985, pp 171–188

Baranger M, Baranger W: La situación analítica como campo dinámico. Revista Uruguaya de Psicoanálisis 4:3–54, 1961–1962

Baranger M, Baranger W: Problemas del campo psicoanalítico. Buenos Aires, Argentina, Kargieman, 1969

Baranger M, Baranger W, Mom J: Process and non-process in analytic work. Int J Psychoanal 64:1–15, 1983

Bion WR: On arrogance, in Second Thoughts: Selected Papers on Psychoanalysis. New York, Basic Books, 1967, pp 86–92

Clarkin JF, Yeomans FE, Kernberg OF: Psychotherapy for Borderline Personality: Focusing on Object Relations. Washington, DC, American Psychiatric Publishing, 2006

De Mijolla, De Mijolla MS: Psychanalyse. Paris, Presses Universitaires de France, 1996

Freud A: The Ego and the Mechanisms of Defense (1936). The Writings of Anna Freud, Vol 2. New York, International Universities Press, 1966

Freud S: The future prospects of psycho-analytic therapy (1910), in The Standard Edition of the Complete Psychological Works of Sigmund Freud, Vol 11. Translated and edited by Strachey J. London, Hogarth Press, 1957

Green A: On Private Madness. Madison, CT, International Universities Press, 1993

Grinberg L: Sobre algunos problemas de técnica psicoanalìtica determinados por la identificación y contraidentificación proyectivas. Revista de Psicoanálisis 13:507–511, 1956

Grinberg L: Projective counteridentification and countertransference, in Countertransference. Edited by Epstein L, Feiner A. New York, Jason Aronson, 1979, pp 169–192

Heimann P: On countertransference. Int J Psychoanal 31:81–84, 1950

Kernberg OF: Borderline Conditions and Pathological Narcissism. New York, Jason Aronson, 1975

Kernberg OF: Object Relations Theory and Clinical Psychoanalysis. New York, Jason Aronson, 1976

Kernberg OF: Severe Personality Disorders: Psychotherapeutic Strategies. New Haven, CT, Yale University Press, 1984, pp 197–209

Kernberg OF: Psychoanalysis, psychoanalytic psychotherapy, and supportive psychotherapy: contemporary controversies. Int J Psychoanal 80:1075–1091, 1999

Kernberg OF: Aggressivity, Narcissism, and Self-Destructiveness in the Psychotherapeutic Relationship: New Developments in the Psychopathology and Psychotherapy of Severe Personality Disorders. New Haven, CT, Yale University Press, 2004a, pp 167–183

Kernberg OF: Contemporary Controversies in Psychoanalytic Theory, Techniques, and Their Applications. New Haven, CT, Yale University Press, 2004b, pp 285–304

Racker H: The meaning and uses of countertransference. Psychoanal Q 26:303–357, 1957

Sandler J: Countertransference and role-responsiveness. International Review of Psycho-Analysis 3:43–47, 1976

Searles HF: Countertransference and theoretical model, in Countertransference and Related Subjects: Selected Papers. New York, International Universities Press, 1979, pp 373–379

Ticho E: The effects of the psychoanalyst's personality on the treatment, in Psychoanalytic Forum, Vol 4. Edited by Lindon JA. New York, International Universities Press, 1972, pp 137–151

Tower LE: Countertransference. J Am Psychoanal Assoc 4:224–255, 1956

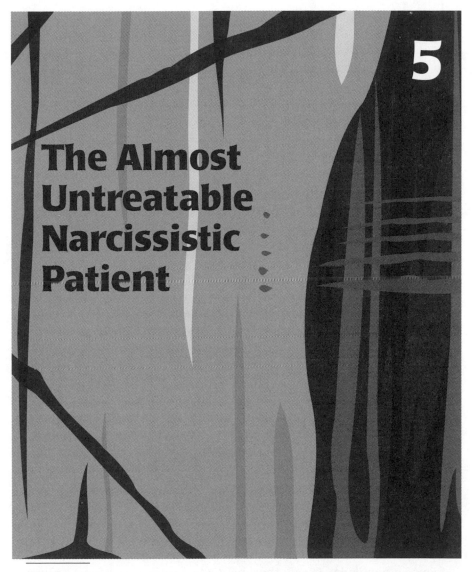

The Almost Untreatable Narcissistic Patient

5

This chapter was first published in *Persönlichkeitsstörungen Theorie und Therapie* 9:131–146, 2006. Stuttgart, Germany, Schattauer, 2005. Used with permission. The final, definitive version of this paper has been published as Kernberg OF: "The Almost Untreatable Narcissistic Patient" in *Journal of the American Psychoanalytic Association* 55:503–539, 2007, by SAGE Publications, Inc., http://online.sagepub.com. All rights reserved. © 2007. Used with permission.

The work reported in this chapter was supported by the Borderline Personality Disorders Research Foundation and its founder, Dr. Marco Stoffel, to whom the author wishes to express his profound gratitude.

In this chapter, I present an overview of the descriptive and psycho-dynamic features that characterize the narcissistic personality disorder, one of the most prevalent and, at times, the most challenging of the severe personality disorders. The typical developments in the transference, and the general techniques available to deal with them in the context of a psychoanalytic therapy, are outlined, followed by the prognostically most negative features these patients may evince. Clinical cases illustrating the predominance of such negative prognostic features are briefly outlined, and ways of dealing with them, as well as the limitations of this approach, are spelled out. The most severe cases of this personality pathology probably are at the very limits of treatability with a psychodynamic approach and, in general, with psychotherapeutic methods. By the same token, it is a most challenging area of exploration of new understanding and therapeutic approaches.

Our shared clinical experience in the Personality Disorders Institute at the Weill Medical College of Cornell University in the treatment of patients with borderline personality organization, which corresponds to the entire spectrum of severe personality disorders, has convinced us that patients with borderline personality organization and a narcissistic personality disorder do have a more serious prognosis than do patients with all other personality disorders functioning on that level and that those who, in addition, present significant antisocial behavior do have an even worse prognosis (Clarkin et al. 1989; Stone 1990). This negative trend culminates in the practically untreatable patients with antisocial personality disorder, who, in our view, represent the most severe cases of pathological narcissism. There are patients with severe narcissistic personality disorder, functioning on an overt borderline level with significant antisocial features, but not presenting an antisocial personality disorder proper, who, at times, do respond to treatment, while others do not. This is the group of patients I wish to explore here, with the focus on particular psychotherapeutic techniques that have proven helpful, as well as on the limits of these technical approaches.

A Brief Overview of the Pathology of the Narcissistic Personality Disorder

In order to keep this summary reasonably short, a certain categorical style is almost unavoidable. I beg the reader's indulgence with this section, which provides the organizing frame for what follows.

The narcissistic personality disorder presents, clinically, at three levels of severity. The mildest patients, who appear "neurotic," usually present indications for psychoanalysis. They typically do consult only because of a significant symptom that seems so linked to their character pathology that anything but the treatment of their personality disorder would seem inadequate. In contrast, other narcissistic patients at that level present symptoms that may be treated without an effort to modify or resolve their narcissistic personality structure. All these patients seem to be functioning very well, in general, except typically presenting significant problems in long-term intimate relationships and in long-term professional or work interactions. A second level of severity of illness of narcissistic personalities reflects the typical syndrome with all the various clinical manifestations to be described below. These patients definitely need treatment for their personality disorder, and here the alternative between standard psychoanalytic treatment and psychoanalytic psychotherapy depends on individualized indications and contraindications. A third level of severity of narcissistic personality disorder functions on an overt borderline level: here, in addition to all the typical manifestations of narcissistic personality disorder, the patient presents general lack of anxiety tolerance and impulse control and a severe reduction in sublimatory functions (i.e., in his or her capacity for productivity or creativity beyond gratification of survival needs). These patients usually show severe and chronic failure in their work and profession and chronic failure in their efforts to establish or maintain intimate love relationships. At this same level of severity, another group of patients may not show overt borderline features but present significant antisocial activity, which, prognostically, places them in the same category as those who function on a borderline level.

All these severely narcissistic patients may respond to a psychoanalytic, transference-focused psychotherapy, unless, for individualized reasons, this approach would seem contraindicated, in which case a more supportive approach or cognitive-behavioral approach might be the treatment of choice (Levy et al. 2005). Patients whose antisocial behavior is predominantly passive and parasitic present less of a threat to themselves and to the therapist than do those others who present severe suicidal and parasuicidal behavior or violent attacks against others. Aggression against others or self is typical for antisocial behavior of the aggressive type, particularly when these patients fulfill the criteria for the syndrome of malignant narcissism. The syndrome of malignant narcissism includes, in addition to the narcissistic personality disorder, severe antisocial behavior, significant paranoid trends, and ego-syntonic, self-directed, or other-directed aggression.

Now, let us review briefly the dominant features of the narcissistic personality disorder as typically represented particularly at the second or intermediate level of severity described (Kernberg 1997).

1. Pathology of the self: these patients show excessive self-centeredness, overdependency on admiration from others, prominence of fantasies of success and grandiosity, avoidance of realities that are contrary to their inflated image of themselves, and bouts of insecurity disrupting their sense of grandiosity or specialness.
2. Pathology of the relationship with others: these patients suffer from inordinate envy, both conscious and unconscious. They show greediness and exploitiveness of others, entitlement, devaluation of others, and an incapacity to really depend on them (in contrast to ongoing need for admiration from others). They show a remarkable lack of empathy with others, shallowness in their emotional life, and a lack of capacity for commitment to relationships, goals, or joint purposes with others.
3. Pathology of the superego (conscious and unconscious internalized value systems): at a relatively milder level, patients evince a deficit in their capacity for sadness and mourning; their self-esteem is regulated by severe mood swings rather than by limited, focused self-criticism; they appear to be determined by a "shame" culture rather than by a "guilt" culture, and their values have a childlike quality. More severe superego pathology, in addition to defective mourning, entails chronic antisocial behavior and significant irresponsibility in all their relationships. In their lack of consideration of others, there is no capacity for guilt or remorse for such devaluing behavior. A particular syndrome—mentioned before, reflecting severe superego pathology, characterized by the combination of narcissistic personality disorder, antisocial behavior, ego-syntonic aggression (directed against self and/or others), and marked paranoid trends, is the syndrome of malignant narcissism.
4. A basic self-state of these patients is a chronic sense of emptiness and boredom, resulting in stimulus hunger and the wish for artificial stimulation of affective response by means of drugs or alcohol that predisposes to substance abuse and dependency.

Patients with narcissistic personality disorder may present typical complications of this disorder, including sexual promiscuity or sexual inhibition, drug dependence and alcoholism, social parasitism, severe (narcissistic type) suicidality and parasuicidality, and, under conditions of severe stress and regression, the possibility of significant paranoid developments and brief psychotic episodes.

General Technical Issues in the Treatment of Narcissistic Personality Disorder

As mentioned before, the indications for various modalities of psychoanalytic and other modalities of treatment vary with the severity of the illness and the individual combination of particular symptoms and character pathology. The general techniques of standard psychoanalysis and psychoanalytic psychotherapy have to be modified or enriched by specific approaches to deal with the narcissistic transference/countertransference binds (Kernberg 1984).

Without further exploring here the general differences between these modalities of treatment and their respective indications, I shall spell out particular issues that typically emerge in the treatment of narcissistic patients and that become especially dominant in treatment encounters with the "almost untreatable narcissistic patients" that we shall explore and, within the entire spectrum of psychoanalytically derived treatments, require certain specific technical approaches to them. Clinical examples summarized in the following section of this chapter illustrate these issues.

A core issue for narcissistic patients is their incapacity to depend on the therapist, because such dependency is experienced as humiliating. Such fear of dependency, often unconscious, is defended against with attempts to omnipotently control the treatment (Kernberg 1984; Rosenfeld 1987). Clinically, this takes the form of the patient's efforts of "self-analysis" as opposed to a collaboration with the therapist leading to integration and reflection. These patients treat the therapist as if he or she were a "vending machine" of interpretations, which they then appropriate as their own, at the same time being chronically disappointed for not receiving enough or not the right kind of interpretations, unconsciously dismissing everything they might learn from the therapist. For this reason, treatment often maintains a "first-session" quality over an extended period of time. Narcissistic patients show themselves as intensely competitive with the therapist and are suspicious of what they consider his or her indifferent or exploitative attitude toward them. They cannot conceive the therapist as spontaneously interested and honestly concerned about them, and as a result of this belief, they evince significant devaluation of and contempt for the therapist.

Conversely, narcissistic patients may also show a defensive idealization of the therapist, considering him or her as "the greatest," but such idealization is frail and can rapidly be shattered by devaluation and contempt. It also may be part of omnipotent control, in that these patients unconsciously attempt to force the therapist to be always convincing and brilliant, as befitting his or her grandiosity, but not superior to them, as that would generate envy. The patient needs the therapist to maintain his or her "brilliance" in order to be protected against the patient's tendency to devalue him or her, which would leave the therapist feeling totally lost and abandoned in the treatment.

A major feature involved in all these manifestations is the patient's conscious and unconscious envy of the therapist and the patient's consistent sense that there can only be one great person in the room, who necessarily will depreciate the other inferior one, which motivates the patient to try to stay on top, with the risk of feeling abandoned because of the loss of the devalued therapist. The envy of the therapist, at the same time, is an unending source of resentment of what the therapist has to give and may take many forms. The most important one is the envy of the creativity of the therapist, of the fact that he or she can creatively understand the patient rather than providing him or her with pat, cliché answers that can be memorized by the patient. Also, the very capacity of the therapist to invest in a relationship, which the patient is aware he or she does not have himself or herself, is envied. The most important consequence of conflicts around envy are negative therapeutic reactions: typically, the patient feels worse following a situation in which he or she clearly acknowledged having been helped by the therapist. Acting out of the envious resentment of the therapist may take many forms, such as playing one therapist against another; an aggressive pseudoidentification with the therapist by playing the therapist's role in a destructive interaction with third parties; and, quite frequently, the patient's constructing a view that he or she alone is the cause of any progress.

The analysis of the constituent, idealized self and idealized object representations that jointly consolidate into the pathological grandiose self of these patients gradually tends to reduce the grandiosity in the transference and the pseudointegration of that pathological grandiose self and brings about the emergence of more primitive internalized object relations in the transference and more primitive affective investments related to them. This development shows clinically in the breakthrough of aggressive reactions as part of such primitive object relations, including suicidal and parasuicidal behavior in unconscious identification with powerful yet hostile objects: the "victory" of these primitive object representations over the therapist may be symbolized by the destruction of the body of the patient.

Chronic suicidal tendencies of narcissistic patients have a premeditated, calculated, coldly sadistic quality that differs from the impulsive, "momentarily decided upon" suicidality of ordinary borderline patients (Kernberg 2001). The projection of persecutory object representations onto the therapist in the form of severe paranoid transferences also may become predominant, as well as a form of narcissistic rage that expresses the patient's sense of entitlement and envious resentment. "Stealing" from the therapist may take the form of learning the therapist's language, in order to apply it to others rather than to the patient, as well as the syndrome of perversity, reflected in the use of what is received from the therapist as an expression of concern and commitment, as a way of expressing aggression against others. In other words, perversity is a malignant transformation of what the patient received from the therapist. The corruption of superego values may be acted out as antisocial behavior that the patient, unconsciously, perceives as caused by the irresponsibility of the therapist and not by himself or herself.

Narcissistic entitlement and greedy incorporation of what the patient feels is denied to him or her may take the form of apparently erotic transferences, demands to be loved by the therapist, or even efforts to seduce the therapist as part of a general effort to destroy his or her role. These are severe complications, very different from the erotic transferences of neurotic patients.

When improvement occurs, typically, the severe envy diminishes, and the capacity for gratitude gradually emerges both in the transference and in extratransferential relations, particularly in the relationship with intimate sexual partners. Envy of the other gender is a dominant unconscious conflict of narcissistic personalities, and the decrease of the envy of the other sex permits a

decrease of unconscious devaluing attitudes toward intimate partners, and the capacity for maintained love relationships improves.
Narcissistic patients may become more tolerant of their own feelings of envy without having to act them out, and, with increased
awareness, tendencies toward defensive devaluation gradually decrease in this process. The development of more mature feelings of
guilt and concern over their aggressive and exploitive attitudes indicates the consolidation of the superego, as well as the deepening
of their object relations. At times, however, that integration may
imply such a severity of the now integrated but sadistic superego
that these patients may experience severe depression at a point
when improvement of their character pathology is evident.

Under optimal conditions, patients who had experienced dominant psychopathic transferences (their conviction of the therapist's
dishonesty or the direct expression of conscious dishonesty and deceptiveness on these patients' part) over an extended period of time
may shift into paranoid transferences, against which the psychopathic transferences, typically, had been a defense. And, later on,
such paranoid transferences (related to the projection of persecutory object representations and superego precursors onto the
therapist) may shift into depressive transferences, as the patient
becomes able to tolerate ambivalent feelings and to recognize his
or her experiencing both intense positive and negative feelings toward the same object (Kernberg 1992).

Perhaps the transference development most difficult to manage
is that of patients with an extreme intensity of aggression, which
may present itself in the form of almost uncontrollable suicidal and
parasuicidal behavior outside the sessions and in chronic sadomasochistic transferences in the sessions. In the latter case, the patient
sadistically attacks the therapist over an extended period of time,
clearly attempting to provoke him or her to respond, in his or her
countertransference, in the same way, only to then accuse the therapist of being aggressive and destructive. In all of this, the patient
experiences himself or herself as the therapist's helpless victim.
This development of a secondary masochistic relation to the therapist may be followed, in turn, by self-directed aggression in which
the patient accuses himself or herself exaggeratedly of his or her
"badness," only, eventually, to revert again to an extremely sadistic
behavior toward the therapist, thus reinitiating the cycle. Here the
technical approach involves pointing out to the patient these patterns of experiencing self or other as either an aggressor or a victim
in the transference, with frequent role reversals.

Another manifestation of severe aggression in the transference is the syndrome of arrogance, quite frequently present in narcissistic personalities functioning on an overt borderline level: the combination of intense arrogant behavior, an extreme curiosity about the therapist and his or her life but little curiosity about oneself, and "pseudostupidity" (Bion 1967). The latter symptom consists in a lack of capacity to accept any logical, rational argument: on the patient's part, the main defensive purpose of this entire syndrome is self-protection against the very awareness of the intense aggression that controls him or her. Aggressive affect is expressed in behavior rather than in an affectively marked representational process.

While these transference developments may evolve in any treatment modality, the advantage of psychodynamic psychotherapies and psychoanalysis, where indicated, is that they may permit resolution of these transference manifestations by means of the interpretative focus. In contrast, supportive and cognitive-behavioral treatments may control and reduce the most severe effects of these transference developments on the relationship with the therapist, but their continued unconscious control of the patient's life continues to be a major problem. Supportive and cognitive-behavioral approaches may reduce, by educational means combined with a general supportive attitude, the inappropriate nature of the patient's interactions at work or in a profession. However, in my experience, work at this level is not sufficient to modify the incapacity of these patients to establish significant love relationships in depth and to maintain gratifying intimate relationships in general. And, not infrequently, the difficult transference developments described above may undermine supportive or cognitive-behavioral approaches. Therefore, when it seems reasonable to conclude that the patient may tolerate an analytic approach, regardless of the severity of the symptomatology, that indication usually is a prognostically positive feature. But, as we shall see in our next section, such an analytic approach has definite limits.

There are references in the psychoanalytic literature, particularly within the Kleinian approach, that indicate successful treatment with nonmodified analytic approaches of some severely ill narcissistic patients (Bion 1967; Spillius 1988; Spillius and Feldman 1989; Steiner 1993). The work of Steiner, particularly, clearly refers to the analysis of narcissistic patients, whom he designates as presenting a "pathological organization," and Hinshelwood (1994) points to the use of this term, within Kleinian literature, for "inaccessible personalities." One problem, however, is that the overall description of such patients in that literature usually lacks sufficiently detailed information about their general symptomatology and personality characteristics, so that it is difficult to compare them to the patients referred to in our work at Cornell University. In addition, the subtle and convincing descriptions in the Kleinian literature of particular interpretations of the transference of these patients convey a sense of effectiveness of these interventions that leaves open, however, the overall question of the long-range effectiveness of the treatment and of indications and contraindications.

We have been strongly influenced by the clinical insights provided by the Kleinian school but are wondering whether their clinical excerpts are mostly focused on successful cases and tend to refer little to nonaccepted, unsuccessful, or interrupted ones. At the same time, however, all analysts tend to mention privately cases they have rejected, considering them as too problematic and unsuccessful ones. In this chapter, in contrast, I focus specifically on the most severe cases within the narcissistic spectrum, in the context of a careful evaluation of symptoms, personality, and long-range developments, and the experience of both success and failure with them.

Typical Presentation of "Impossible" Patients

Usually, negative prognostic features become evident during the initial evaluation of patients, but we are all familiar with cases in which, despite careful history taking and assessment, important data emerge only after treatment has begun, altering our initial diagnostic and prognostic impressions. There are, however, typical manifestations of what may eventually prove as almost insurmountable obstacles to the treatment, which may be identified in the initial evaluation. The following cases reflect such frequent danger signals.

Chronic Work Failure in Contrast to High Educational Background and Capacity

These are patients who have worked for many years below their level of training or capacity and often drift into a "disabled" status so that they must be cared for by their families (if they are wealthy) or the public social support system. Such a chronic dependency on the family or on a social support system represents a major secondary gain of illness, one of the principal causes of treatment failure. In the United States, at least, these patients are high consumers of therapeutic and social services; however, were they to get well, they would no longer qualify for the supports that maintain their existence. These patients come to treatment, consciously or unconsciously, not because they are interested in improvement but to demonstrate to the social system their incapacity to improve and, therefore, their need for ongoing social support. Because they are usually required to be in some kind of treatment in order to get supportive housing, Supplemental Security Income, Social Security Disability, etc., they go from program to program, therapist to therapist. Michael Stone, a senior member of our Personality Disorders Institute at Cornell, has concluded that, for practical purposes, if a patient were potentially able to earn, by working, at least 1.5 times the amount of money that he is receiving from social support systems, there may be a chance that eventually he would be motivated to work again. Otherwise, the secondary gain of illness may carry the day (Stone 1990).

The underlying psychodynamics of this situation vary from case to case. There are patients who would be willing to work if they became immediately the chief executive officer of a major industry or a leader in their profession. They find the need to start out at an "inferior" beginner's position as an intolerable humiliation. There are many patients who prefer to live on social welfare rather than undergo the "humiliation" of working in a subordinate position. In some patients, the dynamics of the unconscious rage at being expected to take care of themselves dominate their lives. These are patients who feel that, because of the severe frustrations or traumatisms that they have endured, they deserve special treatment in life, and to become active on their own behalf would mean to renounce that revengeful expectation.

Consciously, all these dynamics may show only as the emergence of severe symptoms of anxiety or even depression whenever these patients attempt to work. Often, these are patients who have learned by heart all the symptoms of anxiety disorders and claim that they have a chronic anxiety disorder for which they must be in an ongoing medication treatment, but even with the use of medication, the disorder becomes uncontrollable whenever they try to work. This specific emergence of severe anxiety when any work possibilities are contemplated is particularly ominous. There are still other patients in whose pathology antisocial features dominate, and, as long as they have the possibility of exploiting a relative or society, it would seem foolish to them and, therefore, humiliating to work.

This condition of work failure may merge with grandiose fantasies of capacities and success that remain unchallenged as long as the patient does not become part of the workforce: the rationalization of this pattern of social parasitism may include a fantasized profession or talent the patient has and that nobody has recognized as yet: the unknown painter, the inhibited author, the revolutionary musician...often such a patient is perfectly willing to enter treatment as long as somebody else pays for the treatment and will abandon it the day when this payment is no longer available, even if there existed the possibility of continuing the treatment if the patient were willing and able to take on some remunerated employment.

Case 1

The patient, a man in his late forties from a rather aristocratic family in Great Britain, had studied at prominent universities in the United States and gone on to a career in business, in which, despite excellent recommendations and social connections, he failed to progress owing to his haughty, demanding, and subtly irresponsible behavior. Having been bypassed for important promotions, he changed from one firm to another, eventually creating for himself a reputation of someone who could not be relied upon for leading positions. He married a businesswoman whom he had met in one of his employments, originally in an administratively subordinate position to his, but who, through her brilliance and hard work, managed to be promoted to ever more senior positions.

His wife eventually surpassed him in the world of business, whereupon he withdrew from work completely. He started to drink, became depressed, and developed hypochondriacal symptoms that motivated his seeking treatment with internists first, and he was subsequently referred for psychiatric treatment. After brief psychotherapeutic encounters with various psychiatrists, all of whom he dismissed as rather useless, he entered psychoanalysis. At that point, he had not been working for several years. He was living on a rapidly shrinking inheritance and the financially privileged situation of his wife, while resenting bitterly his dependency on her, which he acted out by having multiple brief relationships with other women.

He presented a rather typical narcissistic personality disorder, and his transference to his analyst rapidly evolved into alternating manifestations of intense envy and devaluation. He perceived his analyst as a successful, "cutthroat" businessman, whom he hated, similar to the dominant feelings toward his wife and, at a deeper level, his domineering, self-centered, "aristocratic" mother. At other times, he perceived the analyst as a failing, incompetent, "phony" professional, onto whom he projected that corresponding aspect of his own self-image, while, at such times, identifying himself with the grandiose superiority that he had perceived in his mother. The treatment became a significant source of secondary gain because, as long as he still suffered from depression and insecurity, it made "no sense" to him to work, and he thus could avoid the deep feeling of humiliation in having to acknowledge his professional failure as a consequence of his own behavior. Perhaps more importantly, any attempt to resurrect his career would necessitate taking what he would consider a low-level position, which represented an intolerable humiliation as well. Only after an extended stalemate in the treatment, and following the analyst's insistence upon a return to work as a precondition to continue the treatment, did the situation change, leading to a full deployment of feelings of hatred and humiliation in the transference and allowing for the possibility for working through of his narcissistic structure in this context. His sense of humiliation at having to work at an "inferior" position, the fantasy that the analyst was depreciating him because of that, and the envious resentment of the analyst's "better life" could be worked through gradually and eventually permitted the emergence of gratitude for the analyst's patience and authentic dependency on a loving maternal image. This development in the transference, in turn, led to significant improvement in the feelings toward his wife and his relationship with her. He was greatly improved at termination.

Case 2

A woman in her early twenties, a second-year medical resident, was referred to analysis because of serious problems in her relationships with colleagues, supervisors, and patients. The diagnosis was a narcissistic personality, and she started psychoanalysis with me under an arrangement she had obtained with her father, whereby he would pay for her treatment until her graduation from residency, at which time she would take on the responsibility for her treatment (if it was not completed by then). She made it clear to me from the beginning that she thought this treatment was useless and outmoded, and she was willing to give it a try only as long as she did not have to pay for it.

Analysis of this provocative stance, which, at that time, I considered a manifestation of narcissistic defenses against dependency by devaluing the analyst, opened up complex dynamics of her family background. She described her mother as extremely controlling and yet totally uninterested in what her daughter was involved in and what her feelings were and her father as nice but impotent, who supported his wife completely. But, the patient went on, she had learned to manipulate father and thus to use him to extricate herself from mother's control without confronting her openly. Manipulation, deceptiveness, and ruthless control dominated the interactions of the patient with her parents and a younger sister. I had hoped to gradually work through her devaluation of me through analysis of the transferential replay of the family constellation. When, however, two years later, graduation approached and we reviewed where she was and what the future arrangements for her analysis would be, the patient acknowledged that she had been doing much better in her work, had graduated with an appreciation of her improvement by her teachers, but was nonetheless convinced that all of this she had achieved by herself. She saw "no way" in which the analysis had helped her, and, of course, she would end the analysis the day that her father would no longer pay for it, and that is what happened and serves as an awesome testimony to the power of narcissistic defenses against vulnerability and dependency!

The therapeutic approach to such cases needs to include the reduction or elimination of the secondary gain of illness. Clinically, I would point out to the patient that an active involvement in work and its related interactional experiences and accepting conceptual responsibility for financing the treatment are essential for the treatment to help the patient and that such an engagement is a precondition for the possibility of carrying out a psychoanalytic psychotherapy. Depending on the situation, I might give the patient a period of time, say three to six months, to achieve this goal, with a clear understanding that should it not be possible to achieve it, treatment will be interrupted at that point. This condition constitutes a limit setting that will become part of the treatment frame and, therefore, require interpretation as part of its transference implications from the beginning of the treatment. Practically speaking, these interpretations may focus on the unconscious motivation for the refusal of work, the importance of the gratification of secondary gain, the resentment the patient may experience toward the therapist's threat to the patient's equilibrium, and the self-defeating aspects of the patient implied in denying herself the possibility of well-being, success, self-respect, and enrichment of life linked to a potentially successful and creative engagement in work or a profession.

With this modification technique, it is often possible to overcome this secondary gain of illness; but, in many cases, the patient will find infinite excuses not to carry out any work and even may recruit supportive help from social agencies who may call the therapist's attention to the fact that "excessive demands" on the patient are increasing the patient's difficulties and symptoms, as the patient has revealed to third parties: a social worker or health care manager. In different social systems and health insurance arrangements, secondary gain of illness may appear in different ways, but I have been able to observe these dynamics under a broad variety of social contexts in different countries (e.g., in Austria, Finland, and Germany).

Pervasive Arrogance

This symptom may dominate in patients who, while recognizing that they have significant difficulties or symptoms, obtain unconscious secondary gain of illness by demonstrating the incompetence and incapacity of the mental health professions to alleviate such symptoms. They become super experts in the field of their suffering, diligently research the Internet, check out therapists for their background and orientation, compare their merits and shortcomings, and present themselves for treatment "to give the therapist a chance" but consistently obtain an unconscious degree of satisfaction in defeating the helping profession. They may suffer from symptoms such as chronic marital conflicts, bouts of intense depression when threatened with failures at work or in their profession, anxiety and somatizations, and even significant chronic depression. Such severe, chronic depressions respond only "partially" to whatever psychopharmacological treatment they receive (and even to electroconvulsive treatment that, sometimes, is questionably recommended for patients with chronic and severe characterological depression). Not infrequently, the combination of a psychotherapeutic treatment with psychopharmacological treatment temporarily leads to a surprising improvement, which, in these patients' view, is due to "the medication alone" and the psychotherapeutic treatment is not helpful and becomes unnecessary; later, the medication "does not work anymore."

The sudden shift from frail idealization to complete devaluation of the therapist mentioned before may occur at any point, and, sometimes, a treatment of many months' duration that seemed to be progressing satisfactorily is unexpectedly disrupted because of an intense onslaught of envy of the therapist that triggers a radical devaluation of him or her. The initial evaluation of these patients usually reveals an ego-syntonic arrogance that may evolve into grossly inappropriate behavior and rudeness in some cases or be thinly masked by a surface facade of appropriate tactfulness in others. This characterological arrogance has to be differentiated from the syndrome of arrogance referred to before, described by Bion (1967), that coincides with intense affect storms in the transference and that, in the context of a psychoanalytic psychotherapy in which the patient's relationship with the therapist is firmly established, has a better prognosis.

The pervasive arrogance explored here may be rationalized by the patient in terms of cultural or ideological features, such as a female patient rejecting all male therapists because "they do not understand women," while, in relating to a female therapist, this same patient berates the therapist for being submissive to a world of man's rules, including those that govern a therapeutic relationship. When efforts to undermine the female therapist's therapeutic frame fail, the patient may withdraw triumphantly from the treatment with such a "rigid, subservient" woman. Similar rationalizations may involve racial bias, the patient's assumed differences in political outlook with the therapist, or religious orientations.

Case 3

A woman in her middle forties came to treatment because of a long history of depression (which had not responded to many types of antidepressive medication), chronic suicidal ideation, and several nonlethal suicide attempts that had a somewhat histrionic quality. She had been an office manager in a business operation with responsibility for twenty to thirty persons. She had had a series of similar positions in the past, which followed a recurring trajectory: at first, she was very successful and energetic and impressed people with her intelligence and "getting things done" attitude; but, eventually, she developed conflicts with coworkers and would erupt in temper tantrums, have unexcused absences, and, finally, either resign or be asked to leave her job. At the time she came to our clinic, she had been unemployed for almost one year and was disturbed over the difficulty in finding a position at her level of expertise. She was married and, with great hesitancy, mentioned that because of her husband's impotence, they had not had sex in several years. At the point of history taking, my attempts to elucidate more aspects of this sexual difficulty provoked an irritated reaction and an angry statement that this was her husband's problem and was not relevant to her treatment. She said that she was perfectly satisfied with the marital situation and refused to discuss it any further.

She evinced symptoms of significant depression but not indications of a major depression per se. Her unwillingness to provide much information about herself, beyond symptom reporting, was a first indication of an ongoing negativistic attitude that took the form of depreciatory comments about me from the first session on. She generally demeaned me and the treatment I was offering, while she adamantly insisted on the importance of continuing with the medication she was on (though it was not helping her). I arranged a consultation with the psychopharmacologist on our team, who recommended a shift of medication but continuation of antidepressive medication in combination with psychotherapy with me.

Although she was highly skeptical of our twice-a-week psychotherapy from the outset, she came punctually to all her sessions, complaining that the past sessions had not helped her at all. In fact, as she saw it, it only made her feel worse. Because of a severe breakdown in her capacity to work, in the conflicted relationship with the husband (as it turned out after further inquiry), as well as her general impulsivity and lack of anxiety tolerance, in addition to typical narcissistic features of her personality, I diagnosed her as presenting a narcissistic personality disorder at an overt borderline level.

While attending our sessions regularly, she also eagerly requested sessions and telephone conferences with the psychopharmacologist. In fact, after a few weeks she declared that she was getting better, which she attributed to the medication and the understanding attitude of the psychopharmacologist. In the sessions with me, she talked in a despondent way about her daily activities, evinced a tendency to trivialize her communications, and responded to my comments with a derogatory rolling of her eyes, or challenging questions, attempting to draw me into an argument. She had looked up Internet information about me and showed clear resentment of what she perceived as my many publications by accusing me of using her for my own "experiments," without any consideration of her own interests.

After a few months of treatment, I found out that she had been consulting with other therapists during the time she was in treatment with me and had bought herself a self-help program that she compared with my statements in the hours, concluding, as she eventually confessed triumphantly, that she was learning much more from her tapes than from the hours. I was attempting to focus her attention on her derogatory attitude in the sessions and how this replicated the problems that she had experienced in her work situations, while, at the same time, they perpetuated her sense of being alone and not understood, given the fact that I had become so totally worthless in her mind.

After somewhat less than one year of treatment, and following my return from a vacation, the patient interrupted the treatment telling me that she was doing very well, that medication had helped her, that she had found another job, and that she was ready to proceed on her own. She insisted that she was no longer depressed, that she was functioning well at work, and that her husband was not giving her any problems.

The technical approach to these patients must include a very tactful confrontation and systematic analysis of the defensive functions of arrogance in the transference, pointing out to the patient in the process, from the very start, that given his or her emotional disposition, there is a risk that the treatment will end prematurely because of the devaluation of the therapist. Typically, the patient fears, by projective identification, that the therapist has a similar depreciatory disposition toward the patient, and therefore, if the patent's superiority is challenged or destroyed, he or she will be subject to a humiliating devaluation by the therapist. Whenever possible, it is very helpful, from early on, to interpret the unconscious identification of the patient with a grandiose parental object that often is at the bottom of this characterological disposition (and an important component of the pathological grandiose self). The identification with such a grandiose and sadistic object, on the surface, seems to bolster the patient's self-esteem by protecting the patient's sense of superiority and grandiosity; at the bottom, in this identification, the patient is submitting to an internalized object that stands against any real involvement in a relationship with somebody else that might be helpful and is profoundly hostile to the dependent and true relational needs of the patient.

This arrogant reference system supporting the patient's grandiosity may also be expressed by what, on the surface, appears as an opposite symptom: a patient declares himself to be so bad, or inferior, or damaged, or deficient that nothing is going to change, nobody is going to be of help to him. This surface self-devaluation may be totally resistant to any effort to explore its irrationality, and the patient's attitude of superiority to the therapist emerges precisely in the patient's systematic rejection of the therapist's understanding, his knowing better regarding anything the therapist may express that runs counter to the patient's protests of his inferiority. Here, a real trap for the therapist is to be seduced into what, on the surface, would appear to be a "supportive" attitude, an effort to reassure the patient that he is not so bad, that there is hope, and that he should not be so pessimistic. This approach would only reinforce this transference, in contrast to a systematic interpretation of the patient's arrogant attitude of superiority over the therapist reflected in his systematic refusal to explore his behavior in the transference. Obviously, the profoundly masochistic and self-defeating aspects of the submission to a hostile introject also need to be explored systematically: a negative therapeutic reaction following the patient's sense of being helped by the therapist may reflect this dynamic in the transference.

Destructiveness of the Therapeutic Process, The Expression of a Dominant Unconscious Self-Destructiveness as a Major Motivational System

This group of patients includes what, usually from the very beginning of their evaluation, impresses the experienced clinician as extremely grave conditions. These are patients with severe, repetitive suicidal attempts of an almost lethal nature, suicidal attempts that happened "out of the clear sky," often carefully prepared over a period of time, and even gleefully engineered under the eyes of concerned therapists. Chronic self-destructiveness may also manifest itself, in addition to such suicidal attempts, by self-destructive behavior in what potentially might become gratifying love relationships, a promising work situation, or the opportunity for professional advancement—in short, success in crucial areas of any aspects of life. At times, these patients are seen in relatively early years of adolescence or young adulthood, when many opportunities lie still ahead of them in life. Other cases come to the therapist's attention much later, after many failed treatments, with a gradual deterioration of the patient's life situation, and an apparent search of treatment as a "last resort," which may induce a sense of hopefulness—or an illusion, in the therapist, who believes the patient's life may still change. At times, the patient may very openly state that he or she is committed to death by suicide, defiantly challenging the therapist to see whether he or she can do anything about it. Sometimes this defiant challenge comes to a head early, at the time of setting up of the treatment contract, with the patient refusing to commit himself or herself to such contractual arrangements. Usually the family background of these patients evinces severe and chronic traumatizations, including severe sexual or physical abuse, an unusual degree of family chaos, or a practically symbiotic relationship with an extremely aggressive parental figure.

If antisocial features complicate the picture, the patient may be deceptive about suicidal tendencies, and the chronic lack of honesty and a psychopathic type of transference may preclude any possibility to build up a helpful human relationship with a therapist. For example, one of our patients would ingest rat poison for suicidal and parasuicidal purposes. She was able to smuggle rat poison into the hospital and developed internal hemorrhages. While steadfastly denying the ongoing consumption of rat poison to the therapist, her blood tests showed a continuous increase in the prothrombin time. Eventually, this psychotherapeutic treatment had to be interrupted because of the obvious unwillingness or incapacity to adhere to the treatment contract that committed her to stop ingesting rat poison as a precondition for ongoing psychotherapy. André Green (1993) has described, in connection with the syndrome of the "dead mother," the unconscious identification with a psychologically dead parental object. The unconsciously fantasized union with this object justifies and rationalizes the patient's complete dismantling of all relationships with psychologically important objects. In fact, the onset of this patient's ingestion of rat poison was coincident with a visit to her mother's gravesite.

Unconsciously, the patient may deny the existence of both others and the self as meaningful entities, and this radical dismantling of all object relations may constitute, at times, an insurmountable obstacle to treatment. In other cases, the self-destructiveness is more limited, being expressed not in suicidal behavior proper but in severe self-mutilation that repetitively punctures the psychotherapeutic treatment and signals the unconscious triumph of the forces in the patient that promote self-destructiveness as a major life goal. Such self-mutilation may lead to the loss of limbs or severely crippling fractures but stop short of the risk of immediate death.

Case 4

A music teacher in her middle twenties consulted after a severe suicide attempt, from which she was only saved almost miraculously. After having secretly accumulated an enormous quantity of various types of antidepressants, sedatives, and hypnotics that she stole from her mother (who was on chronic medication because of complex characterological problems and depression), she dug out a grave for herself in the middle of the forest close to her home. It was early winter, with abundant leaves still on the ground. After swallowing all that medication, she lay down to die in that grave, covering herself with leaves. After three days of fruitless search by the police, one more effort in that area led to a police dog finding her still alive.

She had chronically abused drugs, presented chronic characterological depression, and had a long history of manipulation and dishonesty in school and in her family relations, despite her high intelligence and musical capabilities. Clinically, she fulfilled the criteria for the diagnosis of malignant narcissism; that is, a narcissistic personality organization, strong antisocial and paranoid features, and ego-syntonic aggression (directed against herself in the form of chronic, severe suicide attempts and against others in the encouragement of antisocial behavior that might get them into trouble).

Her father was a distinguished philosophy teacher in a prestigious Protestant university, and the high respect he enjoyed in his commu-

nity, a major intellectual center in the South, contrasted sharply with
the chaotic, unconventional behavior both parents engaged in at
home. Such behavior included the parents' playing with each other in
the nude in the bathtub, while inviting their adolescent daughter to
join them in conversation. Father used to play "tricks" on mother that
had a sadistic quality and enjoyed sharing this pleasure with his
daughter. The parents were concerned about their daughter maintaining "formal" behavior in the outside world and with her keeping the
secrets regarding the chaos occurring in the parental home. Chaotic
relationships among the parents, fights and reconciliations, temper
tantrums, and mutual blaming alternated with periods of almost studied indifference of the parents toward their children.

In the treatment, for an extended period of time, the patient
was dishonest about her ongoing use of drugs and her manipulative
efforts to seduce teachers at the musical establishment where she
was obtaining a higher degree. Once that dishonesty (a truly psychopathic transference) and the underlying severely paranoid dispositions emerged strongly in the transference and could be worked
through, she eventually perceived the therapist as no longer an unreliable, dishonest manipulator (a projection of her own corrupt
grandiose self) but as a person who was willing to "stick with" her
and would not abandon her. Only then, she communicated openly
the hatred that she had experienced for him and for everybody who
tried to help her.

In one of her dreams, she was a person in charge of a psychiatric ward, and she had taken the decision to kill all the patients by
gassing them on a day in which all their relatives would be invited to
a garden party. So that, while everybody was celebrating in the gar-
dens, she had the patients killed inside the building. Severe suicide
attempts occurred during the early part of the treatment and ended
only when the origin of this hatred, her wishes for revenge, and the
desperate hope that the therapist would not abandon her could
gradually be interpreted and brought together. This patient improved dramatically after approximately seven years of treatment,
with a complete resolution of the syndrome of malignant narcissism. The process of working through of the transference involved
periods of cheating and lying in her work and in the transference,
forcing the therapist into a "paranoid" stance that she would triumphantly "diagnose" in the sessions. His capacity to tolerate this regression, to remain firmly moral without becoming moralistic, and
to systematically interpret her defenses against guilt feelings in the
transference eventually carried the day.

Alcohol and drug abuse or dependency also may express such
unconscious dynamics. In patients who suffer from these latter conditions, the direct effect of the addiction has to be differentiated from
its dynamic function. In the context of such predominant extreme
self-aggression, that function may be a determined commitment to

self-destruction that well deserves the term of *death drive*. For patients with narcissistic pathology in whom the addiction is self-perpetuating by the physiology of drug dependence, detoxification and rehabilitation in the early stages of the psychotherapeutic treatment may permit the psychoanalytic psychotherapy to proceed. When, in contrast, the function of these conditions is to express a severe and relentless self-destructiveness as the major life goal, repeated periods of detoxification and rehabilitation demonstrate their uselessness and give an indication of the prognostic gravity of the case. Sometimes addictions serve as rationalization for failures in work or a profession that might otherwise threaten the patient's grandiosity: these cases have a much better prognosis than those in which unrelenting self-destructiveness is the major motivation.

This general constellation of extreme self-destructive motivation that, as mentioned before, may be clinically described as a dominance of the death drive needs to be differentiated from a related development—namely, the most severe form of negative therapeutic reaction. Negative therapeutic reaction does not refer to negative transference but to a clear and immediate worsening of the patient's condition whenever the patient feels he or she has been helped by the therapist. The mildest cases of this reaction can be seen in patients with a depressive/masochistic personality structure and unconscious guilt over being helped, a dynamic already described by Freud and relatively easy to diagnose and resolve interpretatively. A more severe form of negative therapeutic reaction is the most frequent type, characteristic although not exclusive of the narcissistic personality disorder, consistent in clinical worsening out of unconscious envy of the therapist's capacity to help the patient: this highly prevalent transference development requires more complex interpretation and working through but still is eminently workable. The most severe form of negative therapeutic reaction, the case we are considering here, reflects an unconscious identification with an extremely aggressive and destructive love object, with the corresponding dominant transference fantasy that only if the therapist were enraged or hated the patient would he or she really and honestly be emotionally involved with him or her. "Only somebody who hates you or wants to kill you really cares for you."

Case 5

I have referred in earlier work (Kernberg 1975) to a patient who developed strong wishes that I should shoot her, with a fantasy that, by murdering her, I would be linked to her, in my mind, for the rest of my life. Under these circumstances, she could die happily, knowing that I would never forget her! To this day, many years later, I am impressed by how strongly the "logic" of that statement impressed me at that time, so much so that, for a moment, I could not find an argument in my mind that would contradict it. This patient improved very gradually, over eight years of treatment, after working through the severely masochistic behavior in the treatment, and her tempting the therapist more than once to discontinue the treatment.

This disposition may emerge in a patient's relentless effort to provoke the therapist into an aggressive disposition or action against the patient, to transform the relationship into a sadomasochistic one. At the same time, this reaction usually is accompanied by desperate efforts to transform the assumedly "bad" therapist into a "good" one, to transform the persecutory object into an ideal one, an effort that fails because of the relentless need to reenact this sadomasochistic transference by repetition compulsion. In contrast to patients whose main motivation is a total dismantling of the object relationship, here there is an implicit recognition that the therapist has attempted to be helpful: in fact, this experience is what triggers this particular negative therapeutic reaction. If the therapist is not provoked to an extent that may, indeed, lead to a disruption of the treatment, the consistent interpretation of this fantasy and unconscious provocativeness may resolve the impasse. One might also say that, as part of the effort to deal interpretively with this whole area of severe dominance of self-destructiveness, efforts to disentangle this kind of relationship from the more extreme ones mentioned before are part of the therapeutic task.

Sometimes the unrelenting need to attack, depreciate, and destroy oneself appears in starkly undisguised forms in patients who are persecuted by constant thoughts of being worthless, useless, and empty; of having wasted their lives; of being uninteresting to anybody; and of being unable to obtain conscious enjoyment of any pursuit or activity, including all sexual experiences. What is striking about these self-accusations and differentiates them from the overvalued or delusional self-devaluations in major depression is the lack of any attempt at justification or rationalization of these extremely harsh judgments of themselves. Typically, the immediate irritation and anger these patients show when they are invited to explain what gives them that sense of worthlessness contrast with depressed patients' efforts to convince the diagnostician of the reasonableness of their self-depreciation.

In the interaction with the therapist, they produce the impression of an irritable and resentful stance rather than the deep sadness or frozen despair that characterizes major depressions. When any achievement or indication of better functioning in some aspect of their lives is pointed out to them, these patients may respond with a rage attack, while denigrating the therapist who dares to make such a statement. By the same token, they relentlessly reject and attack whoever attempts to soothe or encourage them. Over an extended period of time, they tend to reduce and extinguish their working, professional, and social engagements, withdrawing into an empty, monotonous, and parasitic existence.

The gradual development and the chronicity of this syndrome, in contrast to the episodic nature of major affective illness, together with the absence of neurovegetative symptoms and of slowed psychomotor and cognitive processes, also differentiate this constellation from major affective disorders. These patients typically respond slightly or not at all to any antidepressant medication, even to electroshock (when that is applied after nothing else seems to work). The contrast between their chronic self-devaluation, on the one hand, and their grandiose, spiteful, derogatory attitude towards whoever challenges their convictions reflects the primitive grandiosity and arrogance that is part and parcel of their narcissistic personality structure, as well as their unconscious identification with the overwhelming power of a relentless internal destructive force (of which, at the same time, they are the victim). These patients may also be considered extreme cases of what Cooper (1985) described as the masochistic-narcissistic character.

The treatment of these patients is lengthy and complicated and the prognosis reserved. A psychoanalytic psychotherapy usually is the treatment of choice but requires simultaneous attention to the secondary gain involved in the social parasitism that may be part of the syndrome. It often becomes necessary to require, as a condition for treatment, that the patient engage in some activity, limited though it may be, such as a full-time work or an effective advanced study program, together with the patient's firm and reliable commitment to regularly attend all therapeutic sessions. The patient's intense rage with anything coming from the therapist that would seem to have an "encouraging" or "supportive" nature often provides the first opening for the transference analysis, the analysis of the unconscious sense of danger from any nondestructive object relationship as a challenge to the power of the omnipotent, death-pursuing entity that controls the patient's mind and that provides him or her an unconscious sense of superiority as the only meaning in life.

The technical approach to this entire group of patients implies, first of all, to take very seriously the danger of the patient ending up destroying himself or herself physically. The patient's self-destructiveness is an ongoing threat to the treatment, making this danger a selected theme of the interpretive work from the very beginning of treatment. The therapeutic contract that is negotiated with the patient is intended to establish the minimal preconditions that will assure that the treatment not be used as a "cover story" for providing the patient with further freedom or incentives for self-destructive action. This may not be an easy task, as the therapist has to make it very clear that the treatment will not proceed if these minimal conditions for assuring the patient's survival are not met. Such conditions may include, for example, the patient's commitment to immediate hospitalization if suicidal impulses are so strong that the patient believes he or she will not be able to control them or the absolute commitment to stop behaviors that threaten the continuation of treatment and/or the patient's survival.

Once the parameters of the contract have been agreed upon as a condition for treatment, the patient's temptation to break it has to be brought up by the therapist, with an analysis of the unconscious motivation and gratification that such a breaking of the contract would bring about. The triumphal attitude of the patient in threatening the discontinuation of the therapy, in dismantling the therapist's interventions, or in the radical devaluation of the therapy must be interpreted as a corresponding self-destructive effort to destroy any relationship that might be of help. The therapist has to be very attentive to any indication of a more honest approach to the therapist, some indication of a developing dependency, or a "glimpse of humanity" in the patient that shows up in the therapeutic relationship. These positive gains should be highlighted with the patient, along with the anticipation that there may come the danger that the patient will be tempted to destroy them.

It is important not to confuse this entire area of psychopathology with clinical manifestations of an authentic major depression. A major depression would evince indications of severe self-devaluating or self-accusatory ideation, severely depressed mood leading to a frozen indifference, reduction in the patient's psychomotor expression, decreased capacity of concentration, and neurovegetative symptoms. Under these circumstances, the treatment for depression, with an appropriate use of antidepressive medication (and, under specific complicating conditions, such as extreme, uncontrollable suicidal intention, even electroconvulsive treatment) might be the treatment of choice. And of course, the indication for hospitalization has to be considered urgently in such cases. This is not the case for the patient group with the most extreme form of narcissistic psychopathology that we are describing here, in whom such manifestations of major depression are absent, and, to the contrary, a haughty, derogatory, indifferent, or aggressively challenging attitude on the patient's part to the therapist may prevail, if not a gleeful enjoyment because of the therapist's assumed impotence.

By the same token, conscious or unconscious enjoyment of his or her superiority on the part of the patient engaged in dismantling the therapeutic relationship may bring about countertransference reactions of self-devaluation, depression, withdrawal, or angry rejection of the patient on the part of the therapist. Sometimes an overanxious commitment and desperate effort to provide the patient with emotional support may lead to the therapist's sense of exhaustion, and a sudden emotional abandonment of the patient, that he or she may register contentedly. An optimal emotional attitude of the therapist would include a consistent self-exploration of the ongoing commitment to the patient, the willingness to "hang in there" without any undue expectation of success, and a willingness to carry out the work as long as it seems reasonable to do so but not once the conclusion is inevitable that minimal conditions for the continuation of psychotherapy are not available and that, therefore, it must be discontinued.

Such an optimal emotional disposition on the therapist's part may be lost temporarily but, with an ongoing exploration of the countertransference, can be reinstated by a successful integration of the object relations implication of the countertransference into transference interpretations. In addition, it may be helpful to share with the patient the therapist's awareness and acceptance of the fact that the treatment may fail, that the patient may end up destroying his or her life, and that the therapist would be sad if that happened but accepts the possibility that he or she might not be able to help the patient to overcome this danger under the concrete circumstances of treatment. Such an attitude may reduce the secondary gain of the fantasized triumph over the therapist that is frequently one component of the complex transference dispositions of narcissistic patients.

Specialized inpatient services for severe personality disorders permitted, in the past, protection of selected patients from their severely self-destructive behavior during the initial period of psychoanalytic psychotherapy. We regretfully must acknowledge that, with the disappearance—for financial reasons—of the availability of long-term hospitalization in such specialized inpatient services, some narcissistic patients with extremely severe self-destructive and self-mutilating features, or with severe, but potentially still treatable antisocial symptoms, now may only be helped with supportive psychotherapeutic approaches that are limited in their effectiveness.

Predominance of Antisocial Features

Here we are dealing with the aggressive infiltration of the pathological grandiose self, both in cases when this is expressed mostly in a passive/parasitic tendency and in cases when it takes an aggressive/paranoid form (in the syndrome of malignant narcissism). All cases of narcissistic personality disorder with significant antisocial features have a relatively reserved prognosis. Patients with the syndrome of malignant narcissism are at the very limit of what we can reach with psychoanalytic approaches within the field of pathological narcissism. The next degree of severity of antisocial pathology, the antisocial personality proper, has practically zero prognosis for any psychotherapeutic treatment.

Paradoxically, the very severity of the aggressive-paranoid behavior of patients with the syndrome of malignant narcissism, its function to confirm the power and grandiosity of the patient, facilitates the interpretation of this behavior in the transference. Suicidal behavior, for example (that is, self-directed aggression), clearly represents a triumphant aggression toward the family or the therapist or a triumphant "dismissal" of a world that does not conform to the patient's expectations; parasuicidal, self-mutilating behavior may indicate the patient's triumph over all those others who are afraid of pain, lesions, or bodily destruction.

These are also patients who may show the syndrome of arrogance in a restricted sense in the treatment situation, the interpretation of which may effectively resolve it. This interpretive work includes pointing out to the patient his or her intolerance of his or her own intense, envious aggression, which is expressed in behavior or somatization as a way to avoid acquiring full consciousness of it. The pseudostupidity seen in this syndrome through the defensive dismantling of ordinary reasoning and cognitive communication defends against the humiliating possibility of the therapist's interpretative work reaching the patient in meaningful ways. The inordinate curiosity about the therapist's life is a way to control him or her and control any new sources of envious resentment.

The consistent interpretation of the syndrome of arrogance may, in fact, be a key feature in the transformation of the transference from a psychopathic into a paranoid one, a transformation that marks the beginning of the patient's capacity for self-exploration of primitive aggression rather than having to act it out. Helping the patient to become aware of the intensely pleasurable nature of his or her sadistic behavior against the therapist and others is an important aspect of this interpretive work. This requires that the therapist feel comfortable in an emotional empathy with such sadistic pleasure: the therapist's fear of his or her own sadism may interfere with fully exploring this issue with the patient.

Case 6

A woman in her early twenties consulted because of severe, chronic suicide attempts, breakdown at school, and the incapacity to maintain any relationship with a man because of intense rage attacks if her demands were not fulfilled. She had been severely traumatized by chronic physical abuse by her stepmother, but she had maintained an ambivalent friendly though distant relationship with her father. She had been diagnosed as a narcissistic personality functioning on an overt borderline level, and she presented a typical syndrome of arrogance in the transference.

During our twice-weekly sessions of psychoanalytic psychotherapy, she would consistently make fun of me, mimicking how I speak, parroting what she anticipated I would say to her, and at times seeming to be enraged at the mere sight of me. Several times she made menacing gestures toward objects in my office, as if she would destroy or throw them. Her contempt for me was palpable. In spite of her intelligence, and her clear commitment to the treatment (she would not miss a session even during snowstorms), the sessions were filled with these unrelenting attacks and total unwillingness to listen, let alone think about anything I was saying. She perceived me as a carbon copy of her sadistic stepmother.

At the same time, she exhibited an inordinate curiosity about all aspects of my life and my office and would spy on me outside the sessions. She managed to get information about my private life, and my children, by getting herself involved in activities that would provide her with such knowledge and then triumphantly letting me know all she knew about me. It seemed clear to me that she was totally unable to tolerate any reflection about her intense hatred of me as being a projection of what was in her, and because of that projected hatred, she managed her fear by means of triumphant control and surveillance of me. I consistently pointed out that I believed she was not aware of her relentless attacks on me, because they were expressed only in behavior and not in awareness of any feeling. This protected her, I pointed out, against the sense of pleasure in those attacks that she did not dare to confess to herself. This line of interpretation gradually increased her tolerance of her own hatred and marked the beginning of a capacity to acquire an affective representation of the transference relationship expressed in that hatred—namely, her revenge on and yet identification with the abusing stepmother. Eventually, after nine years of treatment, she achieved a full recovery, entered a successful professional career, and established a satisfactory marriage.

Paradoxically, as mentioned before, the situation is more difficult in the case of patients showing passive antisocial behavior, in the sense not only of passive parasitic exploitiveness of others but also of a severe destruction of their capacity for any sense of concern or responsibility for their relationships with significant others. This lack of investment in object relations is different from the active destruction and dismantling of it in the patient group mentioned earlier, who may have a much better integration of superego functioning and evince no overt antisocial behavior. Chronic irresponsibility regarding time, money, and any kind of commitment made with and to others, including the commitment to therapy, are the hallmarks of antisocial behavior of the passive/parasitic subgroup of severe narcissistic pathology. We are all familiar with patients who frequently miss their sessions, come late, and don't pay their bill on time.

Here, rather than being directed at individuals, the antisocial behavior may show more in a parasitic lifestyle through unnecessary reliance on public assistance or family support. In treatment, one finds, with these patients, a chronic dismissal of the relationship with the therapist, often masked by a surface friendliness and "chatty" engagement with him or her that becomes a major issue in the transference and, over time, may convince the therapist that there seems to be no real human relationship going on. The unconscious devaluation of the therapist has such an ego-syntonic quality that even its interpretation may not touch the patient, who may believe that the therapist has completely unrealistic expectations of what human relationships are all about and is either dishonest or a fool and does not need to be taken seriously. In contrast to the other previously mentioned difficult situations, here the surface manifestation of the transference may seem to be pleasant and nonaggressive; the profound tragedy of the dismissal or dismantling of the therapeutic relationship potentially available to the patient may be subtly disguised. The therapeutic focus needs to be on the contradiction between an apparently friendly, calm surface and frequent absenteeism, missed deadlines and commitments, and the absence of any impact of the therapeutic work. It is important not to confuse this group with our next type of patient who, despite relatively better social functioning and psychological organization, has a surprisingly reserved prognosis.

The Repression of Dependency Needs as Secondary Narcissistic Defense

In contrast to the various conditions and circumstances referred to thus far, which usually may be diagnosed in a careful initial assessment of the patient, this next category is very different, in that it appears initially to be much less severe than all the others mentioned so far and that, at least in my experience, it is very difficult to diagnose at the beginning of the treatment. It emerges as a complication that eventually may dominate the entire treatment and make the treatment almost impossible.

Case 7

This patient, a businessman in his middle thirties, consulted because of chronic ennui, estrangement from his wife, and dissatisfaction with his work, although he was at a loss regarding what alternative work or occupation he would like to engage in. His marriage of eight years provided satisfaction that he was carrying out a conventional life within his community, but his relationship with his wife was estranged to the point that he was completely ignorant of and indifferent to what was going on in her life. There was little information about his past. He described his parents as very responsible and dedicated but, however, so engaged in establishing their own business situation as newcomers in this country that they had little time for him.

His main complaint was, in fact, that he had very few memories from the past, from his childhood, or from school, and that was very puzzling to him, given the fact that he had excellent memory for business matters and "facts." The only symptom that he presented, which, again, was puzzling to him, was a fear of injections, or of seeing blood, and he would faint on seeing an accident in which there was any indication of physical damage.

My impression was that this patient presented a narcissistic personality, functioning at a relatively high level facilitated by severe repressive mechanisms that banished much of his entire childhood from conscious awareness. I recommended psychoanalytic treatment, and the patient entered psychoanalysis with me across a three-year period of time, after which period, in agreement with the patient, we decided to shift into a supportive modality of treatment.

The treatment was remarkable for the absence of any emotional relationship, for any emotional dependency of the patient upon me. The patient himself was surprised that he developed no particular feelings in the transference, perceiving me "realistically" as an "agent" who was dealing with his mental health. His associations, in spite of all interpretive efforts, remained at a surface level, with a chronic trivialization of communication that would empty out the hours. In spite of my alertness to and interest in working with narcissistic transferences, I was not able to help this patient gain any deeper understanding about himself. His dominant emotional experience in the sessions, as in life, was a degree of boredom that increased to the extent that it was hard for him not to fall asleep. Eventually, he would spend significant parts of most sessions in deep sleep! Puzzled about this patient, I consulted with senior colleagues, who were similarly puzzled. The fact, however, that some cases similar to this one eventually might show dramatic changes after significant elaboration of their narcissistic pathology kept me hoping for a breakthrough that, unfortunately, never occurred in this case.

I have seen very few patients of this kind over the years, and I would not be able to say which factors may predict whom we can help and whom we cannot. Once in a supportive psychotherapy with me, this patient was able to increase somewhat his availability to his wife and children and accept the "boredom" of his work with more resignation; we agreed to terminate after a period of time in which no further changes occurred, and we both accepted the limitations of the improvement achieved.

This is a relatively rare type of patient, usually functioning at the highest or least severe level of narcissistic psychopathology initially described, in whom repression and other advanced defense mechanisms have developed sufficiently so that the pathological grandiose self is much better protected against the irruption of unconscious envy, against the awareness that all dependent relationships are implicitly humiliating, inferiorizing, and threatening. These patients display a dramatic lack of awareness of their psychological life, often presenting severe forgetfulness about extended periods of their past, their dreams, as well as people who apparently were important in their lives. This stands in contrast to excellent memory for professional or business-related operations and past developments. Although initially, due to their high level of functioning, they may seem to be good candidates for psychoanalysis, in treatment they evince such an incapacity for tolerating their fantasy life, for emotional self-reflection, and for contact with preconscious mental experiences in general that the sessions become remarkably empty and extremely frustrating for the analyst.

Although in the countertransference with all narcissistic patients, the temptation of the therapist to become distracted over extended periods of time, or to fall asleep in the sessions, may be a reflection of the patient's unconsciously treating the analyst as if he or she were not present, this development may particularly affect the countertransference with the patients we are focusing on here. In fact, these patients may themselves feel intense boredom during the sessions, fall asleep for extended periods of time, and then have great difficulty regarding any emotional reflection about the meaning of their falling asleep during therapeutic sessions. By the same token, the descriptions of their life situation are filled with surface interactions that implicitly deny any deeper aspects of relationships.

There is little mention of these cases in the literature, but experienced therapists recognize this constellation in their patient population and the relatively frequent failure of their treatments. Some experienced analysts, in perceiving these manifestations, do decide (often, rightly) that these patients are unanalyzable and recommend alternative treatment methods (not infrequently, with other therapists). Psychoanalytic psychotherapy with these patients rapidly tends to shift into a purely supportive approach, as the apparent concreteness of their narrative leads the focus of the therapeutic interaction toward practical life problems. A supportive psychotherapeutic approach may, indeed, be the treatment of choice for many of these patients, who, in many ways, are functioning adequately, if with significant restrictions in their intimate relationships. If the presenting symptoms are indeed sufficiently mild or restricted, so that a major modification of their character structure would not seem indicated, a supportive psychotherapeutic approach may be optimal. If more severe problems in work and intimacy significantly limit their life, it may be worthwhile to attempt a psychoanalytic approach. Given their clinical characteristics, a standard psychoanalytic treatment may provide greater chances than a psychoanalytic psychotherapy to reduce the massive resistance derived from strongly predominant repressive mechanisms that reinforce and protect the deeper narcissistic defenses against their dependency needs.

Defenses Against the Incapacity to Conceive of the Therapist as Having a Consistent Mental Life

It is probable that this highly complex defensive constellation may only be detected and resolved in the course of psychoanalytic treatment proper, remaining overshadowed in the psychoanalytic psychotherapy of narcissistic patients where the intensity of primitive, split transferences dominates the sessions. What gradually strikes the analyst of these patients over an extended period of time is an alternation of sharply contradictory emotional relations to the analyst, while the patient remains remarkably unconcerned over the extremely contradictory nature of his or her emotional dispositions in the transference and is apparently unable to respond with any increase of concern or reflectiveness to interpretive efforts to resolve the defensive nature of this dissociation.

Case 8

For example, one patient considered the analyst as either "extremely brilliant" or, alternatively, "stupid," "totally indifferent," "corrupt," or "politically biased." This patient would immediately assume that the analyst had fallen asleep if the analyst would remain silent for some time, while, at other times, he complained of the analyst's too intense, penetrating comments regarding the patient's failures and shortcomings. The analyst's exploring any plausible stimuli for these shifting reactions revealed that none of these emotional relations had any basis in reality. Thus, the consideration of the analyst as the "most brilliant thinker" would be expressed in the patient's insistent wish for the analyst to help him with concrete advice regarding political or business problems, about which the patient obviously had at least as much information and knowledge as—if not more than—the analyst, making such requests absurd. Similarly, exploration of the patient's experience of the analyst as either politically biased or retarded, indifferent, or dishonest led to the patient's eventual, if only momentary, recognition that they were unrealistic fantasies. Yet these momentary recognitions of the fantastic nature of all these assumptions did not influence them at all, and they would return in alternative fashion regularly over a period of many months.

Eventually, it became clear that the patient was treating the analyst as if he had no permanent internal life and no consistent, stable, or continuous relationship with the patient. The analyst, in short, was like a robot experiencing isolated feelings, mental brilliance or mental deterioration, dishonesty, rage, or indifference. By the same token, the patient experienced himself as constantly changing, so that the continuity of his verbal communications in the hours seemed to him also a robotlike mechanical behavior that had little relation with his life. The consistent interpretation of the projective identification involved in this process only permitted to resolve it over many months of analytic work. Eventually, he was able to work through this total fragmentation of the experience of himself and of his analyst, achieving a capacity for authentic dependency that, gradually, permitted this analysis to evolve to a satisfactory termination.

This situation might be formulated in terms of La Farge's (2004) description of the "imaginer" and "imagined," mental representations reflecting the patient's view of the analyst and his experience of the view held by the analyst of the patient himself. In fact, the consistent focus on this patient's incapacity to conceive of the analyst as a person with an internal life brought about a gradually increasing, intense anxiety, eventually leading to an entirely new set of complex transference experiences. The patient's chaotic description of his relationship with both parents, remarkably similar to the alternative types of transference developments mentioned before, now could be seen as a profound defense against deeper layers of consciously unavailable internal relationships with them.

This relatively infrequent transference development has to be differentiated from the ordinary narcissistic defenses against envy, the alternation between idealization and devaluation characteristic of narcissistic transferences, and the split-off transference storms of narcissistic personalities functioning on an overt borderline level. The subtlety of sharply contradictory, unchanging, mutually split-off, long-term transference developments only may become clear over an extended period of time. It may be the hidden cause of extended psychoanalytic stalemates and, if not resolved, severely limits the achievements of the psychoanalytic treatment. Attention to such a development and the analyst's raising the question in his or her mind to what extent the patient is concerned over constructing in his or her mind any consistency of the analyst's personality may help to highlight this problem earlier and facilitate its working through.

Some General Prognostic and Therapeutic Considerations

We may summarize the major negative prognostic features that emerge in this overall category of "almost untreatable" narcissistic patients as including the following: secondary gain of illness, including social parasitism; severe antisocial behavior; severity of primitive self-directed aggression; drug and alcohol abuse as chronic treatment problems; pervasive arrogance; general intolerance of a dependent object relation; and the most severe type of negative therapeutic reaction. The evaluation of these prognostic features is facilitated by a careful and detailed initial evaluation of the patient.

For example, regarding the nature of antisocial behavior, it is important to elucidate the extent to which it corresponds to simple, isolated antisocial behavior in a narcissistic personality disorder without other major negative prognostic implications; or to what extent it corresponds to severe, chronic, passive parasitic behavior that augments the secondary gain of illness; or whether what is present is a syndrome of malignant narcissism; or, finally and most importantly, whether we are facing an antisocial personality proper of either the passive parasitic or the aggressive type.

At times, antisocial behavior may be strictly limited to intimate relationships, in which it expresses aggression and revengefulness, particularly when accompanied by significant paranoid features. This may be important when, in the transference, it is directed at the therapist, because, at times, it may create such a high risk for the therapist that treatment under such circumstances might not be wise to attempt. This includes patients whose aggressive, revengeful acting out takes the form of litigious behavior against therapists, initiating a lawsuit against a first therapist while idealizing a second one who is "recruited" into a treatment for the damage done by the first one, in turn to be involved with a lawsuit initiated by the patient while he or she transfers to a third therapist for help, and so on. It may be wise not to accept a patient of this kind for intensive psychotherapeutic treatment while legal procedures related to the involvement with another therapeutic situation are still going on. Some patients with a hypochondriacal syndrome and who are prone to accuse previous therapists for not having recognized the severity of some somatic symptom or illness may be related to this group.

In the case of patients with chronic suicidal attempts, it is extremely important to differentiate suicidal behavior that corresponds to the authentic severity of a depression from suicidal behavior "as a way of life," not linked to depression, and typical for the borderline personality disorder as well as for the narcissistic personality disorder (Kernberg 2001). Here, the differential nature of the suicidal attempts referred to before may be extremely helpful to diagnose the patient's case.

The elimination or reduction of secondary gain of illness is one of the most important and often difficult aspects of the treatment, particularly in setting up the initial treatment contract and a viable treatment frame. The parameters of the treatment contract provide the assurance that the agreed upon treatment frame will protect both parties (and the therapist's belongings and life situation) from patients' acting out that may evolve in the course of the treatment. In the course of the psychoanalytic psychotherapy of all patients with borderline personality organization—and this includes the patients explored in this contribution—the emergence of severe regression in the transference is practically unavoidable and frequently takes the form of efforts to challenge and break the therapeutic frame. In any such challenge, the therapist's physical, psychological, professional, and legal safety takes precedence over the safety of the patient. That means that, while the therapist has to assure the safety of the patient by means of the setting up of the contract and a treatment frame that protects both of them, the therapist's own safety is an indispensable precondition for being able to help the patient, even for setting up conditions that assure the patient's safety. This would seem obvious or trivial, if it were not that so often therapists are seduced into a treatment situation in which their safety is at risk. Concrete conditions, relevant to each individual case, which clearly would indicate discontinuation of the treatment if not fulfilled, must be spelled out and, if necessary, reiterated as part of the treatment arrangements and then, as mentioned before, immediately interpreted regarding their transference implications.

Summarizing the indications for differential treatment approaches mentioned so far, for the mildest cases of narcissistic psychopathology, a focused psychoanalytic psychotherapeutic approach or even a focal supportive psychotherapy may be the treatment of choice and, only if the severity of the corresponding character pathology warrants it, standard psychoanalysis. Standard psychoanalysis would be the treatment approach for the second or intermediate level of severity described before and possibly for some cases of the severe spectrum of narcissistic patients functioning on an overt borderline level who, for individual reason, may make such a treatment possible. For most cases of narcissistic pathology functioning on an overt borderline level or with severe antisocial pathology, the specialized psychoanalytic psychotherapy that we have developed at the Weill Cornell Medical College, namely, transference-focused psychotherapy, is recommended as the treatment of choice (Levy et al. 2005). When individualized preconditions for treatment cannot be met in the initial contract setting (Clarkin et al. 1989), a cognitive-behavioral or a supportive psychotherapeutic approach may be the treatment of choice.

In general, a supportive psychotherapeutic modality based upon psychoanalytic principles is indicated for cases where the patient's need for "self-curing" is so intense that any dependency is precluded, and obtaining active counseling and advice in a supportive relationship may be much more acceptable to the patient (Rockland 1992). When severe secondary gain cannot be overcome, and the patient's prognosis, therefore, would be severely limited with an analytic approach, a supportive psychotherapy focused on the amelioration of predominant symptoms and behavioral manifestations may be helpful. In cases with severe antisocial features that require ongoing information from outside sources and social control, technical neutrality may be too affected to carry out an analytic approach, and a supportive one would appear preferable. For patients who, as a consequence of their long-standing illness, already have suffered such severe regression into social incompetence, all their "bridges burned" behind them, making a realistic adaptation to life much more difficult, a supportive psychotherapeutic approach may be preferable to a psychoanalytic modality of treatment. The latter one would have to face them with extremely painful recognition of having destroyed much of their lives: here the subtle and empathic judgment of the therapist regarding what the patient may be able to tolerate becomes very important.

It needs to be kept in mind that before psychoanalytic knowledge advanced in the understanding of the psychopathology of pathological narcissism and helped us to develop specific techniques to deal with these patients analytically, the prognosis was much more limited for a much larger number of cases than is true today. New developments in the psychoanalytic psychotherapy for those cases of narcissistic personality disorder in which standard psychoanalysis would seem contraindicated have significantly improved our therapeutic armamentarium.

Continuous efforts to explore the cases at the limits of our present psychoanalytic understanding and capacity to help should expand this field further in the future. Given the high prevalence of this kind of pathology and its severe social repercussions in many cases, this is an important task for the psychoanalytic researcher and clinician at this time.

References

Bion WR: Second Thoughts: Selected Papers on Psychoanalysis. New York, Basic Books, 1967

Clarkin J, Yeomans F, Kernberg O: Psychotherapy for Borderline Personality. New York, Wiley, 1989

Cooper A: The masochistic-narcissistic character, in Masochism: Current Psychoanalytic and Psychotherapeutic Perspectives. Edited by Glick RA, Meyers DI. New York, Analytic Press, 1985, pp 117–138

Green A: On Private Madness. Madison, CT, International Universities Press, 1993

Hinshelwood RD: Clinical Klein. London, Free Association Books, 1994

Kernberg OF: Borderline Conditions and Pathological Narcissism. New York, Jason Aronson, 1975

Kernberg OF: Technical aspects in the psychoanalytic treatment of narcissistic personalities, in Severe Personality Disorders: Psychotherapeutic Strategies. New Haven, CT, Yale University Press, 1984, pp 197–209

Kernberg OF: Psychopathic, paranoid, and depressive transferences. Int J Psychoanal 73:13–28, 1992

Kernberg OF: Pathological narcissism and narcissistic personality disorders: theoretical background and diagnostic classification, in Disorders of Narcissism: Diagnostic, Clinical, and Empirical Implications. Edited by Ronningstam EF. Washington, DC, American Psychoanalytic Press, 1997, pp 29–51

Kernberg OF: The suicidal risk in severe personality disorders: differential diagnosis and treatment. J Pers Disord 15:195–208, 2001

La Farge L: The imaginer and the imagined. Psychoanal Q 73:591–625, 2004

Levy KN, Meehan KB, Weber M, et al: Attachment and borderline personality disorder: implications for psychotherapy. Psychopathology 38:64–74, 2005

Rockland LH: Supportive Therapy for Borderline Patients: A Psychodynamic Approach. New York, Guilford, 1992

Rosenfeld H: Impasse and Interpretation: Therapeutic and Anti-Therapeutic Factors in the Psychoanalytic Treatment of Psychotic, Borderline and Neurotic Patients. London, Tavistock, 1987

Spillius EB (ed): Melanie Klein Today: Developments in Theory and Practice, Vols 1 and 2. London, Routledge, 1988

Spillius EB, Feldman M (eds): Psychic Equilibrium and Psychic Change: Selected Papers of Betty Joseph. London, Tavistock/Routledge, 1989

Steiner J: Psychic Retreats. London, Routledge, 1993

Stone MH: The Fate of Borderline Patients. New York, Guilford, 1990

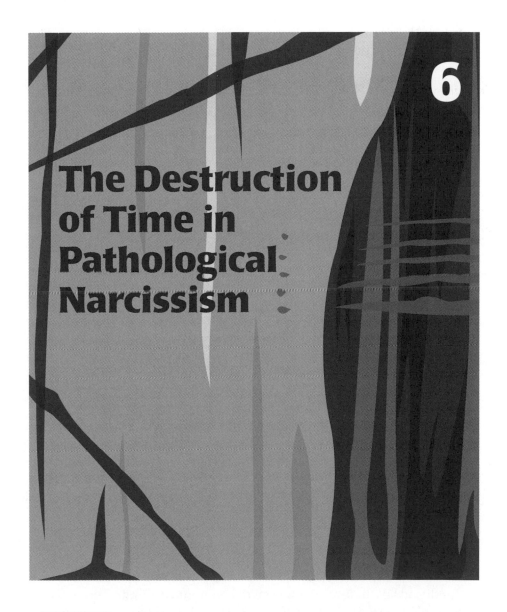

6

The Destruction of Time in Pathological Narcissism

This chapter was reprinted from Kernberg OF: "The Destruction of Time in Pathological Narcissism." *International Journal of Psychoanalysis* 89:299–312, 2008. Used with permission. Copyright 2008 John Wiley and Sons.

This chapter represents work from the Cornell Psychotherapy Research Project supported by a grant from the Borderline Personality Disorder Research Foundation. The foundation and its founder, Dr. Marco Stoffel, are gratefully acknowledged.

In exploring further the technical difficulties in the treatment of narcissistic patients, I focus on their particular relation with the passage of time, their need to deny that very passage. In this context, I explore the changing rhythm of time experience under normal and abnormal circumstances, the changes in time experiences occurring throughout the life cycle, and how narcissistic pathology affects these developments. In the treatment, the tendency to destroy the awareness of the passage of time on the part of narcissistic personalities is expressed in both transference and countertransference developments and may constitute a major challenge for the therapist. At the bottom, in these cases, the pathology of the experience of time reflects the pathology of internalized object relations, a relation explored in the course of this chapter.

Introduction

As Elliot Jacques (1982) pointed out in his overview of psychoanalytic views of the experience of time, it is important to keep in mind the difference between objective time as a scientific concept characterized by the uniformity of linear intervals as defined by the units of measurement of time, on the one hand, and the subjective sense of time, which has very different characteristics, on the other. The subjective experience of the duration of time is irregular and depends on multiple psychological factors.

Throughout the life cycle, a remarkable yet gradual change occurs in the subjective experience of the duration of time. The multitude of early experiences that bombard the infant and small child gradually settle into longer cycles between the past and the future, such as, for example, the long time in between weekends and the endless time between birthdays, thus taking on a quality of "endless time," the correlate to the naturally assumed permanence of childhood. With developing growth and maturity, and a more predictable succession of tasks and personal investments, cycles of past experience seem to accelerate. The expectation of future developments that are now more firmly embedded in consciousness by the individual's own life trajectory, planning, and task investments, matched with active work toward the transformation of such a projected future into the present, decreases the subjective experience of the duration of time so that it seems to be passing more rapidly. There is a clearer sense of what to expect in the future and a sharp linkage between past experience and its expected repetition. The sense of acceleration of the passing of time increases with age and becomes a significant conscious experience in old age (Hartocollis 1983). Now time "flies."

Happy moments, "stellar experiences," while seeming to pass too quickly, nonetheless build up as happy memories, creating a sense of life lived intensely, which extends the sense of duration of time across the life span. The opposite development characterizes traumatic experiences. Severe trauma has multiple influences on the subjective sense of time, depending on the nature and duration of the traumatic experience. In the case of acute, brief situations when the trauma is the product of willful aggression, there will be an almost intolerable sense of extension of time during the traumatic experience itself, with a fixation to the trauma that, by repetitive "flashbacks," extends the subjectively experienced duration of the trauma. The long-range effect of this situation leads to a "time stood still" quality related to reverberating unconscious processes that reduce, retrospectively, the experience of time, particularly that of time lived after the traumatic experience. Thus, for example, a couple who were assaulted, robbed, and controlled with threats to their life over a period of hours had a grossly distorted subjective experience of extension of the duration of the event, with a posttraumatic stress disorder, fixation to the trauma over a period of many months, and a retrospective sense of shrinkage of the time after the trauma over one to three years. It was "as if it happened yesterday."

For extended periods of willfully induced traumatic circumstances—for example, racial persecution, concentration camp imprisonment, or extended periods of physical or sexual abuse—the effect is even more powerful: the dominance of the unconscious consequences of the traumatic situation reduces the capacity for significant new investments and, hence, for the generation of new experiences that otherwise would enrich the experience of passage of time.

In these last examples of cognitive and traumatic influences on the sense of time, the function of memory of an accumulated life experience becomes important. This is, in fact, a complementary dimension of the experience of time, the sense of time lived intensively. The more significant the investment in meaningful and gratifying relationships and activities, the more the moment seems to fly by, but, by the same token, there grows a sense of time having been lived and an enrichment of the total life experience. If, to the contrary, such a meaningful commitment to investments in work,

art, social engagements, and, as we shall see in more detail, intimate relationships is missed, experience of life lived shrinks, and
life itself may seem to be near its end, accompanied by a frightening
sense of the brevity of time lived.

The pathologically persistent dominance of primitive dissociation or splitting operations (that characterize the early stage of development) in the syndrome of identity diffusion characteristic of
severe personality disorders leads not only to the threatening reactivation of dreaded bad experiences that have to be avoided or denied but also to the search for idealized ones that, in turn, cannot be
reactivated fully because the reality of the experience of object relations does not ever totally fulfill that idealized world. All of this reduces the possibility of integrating new experiences and condemns
the individual to repeatedly relive a subjectively unchanging world
of dreaded and fleetingly idealized experiences. As a result, under
such pathological circumstances, repetition compulsion condenses
the sense of lived time, new experiences cannot be integrated normally, and traumatic situations are re-created that require constant attention to the immediate environment and do not permit
new gratifying experiences to build up a significant past. Repetition
compulsion has many sources and functions: but one consequence
relevant here is the implied denial of the passage of time: "nothing
has changed, the repetition indicates that time is frozen." The duration of time shrinks, in contrast to what happens with the deepening of emotional relationships that characterizes normal identity
(the depressive position). This shrinkage of time is even more accentuated in the case of patients with narcissistic personality disorders. Here, the devaluation of significant others as a defense
against unconscious envy is reflected in the dismantling of internalized object relations. The pathological grandiose self is experienced
in isolation, and self-esteem regulation is dependent on the external admiration from others rather than on the security of an internalized world of significant object relations. The failure to develop
significant object relations results in a chronically empty internal
world, depleted of emotionally deep and meaningful experiences,
that condenses, retrospectively, the experience of time: nothing
memorable has happened in the past, except the ongoing efforts to
shore up self-esteem and confirm the grandiosity of the self. The
narcissistic patients will often find themselves "waking up" at age
40, 50, or 60 with a desperate sense of years lost.

In contrast, integrated whole object relations permit the build-
up of a lived past, the sense of duration of time lived expands, and

a desired, imagined future extends it further. Internalized relationships with loved and gratifying others determine the time-framed memories of interactions, real and fantasized, in contrast to the rigid and static memories of stereotyped others with whom no joint history was built up, and no duration of time invested in such interactional sequence is established. Guilt and reparation of past aggression, mourning the lost idealization of the past, and the reinforcement of the sense of a good self by gratifying preconscious and unconscious relationships with significant others fill up life and time. Life, then, is experienced as intense and hopeful; the future holds the expectation for ongoing good experiences, all of which reinforce self-esteem, zestful optimism, and the affirmation of life.

Identity itself develops further in this context, as identity of childhood expands throughout adulthood with the internalization of identifications with significant parental objects at different stages of their life, so that a future can be projected in which one's identity is partially modeled upon the identity of an older generation of strongly invested parental figures and mentors. The acceptance of one's own past and the resolution of early oedipal and preoedipal conflicts permit identification with one's own children, so that the total life experience is enriched by a projected future and a reliving of an accepted past in its creative re-creation and modification with a younger generation. Identity, in short, simultaneously expands toward future and past, and that, in turn, enriches life experience in the sense of life lived intensively, while subjective time expands accordingly.

These developments are relevant for the psychology and pathology of the aging process. The expansion of identity implies the capacity for identification with past and future generations, their interests, struggles, and experiences, and provides a sense of continuity of life. In contrast, the failure of this process to form normal identity with its corresponding time dimension, together with a sense of the shrinking of time in the aging process referred to before, may bring about an increased fear of death. Narcissistic personalities frequently experience, in later decades of life, a sense of not having lived sufficiently, that life has gone by without leaving traces of the past. The experiences of shrinkage of time, in these cases, may bring about an intense and growing fear of death, a sense of unfairness of the brevity of their life as they experience it. This fear is also related to infantile fears of abandonment and loneliness and a deep feeling of the senselessness of life—which predominate when there is an absence of investment in love, work, ideals, children, and values. The functions of ideology, religion, art, and culture as vehicles for creation of values, as well as of human communication and a sense of the continuity of humanity, cannot be internalized fully under circumstances of identity diffusion and the structural dominance of a pathological grandiose self. In contrast, investment in one's own lived history and in the history of those one is involved with and the transcendence of this investment into a general sense of historical continuity provide a reinforcing context to the sense of living and of having lived a full life.

A particularly painful experience of "lost time" may become part of the mourning process, both normal and pathological. Guilt feelings stirred up in the mourning process over not having fully lived the time that was available with the loved person who has been lost (a normal expression of the depressive position) is experienced with much more severity in pathological mourning. In narcissistic personalities, this may take the form of a complete absence of normal mourning, a denial of guilt feelings that cannot be tolerated because of their potentially frightening intensity, or else the emergence of paranoid behavior reflecting the projection of intolerable guilt feelings.

Normal mourning, as Melanie Klein (1940) observed, always involves guilt feelings as an essential aspect of the activation and reworking of the depressive position. The death of a beloved person always illuminates, retrospectively, the infinite number of lost occasions and possibilities of expanding the intimate communication with the lost person, the time that could have been lived together and was not, the feelings of love that were not expressed, in short, the total value of that relationship that could not be actualized under the impact of daily routines not overshadowed by the awareness of death, of a final separation.

Rabbi Moshe Berger (personal communication, June 2006) has stated that all loving relationships are finite, while their loss through death initiates an infinite absence, which only now illuminates all possible aspects and values of the relationship, in contrast to the necessarily limited awareness of them during the deceased loved person's life with us. Only the infinite absence permits us to become fully aware of all the implications, meanings, and possibilities of a finite relationship. Such awareness heightens the regret and guilt over the "waste" of objective time with the loved one and, under optimal circumstances, will induce, in the mourning person, a heightened subjective experience of the time lived with the lost love object. This process is often blocked in the case of narcissistic personalities, for whom the awareness of guilt, regret, and dependency threatens to overwhelm the pathological grandiose self.

Destruction of Time in Narcissistic Pathology

Hartocollis (2003) has described the regressive effects of timelessness induced by free association, and the counteracting effect of the precision, the consistency of duration, and the regularity of the analytic sessions. The unconscious denial of the dependency on the analyst characteristic of narcissistic patients transforms the relationship with him or her into a static, self-indulging focus on internal processes, fantasies, and wishes that are not linked to the time-generating mutuality of a changing object relations. This may not be perceived by the analyst over a period of time. Thus, the regressive effect of the method of free association is significantly increased in the treatment of narcissistic personalities: here the timelessness of analysis lends itself to express one specific aspect of narcissistic pathology. The invitation to free associate, with its explicit discouragement of "prepared agendas" and related moves toward action, is often misinterpreted as an invitation to passivity that narcissistic patients unconsciously translate as a projection of all responsibility on the analyst and a defiant expectation of gratification from him or her...and the analyst's defeat.

The dominant pathology of the time experience of narcissistic personalities derives from the destruction of their internalized world of object relations, a result of the development of a pathological grandiose self that incorporates real and idealized representations of self and others. This leads to the devaluation of others who otherwise would generate envy, and the resulting lack of internalization of gratifying relationships with significant others brings about an impoverishment of the internal world, with its absence of time-bound meaningful interactions in depth. In replacement of such experiences, these patients experience the need for immediate gratification from external sources, be it admiration from others, triumph and success as recognized in the external world that confirms their narcissistic superiority, or, if none of these are available, an escape in depersonalized sexual relationships, drugs, alcohol, or other sources of immediate excitement (Kernberg 1984, 1992).

This stark picture is modified by the fact that many narcissistic personalities do not suffer from such a total destruction of the world of internalized object relations and are able, for example, to obtain narcissistic gratification while making an important investment in relation to their children, onto whom they project their own narcissistic needs. A particular task, talent, or social function at which they excel may generate social recognition and gratification but also provide them with an intrinsic pleasure derived from an investment in such an object. There are, however, cases where, even in the face of apparently well-preserved social functioning, the absence of investment in relationships with others and the resulting sense of internal emptiness are significant features. These cases are often well compensated as long as success at work, a profession, or other social endeavors provide them with adequate narcissistic gratification but who suffer greatly with illness, retirement, or loss of power or recognition. The sense of a lack of lived experiences, with the implicit shrinkage of the duration of time, is an important aspect of their sense of emptiness and fear, an intuition of the waste of time.

In psychoanalytic treatment, narcissistic patients typically evince their defenses against dependency on the analyst by an unconscious devaluation of what they receive from him or her, thus warding off envy of the therapist they need. This process may bring about a stubborn resistance against change, as interpretations fall on sterile ground. Here there is an active, unconscious effort that "nothing should happen," the direct expression of a self-destructive triumph over the analyst, that reinforces the regressive effects of free association in them. It is as if time was standing still in the analysis, and patients typically complain at such points that nothing is helping them. This shrinkage of time, however, may correspond to a still deeper transference development, the unconscious desire that time does indeed stand still: One aspect of the function of the grandiose self is precisely the denial of the passage of time, the fantasy of eternal youth, and the very denial of death as an ultimate threat to their grandiosity. While the fantasy of eternal youth and the denial of death may be a universal manifestation of normal infantile narcissism, in the narcissistic personality it becomes grossly exaggerated, an aspect of the pathological grandiose self that interferes seriously with a realistic adaptation to the objective passage of time. All of this reinforces the function of the unconscious destruction of time in the analytic relationship of such patients, the assertion of their invulnerability to the influence of the treatment, and the defeat of the analyst's work as an expression of unconscious envy of him or her. The emptying out of the narcissistic patient's life experiences during analysis, in fantasy, becomes a triumph over the analyst's capacity to influence him or her. Green (2007) has pointed to the function of repetition compulsion, when it is employed as a form of "murder of time," as an expression of the death drive. This certainly applies to some cases of narcissistic personalities.

One narcissistic patient, a successful businessman, entered psychoanalytic treatment, four sessions a week, because of the incapacity to commit himself to a satisfactory relationship with women. After a lengthy period of indecisiveness regarding marriage, he did marry a woman following a brief infatuation that proved as dissatisfying and "boring" as all other relationships. He presented himself as a shrewd and superior businessman but was easily upset by minor slights or lack of consideration on the part of others and contemptuous of friends and family, particularly of the family of his wife. He was consistently surprised by the intense social life that his wife had with her family, while he felt only resentment and devaluation toward various members of his own family, including his parents. It struck him that he had great difficulty in remembering not only names but also faces and the very existence of people whom he had met throughout his high school and college years and later on during the time of travel abroad and vacations. He had a perfect memory for all aspects of his business, was an expert in a certain historical style of furniture, and could judge authenticity in origins and styles. He was superficially friendly—as long as he felt admired—and although numerous business associates had attempted to establish a more personal relationship with him, he was unable to involve himself in anything beyond direct business negotiations. With a strong sense that his marital life was not satisfactory, he had attempted to establish relationships with other women but soon discovered in them limitations, became bored with them, and went on to the next. His only major symptom, other than a chronic degree of anxiety, was a fear of death and related hypochondriacal concerns and anxious ruminations over his getting old without ever having lived. He had a clear sense that time had passed him by, that he had not really lived, and that his death would mean having been cheated out of life before he had a chance to live it meaningfully.

His success as a major athlete in the past was related to his interest in sports, but once his own active participation was no longer possible, he devalued the interest of the sports he had been involved with as well. He had described his mother as a dominant, overly anxious person; hypochondriacal; and concerned over his, her only son's, health, but he had no memory of any interactions with her other than her controlling his appearance, eating patterns, behavior, and health. My patient despised his father, a rather unsuccessful businessman, and he saw the purpose of his own life in not letting himself be exploited and defeated as he felt his father had been in his business interventions.

In this patient's analysis, the development of a typical narcissistic resistance against involvement in the transference was expressed as a "matter of fact" dominance of immediate, realistic concerns in this patient's life, with almost total absence of any fantasy material, and no reference to, nor curiosity about, the analyst. He saw analysis as an opportunity to resolve his business-related preoccupations and tended to dismiss the interpretations of the analyst as bookish and theoretical. At the same time, he always felt pressed for time, everything had to be resolved rapidly, and he resented the "timelessness" of his sessions, namely, the analyst's patiently listening to free associations instead of indicating courses of action the patient might pursue. He distrusted the value of the analyst's comments as much as the importance of what might come to the patient's mind. Nothing was going on in his analysis, he proclaimed triumphantly, while rejecting most interventions of the analyst. And yet he seemed willing to come to sessions punctually without question. He reiterated his conviction that he had no feelings for the analyst: analysis was a special business dealing....

Thus, fear over the emptiness of time not spent in business considerations or practical life situations coincided with the emptying out of meaningful interactions in his sessions: he was always in a hurry, and nothing seemed to happen in his emotional life. Gradually, focus on his hypochondriacal fear and his fear of death began to uncover his dread over a lack of anything emotionally moving in his life, and eventually intense envy of the analyst as somebody he feared had a rich life experience.

In one session, after complaining at length that nothing was changing in his life, that he was still bored with his wife and dissatisfied with the lack of excitement in everyday experiences, he suddenly laughed and said that he had an image of me sitting puzzled in my chair, unable to help him, yet condemned to be sitting like that for an infinite number of hours. He went on to say that he, actually, was young enough to find new exciting experiences, while I was aging, and time was passing me by while I was stuck in a questionable profession. I pointed out to him that in that fantasy, he remained eternally young with unlimited possibilities, while I, in addition to failing him, would be struck with old age and with good reasons to envy his youth.

The patient became anxious, wondered whether I was angry at him, and, later in the session, realized that, in fact, he had felt angry in the past session because of a new book authored by me that he had discovered on my desk. I then pointed out that it became clearer why, at this point, the thought of lack of progress and waste of time in his analysis had not upset him. Only after many months of this development, after working through his intense envy of the analyst, emerged wishes for an idealized relationship with a powerful father, forbidden because it contained wishes for a homosexual relationship that he was terribly afraid of. Eventually, the tolerance of his homosexual feelings brought back wishes for friendship in his early adolescence and fears of being rejected by another boy whom he was deeply invested in. Now more lively memories of his past could be elicited in his associations. But, behind longing for a previously repressed, dependent relationship with a good father emerged his deep disappointment in mother and distrust and hatred of women. He gradually became aware of a profound resentment of all women because he thought they were so self-sufficient and did not need anybody else that it would be dangerous to look for other than a temporary sexual relationship with them. The conflict around unconscious envy of the analyst now emerged as an expression of his hatred of mother, the deep distrust of depending on her, and the resentment of her power to soothe and to mistreat him. Now the unconscious triumph over me, by asserting my impotence to touch and to change him, could be explored in the hours. Only toward the end of the treatment did oedipal issues of competitiveness with me become prominent, a sense of triumph over me because he was significantly younger than I and, in this context, an awareness of the fear of death as an expression of the projection of his unconscious rivalry wishes to eliminate me and a sense of oedipal defeat.

In the context of these developments, this patient began to experience a profound regret for missed opportunities, friends whom he had rejected, women whom he had not been able to appreciate, and, above all, his neglect and devaluation of his wife's capacity for investment and love that had made him feel terribly envious and inferior. He now began to enjoy his daily life with her that he had taken for granted before, as well as relationships with friends and family. He found new interests in travel with his wife and lost the chronic sense of emptiness together with the fear of death as a confirmation of the uselessness of his life. He no longer was chronically rushing from one encounter to another and could enjoy, for the first time, a contemplative attitude toward his wife and friends.

Another narcissistic patient, also in psychoanalytic treatment, four sessions a week, a man in his middle twenties with an extraordinary talent as a painter and as a specialist in the Spanish language, had spent years in both these fields, earning early recognition and applause, and stimulation to continue in one of these careers but was unable to engage in the work required in order to progress technically or to depend on other experts in order to develop his own technique at a more mature level. His envious resentment of those who would have been able to teach him made him devalue both areas of his expertise and, in the end, abandon them with resentment of those who were successful in them and the painful awareness that he had not achieved anything or obtained any gratification in areas of those talents in which he had invested more than ten years of his life. He consulted because he felt uncertain what profession to select at that point and, in fact, was working in a subordinate function in a field totally unrelated to his learning experiences. He depreciated his present work but could not decide what else to do. He was depressed and neglectful of his appearance. Rather soon in the treatment, he recognized a sense of superiority, of expectations to rise to the top without the effort of a long road ahead of him. Here a sense of destruction of time emerged, in the form of the fantasy that he was going to be eternally young and promising and that, therefore, nothing was lost by avoiding the learning opportunities that would have required, as he saw it, a humiliating sense of not being perfect. This fantasy that he was young and had "all the roads to the future" open to him broke down when confronted with the reality of the success of all those whom he had considered inferior to him and who now were making creative changes in their lives. For a long time, his image of the analyst was one of a passive, "resigned" mediocrity, who could only do the same thing all the time. The awareness that the analyst's interpretations reflected active, creative efforts to understand and to help the patient came as a serious blow; the fact that time advanced, was finite, and could be wasted and lost was a painful new experience.

Still another narcissistic patient, in psychoanalytic psychotherapy, three sessions per week, a woman from an aristocratic European environment who only wished to get involved with leading members of that social group, devalued and dismissed all those lovers who were not part of that group. Now in her late forties, she began to experience the wish to get married and for the first time began to question the haughty way in which she had treated men and her triumphant enjoyment of her seductive capacity without having been able to relate in depth to any of the men she was involved with. Her sense of an empty, wasted life triggered a severe depression that brought her to treatment. That sense reflected her successive abandonment of work and interests she had not been able to sustain because of her envy of those who were ahead of her and the endless repetition of her disappointments in all the men she met—mostly narcissistic personalities whose perceived grandiosity had attracted her at first—and the lack of meaningful, ongoing relationships in depth. She expressed very concretely her terror and sense of loss that she had become forty years of age without having had a sense of really living that long: where had the time gone between a turbulent adolescence through twenty years of routine parties and social engagements?

The most severe cases in which destruction of time becomes dominant are those who almost willfully destroy their opportunities and manage, eventually, to attach themselves to highly destructive partners, with whom they establish a sadomasochistic relationship that, in turn, tends to further reduce their possibilities and potential. Couples of this type may hold onto an eternal repetition of self-defeating fights and mutual accusations, thus neglecting the impoverishment of their life through this fixation to a destructive object. The absence of the sense of the passage of time may be expressed in the unrelenting fixation to a relationship in which the patient binds another person to himself or herself, in an unconscious need to maintain a fantasy relationship that, while destructive to both parties, replaces a real one, sometimes over many years without any real content or interaction. In some cases, what looks on the surface as being in love with an unavailable person turns out to be a disguised self-condemnation to loneliness and emptiness as time seems to collapse in the permanent uncertainty of their lives. Ruminating over months—and years!—over whether they should have engaged or not in a certain love relationship may obscure dramatically their awareness of the passage of time.

In the analysis of patients when the destruction of time is an expression of narcissistic denial of the reality of the passage of time and severely restricts the possibilities of life, unconsciously the patient may repeat the pattern of destructiveness of object relations in the transference by maintaining himself or herself in an analytic situation that, on the surface, is supposed to treat his or her difficulties but that, unconsciously, is used to maintain the equilibrium of narcissistic emptiness and triumph over a parental figure, the analyst who is trying to help the patient get out of this bind. The unconscious use of the destruction of time as a triumph over the analyst while also expressing the fantasy of an available eternity of life to the narcissistic patient may, initially, escape the analyst's attention; the patient may, unconsciously, tease the analyst with apparent changes that prove their lack of substance throughout time. In the early stages of the analysis of such patients, what grabs one's attention is the superficiality of relationships with significant others. The patient may describe the personality of people he or she is involved with in rather behavioral, even categorical, fashion, but it is almost impossible for the analyst to get a real image of such other persons. This feature, of course, is quite typical for all narcissistic personalities, who have an enormous difficulty in an assessment in depth and in the development of significant relationships with others, but here the degree of trivialization of the descriptions, and the endless repetition of the same content, reach a very high degree, so that it is as if the patient has been relating to robots with repetitive behaviors that, for some strange reason, fascinate the patient.

Efforts to raise questions about this kind of information are typically met not only with the patient's sense of puzzlement, fear of being criticized, and need to defend the "realistic" way in which he or she relates to others but also by opening up the transference analysis of similar developments with the analyst, who may be perceived as being interested in the patient for the analyst's own benefit or his or her wishes to be a successful therapist but without any real interest in the patient. The lack of reflection of the patient outside the sessions on what is being discussed in the hours is striking. Any active effort of the analyst to provide some degree of depth to the work acquires the characteristic of a "first session," as if the analysis was just starting at that point. This situation also reflects the patient's subjective timelessness in the hours, as if objective time spent in the hours were magically going to help him or her, even if, in fact, nothing inside the patient really changes. These are also patients who, precisely because nothing is happening in the hours, easily get bored or even fall asleep and, of course, use whatever information they have about "active therapies" of one kind or another to demand a change in the analyst's approach. This feature of the transference may have a discouraging effect on the analyst: it is as if the analysis was starting all over again and again.

The destruction of time may take many forms. Some patients seem to "learn" everything they hear from the analyst and associate with the interpretations in ways that may appear to be confirmatory of them, including the emergence of new, relevant material, conveying an emotional reception of what evolves in the session. But nothing evolves after the session. They maintain perfect memory of what was said, and of their reaction, but do not evince any further curiosity about it, so that, weeks later, the same material may be presented as if it were the first time in which it came up.

At times, the patient questions what had evolved during a particular session but without sharing these questions with the analyst for quite some time. Other people with whom the patient shares what transpired in the session will disagree with the analyst's observations. Or simple "forgetting" occurs, particularly of central points focused upon in the sessions. There are patients who experience a depersonalization during the sessions, as if they were listening and reacting to issues involving somebody else, even being able to communicate this experience to the analyst without any change in it.

The lack of these patients' reflections on their thoughts and feelings, on the analyst's comments, and on their own incapacity to reflect on what they were helped to become aware of in the sessions is a consistent aspect of their relationship to the analyst and his or her interpretations. They may become aware of intense envy of the analyst, and while their envy becomes conscious, their efforts to neutralize it by a lack of response to the analyst's efforts to help them remain unconscious.

The analyst's countertransference may be the dominant instrument signaling an alarm reaction faced with the stagnation of the treatment. The patient's incapacity to depend on the analyst may gradually threaten to undermine his or her commitment to the patient. Aggression in the countertransference may be the only indication of massive projective identification of resentful rage of an envied parental object on the part of the patient. The subliminal expression of such countertransference reaction in interpretive comments may be triumphantly interpreted by the patient as the analyst's "loss of patience" and, therefore, the analyst's problem!

Lengthy stalemates may develop, with the analyst oscillating internally between efforts to find new ways to deal with the stalemate in interpretive fashion and the impulse to set limits to the time in which such a total lack of movement of the treatment should be tolerated. The question, whether the secondary gain of the defeat of the analyst's efforts reinforces the patient's commitment to the denial of the passage of time sufficiently to condemn the treatment to failure may become an acute concern for the analyst. An internal rejection of the patient, reflecting a projective counteridentification with the patient's defensive denial of his or her needs for dependency, may complicate the countertransference.

The solution to this complication is the analysis of the very unavailability to the patient of the analyst as a person, as somebody who thinks, reacts, reflects, and is touched by what is going on in the sessions, and can be generalized to the same unavailability to the patient of everybody else. Very often what can be found at a deeper level is the unconscious identification of the patient with a parental object that treated the patient as an object without an internal life, so that the patient treats the analyst as he or she was treated by the parental object and expects the analyst of course to treat him or her the same way. If the analyst treats the patient very differently from the way the latter was treated in the past, a new world opens up that the patient may experience as painfully illustrating the contrary nature of the terrible deprivation from the past. The pain over a frustrating, empty past childhood is very difficult for the patient to tolerate and may stimulate envy of the analyst for not having been subjected to such a terrible past experience. To begin to depend on the analyst under such conditions may be experienced by the patient as a terribly humiliating defeat, and this reaction may induce regressive cycles of withdrawals and disrupted periods of dependency on the analyst.

Because psychoanalysis is such a long-term treatment, and these patients may be strangely satisfied by regularly coming to the sessions in spite of no discernible progress, all the while giving the appearance of freely associating to varying types of situations, feelings, and understandings, they may unconsciously gratify the analyst's wishes for a dependent relationship on the part of a patient who, apparently, makes no demands and has no expectations for change other than those sudden outbursts of interests in "active treatments." Not infrequently, after a period of time, the analyst may be tempted to move the treatment into a more supportive direction, thus, in turn, gratifying the patient's need to receive narcissistic gratification by this personal "trainer." After a period of time, the development of uneasiness and guilt feelings in the analyst over the growing awareness of an absence of progress may, in fact, paralyze him or her regarding any efforts to "start all over again," that is, to risk the activation of a new "first session," in which the unavailability of the patient to the analyst and of the analyst to the patient can be explored.

Naturally, the general "safety measures" that serve to indicate whether the analysis is progressing, or not, may alert the analyst to what is happening and help him or her face this extremely difficult situation. These measures include the question of what the patient does with the interpretations, how they affect the patient from one session to the next, and what changes, if any, are occurring in the transference and in the countertransference. In this regard, the awareness and the analysis of chronic countertransference developments become relevant in these cases, in which the analyst gradually discovers that nothing seems to be happening except the objective passage of time, without the patient being disturbed by this changeless passage of time.

It is important, faced with a patient in whom active destruction of time seems to be a significant expression of unconscious destructiveness and self-destructiveness, that the analyst tolerate an experience in himself or herself of impatience in every session, while mustering a great degree of patience to deal with the situation over an extended period of time. This impatience within each session might be reflected in a consistent, active effort to deal with the patient's lack of deepening the present object relationship and exploration of what it means in terms of transference and countertransference developments. Such impatience runs counter to a misunderstood overextension of the principle of analyzing "without memory or desire," as Bion (1967) had formulated it in the past. That healthy principle of a neutral analytic attitude runs the risk of here being co-opted into the destructive developments of the transference. I believe that the psychoanalyst has a responsibility to attempt to help the patient, and this responsibility includes an optimal use of the time of each session and is not to be considered a form of "furor sanandis."

The destruction of time as an expression of the destruction of the internalized relationships with significant others may find a dangerous collusion in an analytic approach in which the healthy aspects of the analyst's patience and the long-lasting nature of psychoanalytic treatment are contaminated by the unconscious identification of the analyst with a certain culture of psychoanalytic institutes to extend all educational and supervisory processes to the greatest length possible. The analytic culture in some institutes tolerates and fosters analyses of a duration extending beyond 10 or even 20 years and discourages candidates from "impatience" to graduate and become fully independent. Such cultures may reinforce the delay in diagnosing the narcissistic pathology in analytic treatment we are considering. This may lead to a quiet acceptance of an apparently endless analytic process in which there may be intense fireworks but no real deepening of the emotional investments related by the patient and actualized in the transference/countertransference bind. An unconscious collusion between a narcissist patient and the analyst regarding the "timelessness" of analysis may be particularly dangerous under these circumstances. The destruction of time may, at times, be another expression of the syndrome of the "dead mother" described by André Green (1993), the unconscious identification with and link to a severely depressed mother, experienced as a dead one, which presents itself usually, however, in patients who look much more severely ill on the surface. Typically, in the patients discussed by André Green, the devaluing behavior, the manifest derogatory indifference, and the stubborn rejection of everything the analyst has to offer are quite evident from the beginning of treatment. In the case of narcissistic patients, to the contrary, a surface friendliness, a social easiness, an apparently much more successful social life, and even an apparently intimate one may dominate, so that the destruction of time that goes with a deep unavailability of significant object relations may take time to come to the concerned attention of the analyst.

In conclusion, the destruction of time in narcissistic pathology may serve various functions: the expression of unconscious envy of the analyst, the denial of the unavailability of the grandiose self to any change, and the simple consequence of the unconscious destruction of internalized object relations that would fill objective time with meaning and whose absence shrinks subjective time and condemns the patient to the experience of an empty life.

References

Bion WR: Notes on memory and desire. Psychoanalysis Forum 2:272–273, 279–280, 1967

Green A: On Private Madness. Madison, CT, International Universities Press, 1993

Green A: From the ignorance of time to the murder of time: from the murder of time to the misrecognition of temporality in psychoanalysis. European Psychoanalytical Federation Bulletin 61:12–25, 2007

Hartocollis P: Time and the life cycle, in Time and Timelessness, or Varieties of Temporal Experience. New York, International Universities Press, 1983, pp 215–226

Hartocollis P: Time and the psychoanalytic situation. Psychoanal Q 72:939–957, 2003

Jacques E: The Form of Time. New York, Crane, Russak, 1982

Kernberg OF: Severe Personality Disorders: Psychotherapeutic Strategies. New Haven, CT, Yale University Press, 1984

Kernberg OF: Aggression in Personality Disorders and Perversions. New Haven, CT, Yale University Press, 1992

Klein M: Mourning and its relation to manic-depressive states. Int J Psychoanal 21:125–153, 1940

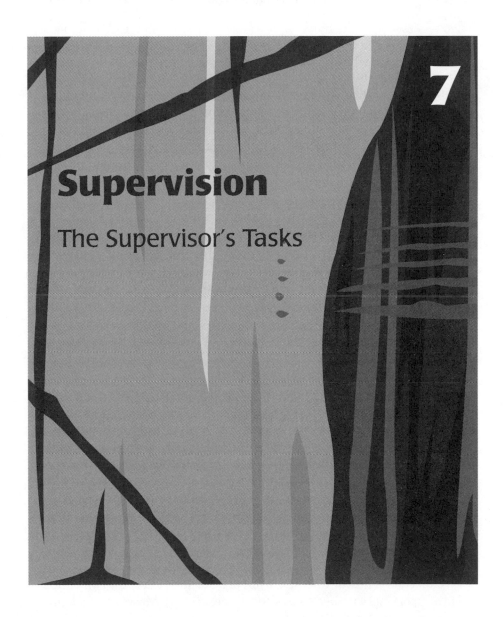

Supervision

The Supervisor's Tasks

In this chapter, I review key aspects involved in the supervisory function of psychoanalytic psychotherapy. They include the capacity to combine a teaching function with an openly expressed evaluating one; a clear, interpretive theory of technique combined with intuitive reaction to the total information of the supervisory situation; a combination of collegiality and honest communication to the supervisee; and the awareness of reciprocal "parallel processes." Reducing the influence of institutional dynamics, particularly those related to authoritarian pressures and paranoid "temptations" in the supervisory situation, is another responsibility of the supervisor. All these tasks also involve discrete understanding and management of countertransference developments in both supervisor and supervisee. Other issues involved include delimitation of responsibilities, utilization of group supervision, the supervisor's management of severe limitation in a supervisee's functioning, and flexible, sophisticated alternative selection of supervisory material. Clinical vignettes represent various typical developments and challenges in a supervisory relationship and illustrate the general principles of supervision spelled out in this chapter.

The Tasks of the Supervisor

A review of the literature on supervision in psychoanalytic psychotherapy and psychoanalysis indicates that the major emphasis is on what the supervisee needs to learn, how this learning can be achieved and evaluated, and what problems the supervisee needs to face and resolve in order to achieve competency as a therapist (Arlow 1963; Blomfield 1985; Greenberg 1997; Junkers et al. 2008; Martindale et al. 1997; Target 2002; Wallerstein 1981). In what follows, I would like to focus on the tasks of the supervisor, what should be expected of him or her, and what are the difficulties that one finds with supervisors rather than supervisees. David, Meyer, and Jacobs (Jacobs et al. 1995) have included this focus on the supervisor in their broad, systematic approach to supervision across the spectrum of psychoanalytically oriented treatments. Here I wish to focus particularly on the specific tasks of the supervisor of psychoanalytic candidates.

Tuckett (2005) and Szecsödy (2008) have contributed significantly on the review of the criteria involved in evaluating a psychoanalytic candidate's psychoanalytic competence. It is generally agreed that a supervisor's responsibilities are to transmit to the supervisee knowledge of the application of psychoanalytic theory to psychoanalytic technique, with particular reference to the skills required to carry out the technical requirements of the supervised case. It is commonly accepted that a collegial attitude be stimulated and maintained, avoiding an authoritarian ambiance that conveys a supervisor's sense of seniority or superiority to the supervisee. The simultaneous function of teaching and evaluating the candidate requires, of course, an honest assessment of the supervisee's work. Some supervisors find it difficult to combine teaching within a collegial atmosphere while critically evaluating the supervisee, and yet that is an essential task of supervision (Junkers et al. 2008). This dilemma is sometimes masked behind the façade of an analytic attitude, whereby the supervisor communicates relatively little to the supervisee, expecting him or her to guess the supervisor's views through carefully formulated hints. That, of course, runs counter to the mutual sharing of experience implied in a collegial attitude in which both participants learn in the process of supervision.

Beyond these commonly accepted tasks, I wish to stress the importance of an integrated view, on the part of the supervisor, of the field to be explored, communicated, and shared, so that the supervisor's concrete recommendations about technical interventions should be embedded in and reflect the application of his or her particular theory of technique. Some might argue that an integrated theory of technique militates against a free-floating attention and an intuitive response to the immediate situation that would capture the communication of unconscious meaning from patient to supervisee, from supervisee to supervisor, and from the supervisor to both supervisee and patient in terms of his or her countertransference reaction.

I propose that there is no reason why such an intuitive process that absorbs, one might say, the total relationship of patient/supervisee and supervisee/supervisor could not be incorporated into a more general frame of reference that would permit the supervisor to transform an intuition into an interpretive remark. Such an implicit frame of reference, of course, is unavoidable as part of the selective focus of what the supervisor sees as essential at any point. The "selected fact" depends not only on immediate intuitive capture of the therapeutic situation but also on the particular theory that orients the focus of the supervisor's intention. One can recognize psychoanalysts with different theoretical formulations in their apparently intuitive reaction to a supervisee's material. Intuition is a form of rapid processing of unconscious and preconscious components from within the theoretical frame of reference in which the supervising analyst has been trained. It might be argued that many supervisors have not formulated such an integrated view that underlies their own interventions, and some may even be reluctant to clarify such a view for themselves. My argument is that this formulation should become an ongoing task for the supervisor; his or her carrying out such a task may become an important contribution to the supervisory process.

A candidate supervisee presented a session of a narcissistic patient with severe difficulties in his relationship with women, who were never good enough for him. In the first part of the session, he had criticized his girlfriend for her neglectful attitude toward her apartment and what he considered her exploitiveness of him. Then, in this session, he had talked, in a desultory tone, about the visit to a friend's house. His friend, he said, was happily married to a stupid woman, enjoyed a rather poorly paid job, but seemed happy with his lot. He then described his serious doubts about continuing the relationship with his girlfriend. My supervisee had interpreted the patient's suspicious attitude about his girlfriend as a projection onto her of his own exploitive feelings and the devaluation of his friend's life situation as a defense against the patient's envy of the friend's capacity for a satisfactory life and love experience. And the patient had listened to these interpretations with his habitual signaling of acceptance of them but without any further emotional elaboration of this material. To my supervisee, it seemed an empty session.

I explored with my supervisee his sense of emptiness of the session, the patient's conveying a sense of both apparent interest in the interpretation and lack of emotional reaction to it, and then suggested that the patient had enacted his defenses against unconscious envy of the analyst in the transference. The unconscious aspects of the conflict with his girlfriend were being enacted in the transference. The patient had been "learning" the meaning of his associations rather than using the analyst's comments as a stimulus for his own associative processes. I used this session to go beyond the concrete analysis of feelings of emptiness in the countertransference to the analysis of the patient's mechanism of intellectualization and "cognitive learning" as an "appropriation," in replacement of an authentic dependency on the analyst. To depend on the analyst meant to this narcissistic patient to accept the need of him, to accept the analyst's freedom to work and to establish a trusting relationship, all of which would cause profound and, so far, probably intolerable envy to the patient. From here, we went into a more general discussion of the importance of conflicts around unconscious envy in narcissistic pathology and its impact on transference developments. This supervisory instance illustrates, I believe, the shift from a concrete exploration of the immediate situation into the more general theory of technique that a concrete interpretation would be based on.

From the viewpoint of the supervisor's task, such an integrated frame of reference is not to be rigidly "superimposed" on his or her intuitive reaction to the material but consciously elaborated and formulated in his or her mind so that it can be called upon to "explain" the reasons for his or her recommended intervention that, at first, seemed to be based on pure intuition. It requires knowledge and intellectual discipline, matched with an internal freedom for intuitive reaction to the material and its unconscious implications. From the point of view of the supervisee's task, learning about the theory of technique that constitutes the organizing integration of the supervisor's intuitive listening and formulations about the material permits the supervisee not only to learn how to deal with a concrete situation but also to learn about the supervisor's way of thinking and the internal frame of reference from which he or she operates and thus facilitates understanding not only about how to intervene in the concrete situation but also how to generalize that learning into a gradually expanding, integrated technical framework. This viewpoint is critical of a not too infrequent situation, in which the supervisor provides the supervisee with wise comments or suggestions that seem to come from a position of profound understanding without leading to the supervisee's possibility of tracing such wisdom back to a general theoretical orientation from within which the concrete formulation would make eminent sense (although that theory might permit other interventions as well).

The supervisor's responsibility to articulate to the supervisee his or her particular theory of technique may create the risk, however, that the supervisor presents his or her position as "the only acceptable" one or that the supervisee reaches such a conclusion, particularly if the supervisor's theory of technique corresponds to one dominant at that institution. The supervisor, while spelling out his or her personal views, also should keep in mind the responsibility to alert the supervisee of alternative ways of conceptualizing the issue under consideration and related, alternative ways to intervene technically. In addition, to stimulate the supervisee to explain his or her own idea of how his or her interpretations function and how they move the therapeutic process forward should reinforce the supervisor's efforts to counter the authoritarian implication of imposing one particular theory of technique.

The supervisor's responsibility to articulate a clear, integrated theoretical foundation of his or her own requires active, ongoing work. It is a creative burden that forces him or her to review critically the interventions and recommendations to the candidate and rework his or her theory of technique throughout time. I believe that the supervisor may be expected to grow in his or her working understanding of psychoanalytic and psychotherapeutic techniques as supervisees present him or her with the infinite novelty of clinical situations that evolve in the interactions between patient and candidate and between candidate and supervisor. Related to this requirement is the importance of the supervisor sharing with the supervisee how he or she would respond to the specific clinical situation that is being interpreted. While focusing on what he or she recommends the supervisee to do, the supervisor might often state what he or she would be thinking and doing under those concrete circumstances.

Institutional Agendas

Supervision takes place, usually, in the context of an organizational institution, be it a psychoanalytic institute, a university outpatient department, or a private or public mental health or hospital setting, all of which have their own structural characteristics, institutional biases, and realistic expectations of learning on the part of the supervisee, as well as other "hidden agendas." "Hidden agendas" usually refer to problems around authority within the institution, legal or financial requirements that determine the boundaries of tolerance of atypical treatment situations and risk aversion of the institution, as well as idiosyncratic rules and regulations of individual supervisors. It might be trivial to refer to this fact were it not that these agendas may powerfully influence the supervisory process, determining, for example, a treatment approach that might be less than optimal because what would be optimal would run into financial and/or political constraints of the institution or activate implicitly ideological struggles within the institution.

For example, if a psychoanalytic institute has a predominantly ego psychological approach, but a supervisee is particularly interested in applying a self psychology approach to his patient, the supervisor might support this, or not, according to the flexibility provided in the teaching programs of that institute and his willingness to depart from his own theoretical beliefs. The practical implication of this issue is that a "parallel process" evolves, not only in terms of the supervisee's unconscious enactment with role reversal of experienced but not understood problems in his relationship with the patient but also that the same process may be activated by subjectively experienced, unresolved conflicts of the supervisor with the institution in which he does the supervision. Here the supervisor enacts the conflict with the institution in a corresponding role reversal with his supervisee. An example of this type of parallel process was seen in the case of a Kleinian-oriented psychoanalytic institute where an intersubjective/relationist approach had developed among a significant group of "rebellious" faculty members. One of the Kleinian supervisors developed a hostile interaction with a supervisee who was interested in the intersubjective/relational approach, so that the institutional dynamic was replayed in the individual supervisory relationship.

The phenomenon of "parallel process" illustrates, better than anything else, the activation of unconscious relations in the supervisory process (Baudry 1993; Kernberg 2006). Unconscious countertransference reactions of the supervisee, usually related to an unconsciously registered but not consciously elaborated aspect of the patient's transference, are enacted in the supervisory situation. Such reactions are then "discharged" with a role reversal in which the supervisee unconsciously identifies himself or herself with that aspect of the patient, while projecting the correspondent countertransference reaction onto the supervisor. The supervisor's alertness to this development, on the basis of diagnosing a specific distortion in the supervisory relationship, may help to clarify the meaning of this transference/countertransference bind, but this process demands an open, honest, collegial relationship.

I believe it is very helpful for the supervisor, aware of institutional conflicts that may be affecting his or her subjective attitude toward the supervisee, to bring this out in the open, at the same time as he or she should feel free to bring out the "parallel process" in the supervisee's relationship to him or her as it might be influenced by an unrecognized or unresolved countertransference problem in the relationship of the supervisee with his or her own patient. In a group supervision at a Kleinian-oriented psychoanalytic institute, a candidate presented a case to me by starting with a recent concrete session. He provided a minimum of preliminary information about the patient's earliest life experiences and went on to read his summary of the session. I interrupted him to say that I was interested in the patient's present difficulties and, particularly, in a brief summary of the patient's present problems in the areas of sexual love, work, or social life. The group reacted quite strongly in reminding me of the advisability to analyze "without memory nor desire." I acknowledged their reaction and expressed to them my admiration of Bion but also pointed to some differences in my approach and wondered whether we could work together sharing both similar and dissimilar ways of approaching the material of the session. The tension in the group decreased noticeably, and I believe we were able to learn from each other. I had the opportunity to illustrate my view about the potential relationship between presently dominant life conflicts and the predominant transference development. Such open exchange in the supervisory process may bring about an honesty that reduces the highly prevalent paranoid fears of the supervisee, particularly in authoritarian organizations, which, in turn, fosters honesty of communication regarding the psychotherapeutic or psychoanalytic process and facilitates countertransference analysis of the supervisee in a nonthreatening, nonintrusive way.

Countertransference Exploration

In this connection, the exploration of the supervisee's countertransference is an important yet delicate aspect of the supervisory process. I believe that it is very important to generate a collegial atmosphere in which the supervisee may feel free to openly explore his or her countertransference reactions, including reactions to the supervisory process of that particular patient. The supervisor may use countertransference analysis to explore aspects of the nature of the patient's transference that may have affected the supervisee's subjective experience but have not been fully understood and elaborated by him or her. The analysis of how the patient contributes to the countertransference reaction of the supervisee is what is important here, while maintaining a tactful respect for the boundaries of privacy of deeper aspects of the supervisee's conflicts that may have been activated in the supervisory situation. Supervision should not become a psychotherapeutic process: when the two become conflated it usually leads to regression in the supervision, tends to blur the clarity of the supervisory process, and may interfere with the collegial aspects of the relationship. It may also foster transference displacement and acting out by a supervisee involved in personal psychoanalysis or psychoanalytic psychotherapy.

As an example, in the case of one psychoanalytic candidate whom I was supervising for the treatment of a severely narcissistic patient who presented instability of object relations, sexual promiscuity, and an unconsciously envious and derogatory behavior toward women, the candidate, a usually secure, open, highly intelligent woman, presented the following information. After telling me that her patient had expressed sexual fantasies about her in a clearly seductive way, she told me that this had made her feel very insecure, and, in fact, she had difficulties in dealing with this patient. On exploring this issue further with her, she finally said: "I have to confess that if I met this man one evening in a bar without any knowledge of him other than that of such a first encounter, I would be tempted to go to bed with him." I commented that she made it clear that he was attractive to her as a man, but, what, in him, made her afraid of him? This led us into the discussion of the controlling aspects of his seductive behavior, his implicit attempt to undermine her authority as an analyst and transform her into the image of a desirable and unavailable woman whom he would be tempted to "conquer," and his usual behavior pattern unconsciously motivated by the envy and hatred of women whom he perceived as teasing him. In short, I expressed my appreciation for her capacity to talk honestly about her feelings with me but focused on the meaning of the participation of the patient in the induction of those feelings and respected the privacy of what particular unconscious tendency in my supervisee might have made her feel particularly attracted to this man.

Some degree of idealization of the supervisor on the part of the supervisee is probably unavoidable under conditions of a good supervisory experience, particularly if the supervisee is simultaneously experiencing regressive reactions in a psychoanalytic treatment. The supervisor needs to keep in mind that in all interpersonal situations in which there exists a role distribution between one who "knows" and one who "needs to know," an implicit deskilling of the student may occur, with his or her attribution of all knowledge and skills to the supervisor and a self-devaluation of the supervisee. The efforts to maintain a collegial attitude by the direct, open, "nonoracular" communication of the supervisor's knowledge and experience may modify the idealization into a bona fide creative, warm professional relationship, in contrast to an idealization process that fixates the supervisee's conviction that the supervisor will always know better and be superior and that a permanent hierarchy will remain in the relationship of the supervisee with that particular supervisor. Such a negative fixation at an idealizing level is not infrequent, particularly in institutions with highly prestigious, powerful, and even "guru"-like figures, whose own narcissistic needs may foster a tendency to surround themselves with admiring students. The encouragement of mutual or peer supervision by groups of trainees who already have some years of experience is one helpful countermeasure: in the process of "intervision," in contrast to "supervision," the trainees may become aware of possessing more understanding and skills than they have been conscious of in supervisions with their revered elders.

Dynamics of Group Supervision

This leads us to the process of group supervision, which may be very helpful toward integrating the developing experience and knowledge of the supervisees, while also providing them with a more realistic awareness of the limitations of the knowledge of the supervisor. In a group situation, there is the opportunity to examine the clinical aspects of a case from many different perspectives, thereby providing a richness and diversity of understanding that does not privilege any one thought above another. At the same time, it is very helpful that the supervisor acquire skills in the field of group dynamics that will permit him or her to utilize the supervisory group situation itself as a teaching instrument. I am referring here to the role distribution that automatically occurs in groups as an expression of the "parallel process" characteristic of the individual supervisory relationship. In practice, an unresolved transference/countertransference fixation in a case presented to the group may elicit different responses in different members of the group that correspond to a distribution of conflictual or split-off aspects of transference and countertransference in that case. The joint analysis by the supervisor of these different reactions to the material on the part of the group may provide an analysis in depth of the dominant transference/countertransference situation that the presenter "discharges" in the group without full awareness of the nature of the issues that he or she is implicitly communicating. This process, naturally, tends to get obscured when the supervisor acts as if he or she were the only source of knowledge regarding the

problems presented in the case under review. In fact, such an assertion of the "last word" by the supervisor may inhibit the communications in the group and, therefore, the learning process.

An interesting expression of institutional dynamics occurs
when the members of a supervision group have, each of them, individual supervisors of the cases that they present to the group. The
same dynamics are also present when a continuous case seminar in
a psychoanalytic institute deals with only one candidate presenting
his or her case in treatment, as long as the individual supervisor of
that candidate does not coincide with the group leader. Under these
circumstances, significant differences of the approaches of individual supervisor and group supervisor may rapidly emerge and challenge the candidate and the group supervisor in many ways.
Rivalries between the two supervisors may implicitly color the interactions in the group, and generally shared anxieties of the trainees over the discrepant views of their supervisors may emerge
timidly or openly. This is an excellent opportunity for clarifying that
to be exposed to different viewpoints has an enormous educational
advantage, in that it forces the student to consider alternative
frames of reference, compare them, and develop his or her own
synthesis.

I supervised a candidate who presented a female patient with a
marked hysterical personality disorder and strong masochistic features in the relationship with her husband and in the transference.
I had helped her to explore the chronic fights of this patient with
her husband as an unconscious expression of profound oedipal
guilt, a submission to a dominant but also deeply frustrated mother
whose own marriage had been a very unhappy one. At one point,
the supervisee presented the patient to a group supervision con-
ducted by another training analyst of my institute. After a few
weeks, it became clear that in that group, the patient's conflicts
with the husband were seen as the expression of profound frustration of the patient's oral-dependent needs in the relationship with
her mother, now enacted in the relationship with the patient's husband.

The candidate was tense and troubled: she told me that the
group supervisor had questioned her interpretive approach and
that much of what was being suggested in the group supervision
made sense to her. My countertransference reaction included a
sense of irritation with the candidate, a sense of competition with
the group leader, and, as I also recognized, a complex condensation
of my oedipal rivalry with the group leader with the candidate's

enactment of her patient's masochistic pattern with me. And, at a different level, I was frustrating the candidate's dependency wishes on me.

I decided to share these interpretations of the institutional situation and their relevance for the understanding of the patient's transference situation with the candidate and invited her to elaborate this situation in her own mind while feeling free to discuss all this with me and to reach her own conclusions in exploring further her experience with the patient.

In fact, as has been pointed out by various authors (Galatzer-Levy 2004; Levin 2006; Shane and Shane 1995), the exposure of trainees to alternative viewpoints in the context of a nonauthoritarian institution fosters the learning process and professional maturation of the trainee. It may be argued that, to the contrary, exposure to such contradictory views may lead to chaos and confusion. This may be true, particularly when there is no forum by which different viewpoints can be aired and compared and instruments provided to the students to arrive at their own synthesis. At this time, in psychoanalytic institutes, it may be a major challenge to decide what basic "common theory of technique" is available to provide a solid ground for the students to permit them to reach educated decisions regarding alternative approaches. One test of the extent to which such a reasonable internal evaluation of different viewpoints has been achieved by the trainee is an assessment of the trainee's ability to evolve an integrated frame of reference for his or her own technical understanding and approaches rather than rely on a chaotic eclectic mixture, based on intuition, of different approaches in different situations that do not give evidence of a common, integrative framework as the basis for which the move into alternative techniques can be justified.

Professional Responsibility

An important issue that often is not fully clarified is the question—who carries the responsibility for the patient? The ideal situation between supervisor and supervisee is one in which both parties are clear that the supervisee carries the ultimate responsibility for the patient. The supervisor has the freedom to recommend one way of handling a situation, whereas the supervisee has the freedom to accept or reject it, using his or her own judgment and with the awareness of the fact that the ultimate professional, legal, and personal responsibility for the patient rests with him or her. In many educational institutions, however, the ultimate responsibility may lie with the institution, particularly from a legal standpoint, and this, then, limits the degrees of freedom that both parties have with regard to ultimate responsibility for the patient. When the supervisor, in representing the educational institution within which he or she is the supervisor, carries the responsibility for the well-being of the patient, his or her responsibility to the patient, the supervisee, and the institution has to be weighed carefully. In most cases, this issue does not impinge on the supervisory process; but when there are serious problems in the functioning of a supervisee, or "impossible cases" that create high-risk complications for the institution, these distributed responsibilities have to be spelled out clearly and openly, with the understanding that the supervisee may have to, under certain circumstances, do what the supervisor is instructing be done in the case. The extent to which this is a problem depends, naturally, on the particular ideological and legal culture in which the educational institution operates. In the United States, with its highly litigious culture, this issue becomes very important with problematic cases. The main point here is that the extent to which responsibility for the patient rests on one or another professional, or is shared by them and an institution, be clearly communicated.

A psychoanalytic candidate treated a patient with a severe personality disorder in analysis as part of his group practice within a university hospital. At one point, the patient became acutely suicidal. It seemed to me, the supervisor, that this was not a suicidal tendency linked to a depressive reaction but a characterological pattern that needed to be analyzed rather than treated with a preventive hospitalization. However, I was concerned about whose responsibility it was to make that decision. I would have been willing to document this approach as part of my responsibility, but it was not my patient. The candidate was part of an institutional system— the hospital—that had a very conservative view of such situations.

After clarifying the various responsibilities involved, the supervisee and I decided that he would use his administrative supervisor in the hospital as consultant on this case, and my supervisee would make the decision about the strategy to follow in the light of that consultation. I committed myself to help him whatever the course of action would follow.

This leads us to the question of limitations in the candidate's professional functioning and the responsibility of the supervisor under such circumstances. The need for honesty with trainees who, for a variety of reasons, are not able to achieve the minimum required learning is an essential requirement for the supervisor. Situations in which supervisors internally give up on a supervisee without honest and courageous communication about it directly to the supervisee are not infrequent. The supervisor has a responsibility to the institution and to the profession as well as to the supervisee and the patient. The following are frequent cases in which such painful moments of truth may emerge.

Supervisees' Pathology

First, in the case of supervisees with limited intellectual capacities, there is a great reluctance to acknowledge the possibility that, particularly in the course of advanced psychological and/or medical training, supervisees who have been able to reach the point of specialization in psychotherapy or psychoanalysis may not have the intellectual capacities to carry out such work. It is, of course, difficult to differentiate lack of emotional introspection and of depth of awareness of human feelings as an expression of character pathology from cognitive factors per se, and the supervisor, without the availability of corresponding psychological testing, or alternative sources of information, may not be in a position to make this differential diagnosis. The usual assumption is that the supervisee is emotionally incapable of achieving adequate competency. The safe way to reach such a conclusion, of course, is to provide the supervisee ample opportunities to learn in the supervisory sessions, patiently repeating the same issues while evaluating to what extent a learning process is taking place. The supervisor is responsible for remaining alert to what happens to his or her contributions, to what extent they are like seeds planted that lead to new growth, or to what extent they resemble seeds that perish in the desert. Individual supervisors may disagree on the length of time that is reasonable for a supervisee to demonstrate certain core competencies, but there comes a point when failure to learn may have to be addressed. When it becomes evident that issues that have been repeatedly clarified in the supervisory situation do not bring about change, and that the same problems emerge again and again, this should, of course, be shared openly with the supervisee.

The following case was one of the most painful experiences in my functions as supervising analyst. The candidate belonged to a small minority population, who had been able to obtain a full education in medicine and psychiatry, helped, it must be said, by the efforts of a particular agency throughout her life to achieve this goal. She was a warm, responsible, engaging person who was received with open arms at an international institution particularly interested in fostering high-level education for this minority group, including analytic training.

I was one of three visiting supervising analysts (from a different country) at the international institution who supervised her work, and my impression was that she could not achieve any learning from her interaction with me. Over almost two years of supervision, I had a sense that I had to repeat the same suggestions over and over again and that, while she almost desperately tried to use what I had said in the following sessions with her patient, this knowledge would leave no long-term traces. I discussed the situation openly with her, more and more frequently throughout time, and she was very straightforward in conveying her difficulty to transfer general principles from one situation to another. I could not diagnose any major characterological difficulties in her and, after a time, consulted with the other two supervisors about this situation. All three of us had exactly the same experience. We all wanted to help her but could not. We studied her past records and discovered that she had significant learning difficulties all along, being able to get to this advanced stage of her professional career by extremely hard and consistent work. She had a fine memory, which had helped her through all educational experiences, including medical school.

Our conclusion was that she had some kind of cognitive limitation or impairment and, finally, recommended to her a shift in her career, a neuropsychological examination if she were interested, while suggesting a suspension of her analytic training at that international institution.

A frequent situation that may lend itself to confusion with the previous one is the case of supervisees with significant narcissistic pathology, who, although eager to learn whatever new knowledge is offered to them, soon become convinced that they have absorbed it all and that there is nothing new that the supervisor now may offer them. This type of supervisee tends to show an excessive degree of idealization at the beginning, followed by subtle devaluation of what he or she has received. They seem to absorb what the supervisor offers as simple or clever formulas that are useful in this very fashion but lack an authentic expansion of the supervisees' own elaboration and development of that material. Sometimes severe narcissistic pathology shows in excessive enthusiasm with some new, "original" developments that seem to be offered by a certain supervisor, followed by disappointment or disillusionment, and then by the search for another new, magical approach with somebody else, leading to the surprisingly radical shifts in approaches by some candidates that, at the end, reveal a superficial acquisition of such new theories of technique.

Supervisees with significant emotional immaturity, whose personal chaos not only distorts their capacity to listen to patients but also does not permit them to integrate new learning in a significant way, constitute another source of frustrating supervisory situations. However, the gradual conflict resolution and personal growth in a psychoanalytic or psychotherapeutic treatment of the trainee may improve the supervisory experiences significantly.

The key challenge in all limitations to learning is to determine the cause. To what extent is the supervisor or his or her attitude or approach part of the problem? To what extent is it personality or intelligence of the supervisee that constitutes significant limitations?

We must acknowledge that sometimes significant psychopathology of the supervisee may remain undetected even by very experienced supervisors. From that viewpoint, the simultaneous supervision of trainees by several supervisors significantly improves the possibility of diagnosing difficulties and resolving them in the educational process. Such an arrangement, of course, is not possible in the private supervision of an independent mental health professional by another one but should become possible in institutional settings, particularly in departments of psychiatry and even more so in psychoanalytic institutes, where the educational structure is so much focused on supervision. Regular meetings of supervisors to discuss supervisees, particularly those who seem to present problems, may help to clarify issues that, for the individual supervisor, may take much more time to grasp.

For example, I supervised a fourth-year (!) psychiatric resident who was treating a very ill borderline patient, and I found it impossible to get a clear view of the patient, in spite of the fact that the supervisee seemed very clear in what he was saying, seemed to have understanding, and was being quite open. But the patient was getting worse by the day, with all kinds of complications emerging in the patient's life, in the relation of the patient with the therapist, and in the relation of the therapist with other mental health personnel connected with that patient's treatment. I was tempted to see the patient myself in order to clarify what made it so difficult to get a live picture of the patient throughout the supervisory process. I decided to discuss this with the supervisory group connected with this supervisee's progress and found out, not only that everybody had the same difficulties with him but also that there were very serious questions about the ethical behavior of this resident. In the middle of our discussions, this resident disappeared from the map, abandoned his functions without formal resignation, and had to be formally dismissed from the program. Another fourth-year resident was invited to continue the treatment of this patient, and after a few weeks of supervision, I had a clear sense of understanding what kind of person the patient was and what the main conflicts were that had to be explored at this time, and all the complications in the relationship of the patient with other professional staff and in the patient's life started getting resolved, and a transference/countertransference bind established with the new therapist could now be meaningfully explored in the supervisory sessions. I had missed, in short, the severely antisocial features of the first resident and his capacity to convey a pseudomature understanding that in fact reflected consistent distortions in the information that I had been receiving from him.

Supervisory Material

In this connection, it is also helpful for the supervisor to combine flexibility in letting the supervisee choose in which form he or she wishes to present the case to the supervisor with the requirement that, in turn, the method of selection of supervisory material be flexibly shifted, thus surveying information regarding tactical and strategic interactions and interventions. I am referring here to the typical observation that the study of a brief segment of one session, of an entire session, of a sequence of sessions, and of development in the treatment over a period of weeks typically reveal the same structure; in other words, the same transference/countertransference pattern and dominant defensive operations throughout those very different time spans. The macro cosmos of the session reproduces the micro cosmos of the interaction in a brief segment of it. The shift from studying segments of a session to studying what happens over weeks and vice versa provides a third dimension to the evaluation of the material and of the learning process of the trainee. There are many supervisors who insist on receiving no written notes but only subjective information from the supervisee on the basis of brief summaries he or she has made for himself or herself, whereas other supervisors require detailed process notes of verbal interactions in their natural sequence. Again, flexibility and change of approaches throughout time in this regard would seem optimal.

Informal, verbal communication on the part of the supervisee provides rather imprecise information about the concrete therapeutic dialogue but excellent information about the supervisee's general understanding, attitude, and parallel process. Detailed written material, stemming from written notes or audio recording during the hours, provides a more accurate reflection of the dialogue and of the therapist's intervention but may miss out on the subtleties of emotional interactions that are communicated by means of the parallel process. Direct listening to audiotapes of sessions conveys more clearly the emotional interaction and gives a very full sense of what has been happening in the session, but because of the slowness of the process of replicating the timing of development in the sessions, it is usually necessarily limited to listening to segments of a particular session.

The observation of videotapes of psychotherapy sessions provides maximum information on content and attitudes and permits making significant judgments regarding transference and countertransference by means of the shifting nonverbal behavior of patient and therapist. A limitation, of course, derives from that related to building videotaping into the therapy in such a naturalistic way that it does not distort the therapeutic process significantly; videotaping also reduces the manifestation of the parallel process in the supervisory sessions: the supervisee is cast into a passive spectator role. However, all in all, it may be the best source of information about the overall functioning of the therapist, and often there are surprisingly marked differences between what the therapist reports and what one can see on videotapes. Perhaps the main problem with videotaping is that in the case of psychoanalytic treatment, in which most information is really the communication of the patient's subjective experience by verbal means, relatively little nonverbal, visually observable interaction occurs in the sessions, which makes videotaped psychoanalytic sessions extremely boring, to the extent that the supervision may become a self-defeating process. In contrast, in the case of psychoanalytic psychotherapy, particularly with severely regressed patients, in which intensive behavioral face-to-face interactions between therapist and patient are registered, videotaping, in our experience at the Personality

Disorders Institute at Cornell, is by far the most effective way of facilitating the supervisory process.

In this connection, it needs to be recognized that the bias against videotaping psychoanalytic sessions is so strong in psychoanalytic circles that this entire area of exploration of the supervisory process may even be shocking to some psychoanalytic colleagues. This is not the place to clarify these issues on the basis of the experiences in various research-oriented organizations that have confirmed the possibility of psychoanalytic work under such circumstances, because, in practice, as mentioned before, videotaped psychoanalytic sessions usually are not a helpful supervisory instrument, even if they are helpful for certain research purposes. But I may mention that, on the basis of the clinical and research experience of thirty years, patients quite readily accept ongoing video recording if they have been appropriately informed and assured of the confidentiality of those recordings, and the psychotherapeutic process is remarkably little affected by these arrangements. In our experience at Cornell, therapists just beginning their professional careers have significant initial difficulty with video recording, owing to their own self-consciousness, but they too quickly forget that the camera is there.

General Characteristics of Competence

A research finding regarding the competence of therapists carrying out psychoanalytic psychotherapy may be relevant. Although this finding applies to psychotherapy rather than psychoanalytic supervision proper, I believe it may also be relevant in psychoanalytic supervision.

Our work at The Personality Disorders Institute at the Department of Psychiatry at the Weill Medical College of Cornell University and the Westchester Division of the New York Presbyterian Hospital has provided us with important learning regarding the overall desirable personality qualities of therapists and the development of therapeutic skills in psychoanalytic psychotherapy with severe personality disorders. Here I shall limit myself to point to our conclusion that four relatively easily evaluated qualities of therapeutic interventions in psychoanalytic psychotherapy define the quality of psychotherapeutic work on the part of our trainees—namely, third-year psychiatric residents and beyond and first-year postdoctoral psychology fellows and beyond. These are the four factors: 1) the relevance of the therapist's comments to the dominant affective issue evolving in the session; 2) the clarity with which interpretive interventions are formulated; 3) the depth to which those comments penetrate into the dominant conflicts of the patients, particularly the unconscious layers of defense and impulse involved in the conflicts activated in transference and countertransference; and 4) the speed with which the trainee is able to carry out such interventions. This last feature may seem surprising, but the dissociative nature of communications in patients with severe personality disorders and the prevalence of enactment and acting out in the sessions, as well as the prevalence of nonverbal behavior over what patients communicate verbally about their subjective experience, all combine to bring about rapid shifts in the content of the hours that require rapid interventions rather than patiently waiting for the material to clarify itself throughout time.

When everything goes well, it should be possible, throughout time, for the supervisor as well as for the supervisee to construct in their minds an integrated picture of the personality of the patient, a three-dimensional awareness of the present vicissitudes of the patient's conscious and unconscious life experiences and their relation to significant aspects of his or her past, to experience directly what areas are now affectively dominant in the sessions that have to be approached and what areas of the patient's life experience are glaringly absent in the treatment situation and require an active focus on them. Mutual learning may occur as supervisee and supervisor express freely their views and questions about the patient. For the supervisor, the growing independence of good work of the supervisee, such as the supervisee's capacity to convey new information and to provide new leads to the supervisor, is a very gratifying experience of having contributed to the supervisee's autonomous growth. I have found it very helpful to shift the rhythm of intensity of contributions on my part to the supervisory process, from periods when I might very actively try to convey information and influence the therapeutic process to other times when I might sit back and be on the learning process of what is going on with the patient and what are the new contributions the therapist may make. Good supervision becomes an extremely interesting learning process for both participants; failing supervision can be a trying experience for the supervisor to which he or she should not react masochistically (or sadistically!). Throughout time it will become clear to what extent the trainee is developing his or her own frame of reference, integrating knowledge received from the supervisor without a process of "surface imitation" that is often misread as identification with the supervisor.

A psychiatrist would present her case to me with some general reflection about what struck her most in a particular session or over a particular time. She might reflect on alternative ways to handle the material that she presented to me, show very openly expressed uncertainties or doubts, and be able, looking back at a set of sessions over a more extended time period, to venture hypotheses about where the treatment was going or in what way she was changing her view about a particular development.

I had the growing feeling, during that supervision, that an experienced colleague was presenting a case to me. Not infrequently, I was surprised and stimulated by the originality of her interventions. I was learning in the process, and I told her so. Not surprisingly, she wrote a series of papers on the technical issues presented by the patient, making an original contribution to this field.

Köerner (2002) has defined the objectives of psychoanalytic education as the development of the candidates' knowledge, technical skills, and analytic attitude: all three can be observed throughout time in the course of the supervisory process and facilitate a realistic evaluation of that process, an evaluation that, as mentioned before, needs to be shared fully and openly with the candidate and open to the candidate's reactions regarding the supervisor's views. The supervisor's self-reflective function may be shared, over time, in an increasing degree with the supervisee, so that the supervisor's speculations, uncertainties, and alternative possible formulations regarding the patient can be made available in more direct free and open ways to the supervisee, facilitating his or her identification with the self-reflective attitude of the supervisor, which, in turn, broadens and deepens the nature and pleasure for her or him in the supervisory process. Last but not least, the supervisor may convey to the supervisee the need to be very patient over time in tolerating the repetition of the severe problems again and again, the same transference developments of the patient, without losing patience, while maintaining an attitude of alertness and therapeutic "impatience" in every session. And this, of course, also holds for the supervisory process: the need to be patient throughout time but to attempt to use maximally every supervisory hour, alert to the defensive operations and obstacles that may block that process.

References

Arlow JA: The supervisory situation. J Am Psychoanal Assoc 11:576–594, 1963

Baudry FD: The personal dimension and management of the supervisory situation with a special note on the parallel process. Psychoanal Q 62:588–614, 1993

Blomfield O: Psychoanalytic supervision: an overview. Int Rev Psychoanal 12:401–409, 1985

Galatzer-Levy R: Chaotic possibilities: towards a new model of development. Int Rev Psychoanal 85:419–442, 2004

Greenberg L: On transference and countertransference and the technique of supervision, in Supervision and Its Vicissitudes. Edited by Martindale B, Mörner M, Rodriguez MEC, et al. London, Karnac Books, 1997, pp 1–24

Jacobs D, David P, Meyer DJ: The Supervisory Encounter. New Haven, CT, Yale University Press, 1995

Junkers G, Tuckett D, Zachrisson A: To be or not to be an analyst—how do we know a candidate is ready to qualify? Difficulties and controversies in evaluating psychoanalytic competence. Psychoanalytic Inquiry 28:288–308, 2008

Kernberg OF: The coming changes in psychoanalytic education: part I. Int J Psychoanal 87:1649–1673, 2006

Köerner J: The didactics of psychoanalytic education. Int J Psychoanal 83:1395–1405, 2002

Levin CB: "That's not analytic": theory pressure and "chaotic possibilities" in analytic training. Psychoanalytic Inquiry 26:767–783, 2006

Martindale B, Mörner M, Rodriguez MEC, et al (eds): Supervision and Its Vicissitudes. London, Karnac Books, 1997

Shane M, Shane E: Un-American activities and other dilemmas experienced in the supervision of candidates. Psychoanalytic Inquiry 15:226–239, 1995

Szecsödy I: Does anything go in psychoanalytic supervision? Psychoanal Q 28:373–386, 2008

Target M: Psychoanalytic models of supervision: issues and ideas. Presented at the European Psychoanalytic Federation Training Analysts' Colloquium, Budapest, Hungary, November, 2002

Tuckett D: Does anything go? Towards a framework for a more transparent assessment of psychoanalytic competence. Int J Psychoanal 86:31–49, 2005

Wallerstein RS (ed): Becoming a Psychoanalyst: A Study of Psychoanalytic Supervision. New York, International Universities Press, 1981

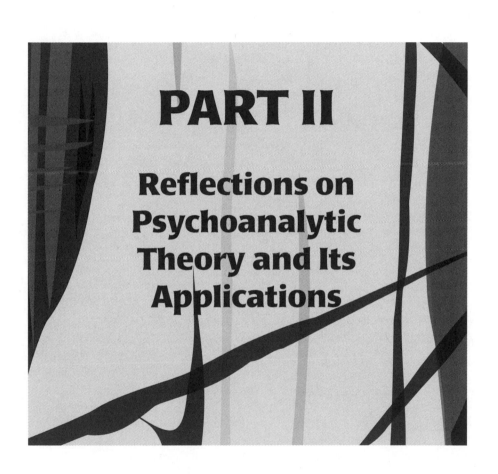

PART II

Reflections on Psychoanalytic Theory and Its Applications

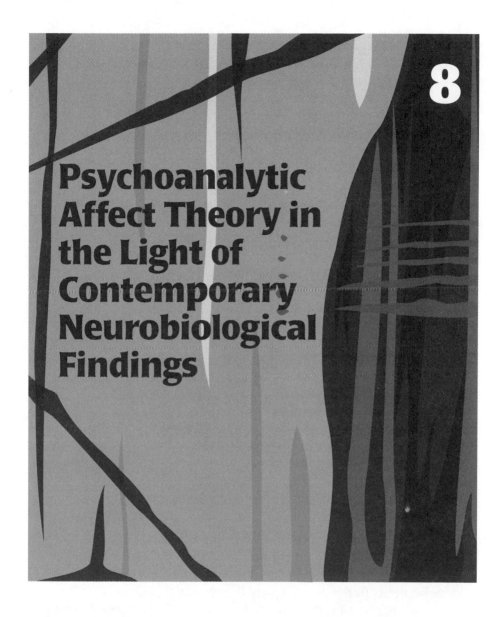

8

Psychoanalytic Affect Theory in the Light of Contemporary Neurobiological Findings

Presented at the Delphi International Psychoanalytic Symposium, Delphi, Greece, October 27–31, 2004. This chapter was reprinted from Kernberg OF: "Psychoanalytic Affect Theory in the Light of Contemporary Neurobiological Findings," in *Beyond the Mind-Body Dualism: Psychoanalysis and the Human Body.* Edited by Zacharacopoulou E. Amsterdam, The Netherlands, Elsevier Health Sciences, International Congress Series Vol. 1286, March 2006, pp. 106–117. Copyright Elsevier 2006. Used with permission.

In this chapter, I explore the relation between contemporary developments in neurobiology and the psychoanalytic "dual drive" theory of motivation. The chapter presents a capsule review of the evolving affect theory in neurobiology and proposes that affects are a primary motivational system that occupies a boundary function between neurobiological and symbolic, intrapsychic structures. It is proposed that the integration of positive and negative affect dispositions constitute the components, respectively, of "libido" and "aggression" as the hierarchically supraordinate intrapsychic drives. Throughout this chapter, the relationship between affect activation and the establishment of internalized object relations—the "internal working models" of attachment theory—is explored: affective memory (always?) includes a corresponding representation of self and other ("object").

On principle, most psychoanalysts would agree that the advances in the neurosciences are of great importance to psychoanalysis. Psychoanalytic theory, after all, is based on the assumption that psychological functioning is profoundly influenced by the central nervous system, and the motivational system postulated by Freud's dual drive theory is based on the assumption that the drives represent the demands for work made by the body to the psychic apparatus. The fact that, as Freud clearly saw, affects and representations are the observable, clinical expressions of the drives places affect theory and neurocognitive science in a central place as far as the entire theoretical structure of psychoanalysis is concerned. Affects and representations constitute the components of unconscious fantasy and are the available evidence of unconscious intrapsychic conflict. Affects and representations are central in the clinical situation: in fact, in contemporary object relations theory, self- and object representations relating to each other within the frame of a predominant affect are the building blocks of the tripartite structure and determine all intrasubjective and intersubjective developments in the psychoanalytic situation.

In principle, then, psychoanalytic interest in the development of the neurosciences is clear and unambiguous. Practically speaking, however, there appears to be some ambivalence behind this openly expressed interest. The fear that new scientific developments in neurobiology and other sciences may challenge aspects of Freud's theoretical framework and oblige us to reexamine basic psychoanalytic theory may lead to a distortion in the psychoanalytic approach to the neurosciences. Our temptation may be to endorse findings that confirm long-cherished theories and to reject new information that would oblige us to reformulate them. I believe that it is reasonable to be alert to such a risk.

What follows is an overview of my proposals, developed in recent years, to reformulate the relationships between affects, drives, and the organization of self- and object representations that constitute the building blocks of the tripartite structure. Empirical research on neurocognitive functions, and functional magnetic resonance imaging studies carried out at the Personality Disorders Institute of the Department of Psychiatry of the Weill Medical College of Cornell University, have further influenced my exploration of affect theory and of affective developments in severe personality disorders (Silbersweig et al. 2007). The enormous developments in neuropsychological studies of affect by Tomkins (1963, 1970), Ekman (1985), and Krause (1990), on the one hand, and in the neurobiological studies of Depue and Zald (1993), Damasio (1994), and, particularly, Panksepp (1998), on the other, have provided us with new approaches to affect theory that provide a frame for the biological studies mentioned, in conjunction with the study of specific neurotransmitters and brain structures involved in affect activation and affect regulation. Earlier studies on the development of affect expression in infants, the role of affective attunement in normal and pathological attachment, and the study of affective communication in mammals are other areas of research that are enriching this field—and partly engaged in by psychoanalytic researchers (Fonagy and Target 2003).

At the same time, it is important to keep in mind that psychoanalysis itself has been evolving in its approaches to affect theory. The relationship of affects to drives and object relations emerges strongly in the work of Brierley (1937/1951), Winnicott (1965), Rapaport (1953), Klein (1940/1948), Jacobson (1953/1971), Mahler et al. (1975), Bion (1967), and Green (1977/1986). I think we have the exciting task to bring together, wherever possible, developments within the psychoanalytic and the neurobiological realm.

Freud's Affect Theory and Later Psychoanalytic Development

David Rapaport (1953), in his excellent synthesis of the development of Freud's thinking regarding the role of affects in the context of his theory of drives, pointed to three stages of Freud's formulations. Until 1915, Freud treated affects as approximately equivalent to drives and described the function of such unconscious affects or drives as central in the development of unconscious intrapsychic conflict. In his 1915 formulation of drive theory (Freud 1915/1957), he specified the relationship between affects and drives, proposing that drives were the fundamental motivational system, at the border between the physical and the psychic, and that drives could be known only by their expression through representations and affects. He further proposed that libido as a drive included the integration of partial instinctual impulses, implying that this integration occurred in the intrapsychic realm.

Freud now differentiated drives from instincts and stated that the latter were biological functions, discontinuous, and species specific, in contrast to the highly individualized nature of psychic drives. Drives were subject to postponement and modification, while instincts required immediate gratification. We might say that in his view, instincts were related to immediate consummatory action, particularly in the areas of fight, flight, feeding, and sexuality, while drives constitute a continuous presence as unconscious motivation and lend themselves to displacement, development, and modification.

In 1923, Freud (1923/1961) established his third and final theory of the relation between drives and affects, now considering affects, particularly anxiety, as ego dispositions, reflecting channels for affect expression and thresholds of affect activation. In short, the relationship between drives and affect became more and more distant in Freud's thinking. This was reflected in the psychoanalytic literature through the 1930s, when Marjorie Brierley (1937/1951) pioneered the awareness that what is being dealt with in the psychoanalytic situation is mostly affect and that psychoanalysis needed to develop a theory of affects and their relation to transference activation.

Throughout all those years, when Freud's second theory of affects, which implied that affects were discharge processes of drives, dominated the psychoanalytic literature, analysts argued about whether it was reasonable to talk about repressed affects. It is of interest that Freud's theory of affects as discharge processes corresponded exactly to what was dominant in the neurobiological theories of affects of that time—namely, the James-Lange theory that postulated that affects were primarily peripheral manifestations of the central nervous system and were only secondarily recognized by the conscious experience of bodily expression of affects that would then imprint the specific nature of the affect (James 1884). This theory was replaced in neurobiological thinking in the 1920s by the Cannon-McDougall theory of affects as central subjective states of which the peripheral neurophysiological manifestations were an expression (Cannon 1927; McDougall 1928). That shift in neurobiological thinking occurred as a parallel development to the psychoanalytic thinking from the 1930s to the 1950s, when Edith Jacobson (1953/1971), in a crucial contribution to psychoanalytic affect theory, proposed that affects were not only discharge states but also part of the structural organization of the intrapsychic life.

Jacobson proposed that affects link the representations of self and objects or rather that they are always activated in the context of the relationship between self-representations and object representations and, as such, constitute the affective expression of drives, while self- and object representations themselves constitute the representational aspect of drives. The radical transformation of Freud's theory regarding the manifestation of drives in the form of affects and representations formulated by Jacobson was not, I believe, fully understood by the psychoanalytic community in the 1950s and 1960s. Jacobson's proposals have only begun to dominate psychoanalytic thinking in the context of new developments in neuropsychology and infant research, the latter, in turn, strongly influenced by psychoanalytic thinking. Jacobson had already proposed that affects were both states of pleasurable and unpleasurable tension and discharge phenomena and that the cognitive aspects of affects always involved self- and object representation. Affects, she proposed, could be differentiated into primitive and elaborate ones that she designated as feelings or emotions. Piaget's (1954/1981) studies of developmental psychology also led to his conclusion that all affects have cognitive implications, in contrast to the traditional separation in academic psychology of affect and cognition. The Cannon-McDougall theory of affects as central subjective states was further developed by Magda Arnold (1970a, 1970b) in the 1960s in her proposal that affects are the basic motivational system consisting of an appraisal of the environment and the desire either to approach rewarding perceptions or to withdraw from aversive or dangerous ones. She tentatively mapped out the brain structures and systems involved in affect activation, linking neuropsychological and neurophysiological developments.

From a completely different neuropsychological orientation, the path-breaking work of Sylvan Tomkins (1970, 1984) led to the

understanding in the 1970s that affects constitute both an amplification system of organismic experiences of pleasure and pain and,
importantly, a communicative system that signals that organismic
state to the environment. Paul Ekman (1984, 1985) elaborated
Tomkins's focus on this crucial function of affect states in a systematic mapping of a broad spectrum of universal facial expressive
patterns of affect states. Rainer Krause (1988, 1990), interested in
the nature of conscious as well as unconscious communication,
particularly in the context of the psychotherapeutic process, systematized the findings regarding facial expressions of affects as
part of the total interpersonal communicative process in normality
and pathology. Krause formulated the proposal that affects constitute a philogenetically recent regulatory system, the biological
function of which is the regulation of the contact between infant
and caretaker, and described the suppression of lower, consummatory action instinctive behaviors by affect activation. He clarified
that communication through the facial motor system and other psychomotor behaviors is constitutionally wired in and also corresponds to an inborn disposition to read such affect expression in
other human beings: mothers can "read" their infant's affect expression without any "learning experience."

In a parallel development of research on affect expression in infants, Izard (1971), Emde (1983), and Stern (1985) described the
typical expression of basic affects in the human infant, particularly
anger or rage, joy or elation, crying or sadness, fear or anxiety, the
startle expression of interest or surprise, the aversive expression of
disgust, and the more complex, later expressions such as those of
pride, shame, guilt, and contempt (Kernberg 1992). Daniel Stern
(1977/2003), in his description of stages in the development of a
subjective self and of intersubjectivity, advanced the study of affect
expression; Emde (1987) saw the mother-infant relationship as a
basic matrix for longitudinally stable patterns of behavior and affects as positive or negative facilitators or inhibitors of such patterns.

Gradually, a complex pattern of affective components has been
described, leading to the contemporary concept of affects as a combination of subjective experiences of pleasure and pain, psychomotor patterns, particular facial expression as a communicative
function, neurovegetative patterns of discharge, and crucial cognitive framing that involves representations of self and others. The
study of normal and pathological attachment initiated by Bowlby
and by Main (1995) helped to further develop our understanding of

the organization of early affective experience and expression, culminating in the proposal by Fonagy and Target (2003). They proposed that mother's capacity for empathic reading of the infant's
affective state determines a congruent, affective response on her
part, combined with "marking" of the infant's affective state, in the
sense of communicating a differentiation between the affective experience of her infant and her own affective state as are the preconditions for normal affective organization in the infant's mind. In
contrast, when either congruence or marking is missing, this leads
to an incapacity of the infant to differentiate and organize his or her
own affect state.

Affect Theory in Contemporary Neurobiology

The advances in the neurophysiological studies of affect development of the 1980s and 1990s have added fundamental knowledge
to this field and possibly permit us at this point to begin linking neurobiology, neuropsychology, and psychoanalytic understanding. As
mentioned before, the neurobiology of affects advanced significantly with the central theories of affect that started with Cannon
and McDougall and then led to Magda Arnold's definition in the
1960s of affects as primary motivational systems. James Papez
focused on the central function of the limbic brain system in the
activation of affects, and although the "Papez circuit" as originally
described was only partially correct, his basic focus on the thala-
mus as center of sensation, the hippocampus as center of memory,
and the hypothalamus as the center of affect activation proved to be
essentially correct (Panksepp 1998). The enormous advances of
this field have focused on particular functions of the various components of the limbic system and related central nervous system
structures.

The existence of both general and highly specialized neurotransmitters related to affect activation, facilitating the activation
and integration of affect-related systems by chemical neurotrans-
mission and of specialized neural centers and circuits dealing with
various affective systems, has expanded our knowledge in depth of
the interaction between neural and neurochemical systems. The
hypothalamus centrally controls homeostatic bodily systems and is
also involved in both positive or rewarding and negative or aversive

affect activation through its respective connection with the mesolimbic region and the periaqueductal gray. The hypothalamus receives multiple somatic information and regulates indirectly the somatic response to affect activation.

From the viewpoint of psychopathology, the amygdala has a central function in the activation of negative affect, the lateral region with the fear response and the medial region with the rage response. Connections between the amygdala and the prefrontal and preorbital cortex and the anterior part of the cingulum that processes cognitive information provide the cognitive context to affect activation, in this case, to negative affect states originated from the amygdala. Connections of the amygdala and of the prefrontal-preorbital regions with the hippocampus provide the contextual affective information that is stored in the hippocampus and, in turn, facilitates the modulation of subsequent affective responses in the light of this affective memory. The neocortex processes both the declarative or semantic memory processed by the thalamic-cortical axis and the affective memory, which, originating from reward and punishment circuits in the hypothalamus, then generates or connects with the specialized areas and systems expressing specific affect states referred to before. What is most important here, from the viewpoint of psychoanalytic affect theory, is the present knowledge of specialized neurobiological systems that specifically, and separately, process positive and negative affects and integrate immediately cognitive contextual and control systems with affective experience: affect and object relations are integrated as part of the process of affect activation.

The brain neurotransmitters include many with global effects, such as the amino acids glutamate and gamma-aminobutyric acid (GABA) and the biogenic amines serotonin, dopamine, and norepinephrine. The most interesting and not yet fully explored neurotransmitters are neuropeptides involved in specific affective responses, such as the thyrotropin-releasing hormone related to arousal and playfulness; adrenocorticotropic hormone (ACTH), involved in stress and attention; oxytocin, involved in male sexual arousal; vasopressin, involved in male sexual arousal, dominance, and social memory; prolactin, involved in maternal motivation and social feelings; luteinizing hormone releasing factor, involved in female arousal; and beta-endorphins, involved in pain, pleasure, and social feelings. It is likely that many of the specific effects of these and other related hormones, yet to be explored, will yield important understanding.

In summarizing our present knowledge about the interaction of the central nervous system's structures and neurotransmitter systems, Panksepp (1998) has described the following major neurochemical maps of the brain: 1) the stress response, mediated through the HPA system (the hypothalamic-pituitary-adrenal cortical circuit) involved in stress response and attachment; 2) the appetitive motivational system, which includes the opioid and dopamine systems related to pleasurable experience, the hypothalamic control system (both the reward-seeking system of the lateral hypothalamus and the homeostatic detectors of the medial hypothalamus), the serotonin-dominated activity and intensity of rage response, and the related testosterone system, all of which are mediated by lateral and medial hypothalamic centers: the medial amygdala is central in the activation of the rage response; 3) the fear system, activated by the lateral amygdala, while rage is centrally determined and controlled and then is related to the hypothalamic centers and periaqueductal gray; there are separate circuits for anxiety and panic, reflecting a different reaction in fearful anxiety and separation anxiety; and 4) the neural control of sexuality, related to stimuli emerging from limbic brain areas, including the septal area, the stria terminalis, and the preoptic area, all of which converge through the anterior hypothalamus into the medial forebrain bundle of the lateral hypothalamus. The neuropeptides vasopressin and oxytocin have influence on the sexual response in a different way in males and females, and, as mentioned before, affective memory regarding sexual affects and experiences stored in the hippocampus powerfully influences the sexual response.

In summary, while the frontal areas, the prefrontal and preorbital cortex, are the planning cortex areas related to the working memory that integrates affects and perception of the present environment of the organism, the amygdala is central in the activation of affects, particularly negative affects that dominate in psychopathology and, through its connection with cortex and hippocampus, leads to the storage of affective memory in the hippocampus.

Toward an Encounter of Psychoanalysis and Neurobiology

The implications of these developments in the neurobiological understanding of affect activation for psychoanalytic theory and psychoanalytic understanding of psychopathology are fundamental. To begin, there is evidence that genetic disposition toward abnormality of the major neurotransmitters, particularly the serotonergic, dopaminergic, and noradrenergic systems, will influence not only affect development but also psychopathology in general. A generalized decrease of functioning of the serotonergic system is related to excessive aggressive affect and self-directed aggression. Silbersweig, director of the neuroimaging program at the Department of Psychiatry of the Weill Cornell Medical College, working with the research program on borderline personality disorder at the Personality Disorders Institute of that department, found in his functional magnetic resonance imaging studies that borderline patients present a hyperactive amygdala response when confronted with affectively negative semantic stimuli and, a first discovery in our neuroimaging laboratory, a primary inhibited response of the prefrontal area related to cognitive control of activated affect (Silbersweig et al. 2007). This indicates a neurobiological predisposition, in borderline patients, to both excessive aggressive affect activation and a primary inhibition of cognitive framing of activated affect.

In a randomized controlled trial comparing dialectic behavior therapy (DBT); transference-focused psychotherapy (TFP), a specific psychoanalytic psychotherapy for borderline patients developed at our institute; and supportive psychotherapy based on psychoanalytic theory, all three treatments manualized and carried out by experts in these respective fields, we found that only TFP improved reflective functioning. That is, we found a significant increase in the capacity for differentiated conceptualization of self and object representations, an awareness of mental experiences in the self and in others, and the capacity to reflect about them in the TFP treatment condition. This specific effect of psychoanalytic psychotherapy was accompanied by an increased capacity to maintain cognitive sets and a reduction of impulsivity in carrying out motor tasks evaluated by neuropsychological tests, suggesting specific neurobiological effects of psychoanalytic psychotherapy (Clarkin et al. 2001, 2005).

From the viewpoint of psychoanalytic theory, the genetically determined and constitutionally given capacity to react affectively to bodily and environmental stimuli, with separate affective systems for pleasurable and aversive affect development, indicates the biological basis for the overall classification of the affective system into positive or rewarding and negative or aversive affects. The fact that separate emotional systems are neurobiologically determined by specific integration of neurotransmitters and brain structures points to the original biological independence of primary affects; for example, the separate systems for panic-separation and for fear-anxiety, as well as those for joyful socialization and for sexual excitement. These data provide the basis for a developmental model of the original affective dissociation into a positive or rewarding and a negative or aversive affective memory system and the later affective integration that gives rise to the complex emotions under the effect of overall psychological development. The immediate integration of affect into a cognitive context provides the neurobiological basis for the contemporary psychoanalytic theory of attachment and, even more importantly, points to the indissoluble integration of affect and cognition from the beginning of life.

This brings me, finally, to my own theoretical developments regarding the place of affect theory in contemporary psychoanalytic thinking. What follows is a summary of my present views of this subject.

I start from contemporary instinct theory in the biological sciences, particularly the work of Lorenz, Tinbergen, and Wilson (Krause 1990), conceptualizing instincts as the overall organization of behavior patterns involving hardwired instinctive patterns of perception and motor behavior that are organized by the activation of trigger mechanisms released under changing environmental stimuli. These instinctive dispositions are inborn behavior patterns common to the species, and their sequential integration and overall organization depend on the experience of the individual animal. Transferring this conceptualization to the psychoanalytic concept of drives, it needs to be stressed that Freud had a clear sense of the differences between biological instincts, common to the species, that are discontinuous and lead to immediate consummatory behavior, on the one hand, and drives, that he considered as highly individualized, continuous, occupying a space in between body and mind, and characterized by developmental features and integration of partial drives, on the other. It is true, of course, that he referred mostly to libido, and his theory was never fully worked out for aggression.

I have proposed that affects are the hardwired, instinctive components that are organized under the influence of intrapsychic developments into two overall drives as hierarchically supraordinate intrapsychic motivational systems, namely, libido and the death drive. The integration of all positive or rewarding affects into libido and of all the negative or aversive affects into the aggressive drive would then determine the overall motivational system that is involved in unconscious intrapsychic conflict and constitutes the dominant motivational system of psychological functioning in normality and pathology (Kernberg 1992, 2004).

I need to add that, regarding the concept of the death drive, I have proposed that the original function of the aggressive drive is related to the unconscious need to destroy, induce suffering, and control bad internal and external objects and that only when, under pathological conditions, this drive is directed mostly against the self would it deserve the name of the death drive. This view is consonant, I believe, with André Green's (1993) recent formulations regarding the death drive and its characteristic tendency toward deobjectivization. My view of the relation between affects and drives also is close to the formulations of Rainer Krause (1998) within affect theory; to Serge Lebovici (Lebovici and Soulé 1977), on the basis of his infant-mother observations; and to Laplanche (1992), who has described the transformation of body surface eroticism into the unconscious erotic aspects of the mother-infant relationship under the influence of mother's "enigmatic" messages.

This formulation of the relationship between affects and drives must be complemented with consideration of the immediate integration of affect states, from birth on, into the relationship between self and object, the dyadic and triadic object relations from the beginning of life. I have proposed that the cognitive contextualization of affect states is precisely their integration into a perceived relation between self and other, with the subsequent internalization of that relationship within the frame of the corresponding affect. This determines the nature of the storage of affective memories, particularly in the hippocampus and, progressively, also in the declarative conscious and preconscious memory system related to the thalamic-neocortical system. Here I started from Edith Jacobson's (1953/1971, 1964) affect theory, complemented by the British object relations theories of Fairbairn (1954) and Melanie Klein (1946, 1952).

While Fairbairn systematically described the organization of intrapsychic structures on the basis of libidinal and antilibidinal self and object relationships, Melanie Klein provided, I believe, the most comprehensive analysis of the early stage of development, which precedes the capacity for integration of idealized and persecutory "all good" and "all bad" internalized object relations, namely, the paranoid-schizoid position, and the later stage of integration of these idealized and persecutory object relationships, the depressive position, with the consequent consolidation of the tripartite structure, brought about by the crystallization of the superego. While none of these major contributors to contemporary object relations theory formulated an integrated view of the transformation of primitive internalized object relations into the tripartite structure of the mind, I believe that such a developmental model flows naturally from the contributions of Fairbairn, Jacobson, and Melanie Klein. I have described in earlier work how ego, superego, and id are constituted by different types of internalized object relations.

Another implication of these formulations is that the deepest layers of psychic experience that will organize the psychic apparatus are represented by peak affect states of a positive or negative quality, in the context of which the deepest aspects of the relationships between self and others are internalized, presumably initially into procedural memory, and only later as declarative or preconscious memory. However, insofar as the activation of peak affect states probably corresponds to early states of consciousness as well, I assume that the deepest layer of human experience had originally preconscious qualities and only gradually are incorporated into the developing system of the id or dynamic unconscious. Insofar as processes of progression and regression may reactivate remnants of these earliest experiences and become condensed with later ones, the characteristic absence of time and space considerations of the id would be a logical consequence of such condensations. In the end, the dynamic unconscious would consist of repressed relations between the self and its objects and, specifically, of desires for specific relationships as well as repressed fears and terror of certain relationships, thus determining unconscious fantasy in its motivational aspect. Edith Jacobson (1964), in her comprehensive analysis of the development of the superego, has spelled out the transformation and integration of internalized object relations into superego and id structures, which she contrasts with the original, undifferentiated ego-id, a point of view that underlies my developmental model as well.

The developmental model presented in my formulations implies the integration of neurochemical and neural substructures at a neurobiological level that, in turn, evolve into more complex neurobiological structures of affects that emerge with an intrapsychic component, the subjective experience of pleasure and unpleasure. This psychic component of affects is integrated with the cognitive, psychomotor, communicative, and neurovegetative features of affects referred to before. Psychic substructures, in turn, such as the specific affects of the libidinal and the aggressive series, are integrated, on the basis of symbolic processes, into the overall motivational systems of the dual drives. At the same time, self- and object representations are integrated, on the basis of similar symbolic processes, into the complex concepts of self and significant others. In short, neurobiological substructures are integrated into broader structures with intrapsychic aspects that, in turn, constitute psychic substructures that are integrated into broader intrapsychic structures.

But all these integrative processes raise major questions that, at present, cannot yet be answered: one of these questions is, what are the neurobiological correlates of such development of ever more complex intrapsychic structures?

The pioneering work of Gerhard Roth (2001) has proposed that the concept of self is constituted by several components that develop in different maturational stages, such as the fundamental reflection regarding one's position in space, the organization of the body image, the procedural and the declarative memory of past experiences, the linguistic memory, and the perception of self as a reflecting agency. All of these aspects of the subjective self represent processes in different areas of the brain that are activated simultaneously at points of self-reflection. In other words, our very concept of the self, a stable intrapsychic concept under normal conditions, is reflected in the momentary flickering or lightening up of seven or eight brain areas that conjointly provide the neurobiological correlate of that intrapsychic process. The mechanisms by which such an integrated activation may occur, the deepest influence, we might say, of the mind over the body, are yet completely unknown.

Another problem, related particularly to the treatment of posttraumatic stress syndrome, is the extent to which the intrapsychic processes that determine the symbolic elaboration of primitive defensive operations and the advance from the paranoid-schizoid into the depressive position do change the original, traumatic memory structures and their effects on the central nervous system or to what extent they bypass them by higher-level cortical operations that do not touch those first experiences. It seems reasonable to suggest, on the basis of present empirical evidence, that intrapsychic changes mediated by symbolic processes such as psychoanalytic treatment may affect processes and organization at a neurobiological level in the same way as significant alterations in the neurobiological sub-systems represented by neurotransmitters and brain centers pro-foundly affect psychic functioning.

In this context, the psychoanalytic session as a research instru-ment facilitates confirmation of the fact that, in primitive affective outbursts, we do see the full gamut of affective components: sub-jective experience, cognitive implications, facial expression, asso-ciated psychomotor movements, and neurovegetative discharge, while in the case of specific types of psychopathology, primitive unity is secondarily disrupted by defensive processes. These pro-cesses include the repression of the subjective affective experience in the obsessional personality, the repression of the cognitive con-textualization of affect in the hysterical personality, and the general loss of depth of affective quality under conditions of severe destruc-tion of internalized object relations in the case of narcissistic pathol-ogy. And, of course, the dissociation of affects into their primitive, idealizing, and persecutory types under conditions of predomi-nance of splitting and related defensive operations signals the ac-tivation of primary affect states directly related to their original neurobiological organization. More recently, these findings have been expanded by observations of the pathological distortions of af-fective experience in the cases of borderline personality organiza-tion, in which affects that cannot be tolerated intrapsychically are expressed exclusively by their psychomotor and/or neurovegetative aspects, sometimes in violent behavior, while the patient remains blind to the very affective implication of that behavior. Here, we do have illustrations how symbolic experience related to unconscious intrapsychic conflict may distort the very neurobiological structure of affect expression or reactivate its earliest activations. The awareness of the effect of pathological attachment on affect devel-opment gives complementary evidence in this regard.

In conclusion, affect theory is a crucial aspect of psychoanalytic theory and practice that opens the road toward the encounter with the neurobiological studies of affect and thus promises to clarify one of the fundamental boundaries of the relation between body and mind. The study of the development of symbolic cognitive pro-cesses, undoubtedly, is another one of these fundamental bound-aries, and this is also true for the study of consciousness. It is rea-sonable to expect that psychoanalytic advances in these other areas will also contribute to points of encounter with neurobiology for mutual illumination and development of these two basic sciences of the human being. But the development of psychoanalysis as a science cannot rest on the specific instrument of the psychoanalytic treatment alone. It will require basic reorientation and retooling of psychoanalytic education in order to foster the development of psychoanalytic scientists and researchers, new research instruments and methods, and an active and consistent immersion in the developments of the sciences at the boundary of psychoanalysis.

References

Arnold MB: Brain function in emotion: a phenomenological analysis, in Physiological Correlates of Emotion. Edited by Black P. New York, Academic Press, 1970a, pp 261–285

Arnold MB: Perennial problems in the field of emotion, in Feelings and Emotion. Edited by Arnold MB. New York, Academic Press, 1970b, pp 169–185

Bion WR: Second Thoughts: Selected Papers on Psycho-Analysis. New York, Basic Books, 1967

Brierley M: Affects in theory and practice (1937), in Trends in Psychoanalysis. London, Hogarth Press, 1951, pp 43–56

Cannon WB: The James-Lange theory of emotions: a critical examination and an alternative theory. Am J Psychol 39:106–124, 1927

Clarkin JF, Foelsch PA, Levy KN, et al: The development of a psychodynamic treatment for patients with borderline personality disorder: a preliminary study of behavioral change. J Pers Disord 15:487–495, 2001

Clarkin JF, Levy KN, Schiavi JM: Transference focused psychotherapy: development of a psychodynamic treatment for severe personality disorders. Clinical Neurosci Res 4:379–386, 2005

Damasio AR: Descartes' Error: Emotion, Reason, and the Human Brain. New York, Avon Books, 1994

Depue RA, Zald DH: Biological and environmental processes in nonpsychotic psychopathology: a neurobehavioral perspective, in Basic Issues in Psychopathology. Edited by Costello CG. New York, Guilford, 1993, pp 127–237

Ekman P: Expression and the nature of emotion, in Approaches to Emotion. Edited by Scherer KR, Ekman P. Hillsdale, NJ, Erlbaum, 1984, pp 319–343

Ekman P: Telling Lies: Clues to Deceit. New York, WW Norton, 1985

Emde RN: The prerepresentational self and its affective core. Psychoanal Study Child 38:165–192, 1983

Emde RN: Development terminable and interminable. Plenary Presentation at the 35th International Psychoanalytical Congress, Montreal, Canada, July 27, 1987

Fairbairn WRD: An Object Relations Theory of the Personality. New York, Basic Books, 1954

Fonagy P, Target M: Psychoanalytic Theories: Perspectives From Developmental Psychopathology. Philadelphia, PA, Whurr, 2003, pp 270–282

Freud S: Instincts and their vicissitudes (1915), in Standard Edition of the Complete Psychological Works of Sigmund Freud, Vol 14. Translated and edited by Strachey J. London, Hogarth Press, 1957, pp 111–116

Freud S: The ego and the id (1923), in Standard Edition of the Complete Psychological Works of Sigmund Freud, Vol 19. Translated and edited by Strachey J. London, Hogarth Press, 1961, pp 12–66

Green A: Conceptions of affect (1977), in On Private Madness. London, Hogarth, 1986, pp 174–213

Green A: Le travail du négatif. Paris, Les Editions de Minuit, 1993

Izard CE: The Face of Emotion. New York, Appleton-Century-Crofts, 1971

Jacobson E: The Self and the Object World. New York, International Universities Press, 1964

Jacobson E: On the psychoanalytic theory of affects (1953), in Depression: Comparative Studies of Normal, Neurotic, and Psychotic Conditions. New York, International Universities Press, 1971, pp 3–47

James W: What Is an Emotion? Mind 9:188–205, 1884

Kernberg OF: Aggression in Personality Disorders and Perversions. New Haven, CT, Yale University Press, 1992

Kernberg OF: The concept of drive in the light of contemporary psychoanalytic theorizing, in Contemporary Controversies in Psychoanalytic Theory, Techniques, and Their Applications. New Haven, CT, Yale University Press, 2004, pp 48–59

Klein M: Notes on some schizoid mechanisms. Int J Psychoanal 27:99–110, 1946

Klein M: Mourning and its relation to manic-depressive states (1940), in Contributions to Psycho-Analysis, 1921–1945. London, Hogarth, 1948, pp 311–338

Klein M: The origins of transference. Int J Psychoanal 33:433–438, 1952

Krause R: [A taxonomy of affect and its use in understanding "early" disorders] (in German). Psychother Psychosom Med Psychol 38:77–86, 1988

Krause R: Psychodynamik der Emotionsstorungen, in Psychologie der Emotion. Göttingen, Germany, Verlag für Psychologie, Dr. C.J. Hogrefe, 1990, pp 630–690

Krause R: Allegemeine psychoanalytische Krankheitslehre, Vol 2: Modelle. Stuttgart, Germany, Kohlhammer, 1998

Laplanche J: Seduction, Translation, Drives. Edited by Fletcher J, Stanton M. Translated by Stanton M. London, Institute of Contemporary Arts, 1992

Lebovici S, Soulé M: La connaissance de l'enfant par la psychanalyse, 3 édition. Paris, PUF, Coll Le Fil Rouge, 1977

Mahler MS, Pine F, Bergman A: The Psychological Birth of the Human Infant. New York, Basic Books, 1975

Main M: Recent studies in attachment: overview with selected implications for clinical work, in Attachment Theory: Social, Developmental, and Clinical Perspectives. Edited by Goldberg S, Muir R, Kerr J. Hillsdale, NJ, Analytic Press, 1995, pp 407–474

McDougall W: Emotion and feeling distinguished, in Feelings and Emotions: The Wittenberg Symposium. Edited by Reymert ML. Worcester, MA, Clark University Press, 1928, pp 200–205

Panksepp J: Affective Neuroscience: The Foundations of Human and Animal Emotions. New York, Oxford University Press, 1998

Piaget J: Intelligence and Affectivity (1954). Palo Alto, CA, Annual Review Press, 1981

Rapaport D: On the psychoanalytic theory of affects (1953), in The Collected Papers of David Rapaport. Edited by Gill MM. New York, Basic Books, 1967, pp 476–512

Roth G: Fühlen, Denken, Handeln wie das Gehirn unser Verhalten steuert. Frankfurt, Germany, Suhrkamp, 2001

Silbersweig DA, Clarkin JF, Goldstein M, et al: Failure of frontolimbic inhibitory function in the context of negative emotion in borderline personality disorder. Am J Psychiatry 164:1832–1841, 2007

Stern D: The First Relationship (1977). Cambridge, MA, Harvard University Press, 2003

Stern D: The Interpersonal World of the Infant. New York, Basic Books, 1985

Tomkins SS: Affect, Imagery, Consciousness: The Negative Affects, Vol 2. New York, Springer, 1963

Tomkins SS: Affect as the primary motivational system, in Feelings and Emotions: The Loyola Symposium. Edited by Arnold MB. New York, Academic Press, 1970, pp 101–110

Tomkins SS: Affect theory, in Approaches to Emotion. Edited by Scherer KR, Ekman P. Hillsdale, NJ, Erlbaum, 1984, pp 163–196

Winnicott DW: The Maturational Processes and the Facilitating Environment. New York, International Universities Press, 1965

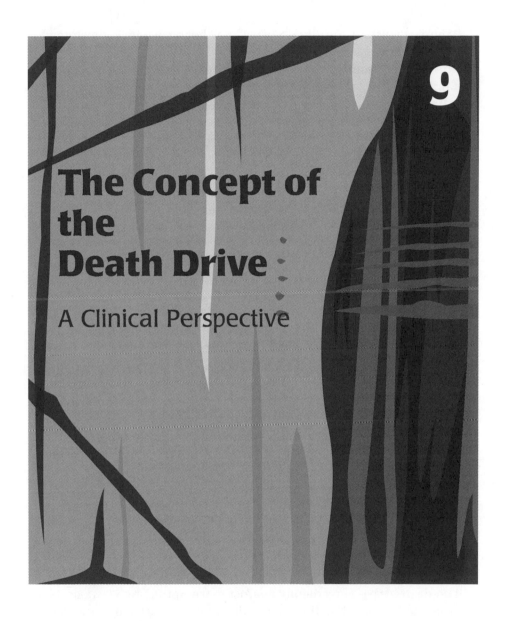

The Concept of the Death Drive

A Clinical Perspective

This chapter was reprinted from Kernberg OF: "The Concept of the Death Drive: A Clinical Perspective." *International Journal of Psychoanalysis* 90:1009–1023, 2009. Used with permission. Copyright 2009 John Wiley and Sons.

Freud's theory of the "death drive" has been seriously questioned within recent psychoanalytic literature and largely rejected outside the psychoanalytic field. From a psychiatric and psychodynamic viewpoint, however, the symptoms he described as clinically reflecting the death drive require further exploration regarding the widely prevalent tendency to self-destruct. The phenomena of repetition compulsion, the syndromes of sadism and masochism, the negative therapeutic reaction, suicide in both severe depression and nondepressed severe personality disorders, and, last but not least, destructive and self-destructive behavior as part of group processes all evince self-destructiveness as a major, sometimes completely domineering, motivational system. In this chapter, I explore these syndromes and their descriptive and dynamic features and conclude that they reflect, indeed, an overwhelming dominance of negative affects organized as self-destructive aggression. These developments justify, in the author's view, the clinical concept of a "death drive," not as an inborn disposition but as the consequence of pathological development of severe aggression, channeled, for developmental reasons, against the self.

I believe that it is quite evident that the two major controversies that have been raised by Freud's monumental discoveries are his theory of libido or the sexual drive and his theory of the death drive, representing, respectively, the struggle between life as centered in erotic impulses and aggression. Freud considered both drives as the fundamental motivational principles determining unconscious conflict and symptom formation (Freud 1920/1955). In a broader sense, they were what drive human beings toward the search for gratification and happiness, on the one hand, and to severely destructive and self-destructive aggression, on the other. Freud's stress on the infantile origins of sexual orientation, infantile sexuality, and particularly its sadomasochistic components has raised shock, opposition, and efforts at denial in the general culture (Freud 1905/1953). The death drive runs deeply against more optimistic views of human nature, based on the assumption that if severe frustrations or trauma were absent in early development then aggression would not be a major human problem.

These perennial cultural reactions toward Freud's theories are mirrored within the psychoanalytic community proper. Recent tendencies, particularly in American psychoanalysis, reflected by the relational approach, tend to deemphasize both infantile sexuality and aggression, in contrast to their centrality in the psychoanalytic focus in European and Latin American psychoanalytic contributions (Kernberg 2001). Additionally, Freud's concept of the death drive has been questioned within American ego psychology, and the debate about whether aggression is primary or a secondary response to trauma and frustration permeates the psychological field widely beyond psychoanalysis proper.

In this chapter, I wish to focus exclusively on the controversies surrounding Freud's theory of the death drive. The affective and symbolic systems that jointly constitute the main components of libido will be explored in Chapter 11. The importance of the controversy regarding the death drive relates directly to the social and cultural problems of the 20th century and the beginning of this new century. The fundamentalist regimes of the last century were unprecedented in their primitive and brutal aggression, both systematic and daily. The tens of millions killed in the name of German National Socialism and Marxist communism are beginning to be replicated under new banners in this century. But no society, no country is free of the history of senseless wholesale massacre of imagined or real enemies. The relative ubiquity of these phenomena throughout the history of civilization cannot be ignored. The question of the existence of the death drive as part of the core of human psychology is, unfortunately, a practical and not merely a theoretical problem (Kernberg 2003a, 2003b).

To begin, regarding Freud's theory of motivation: the study of the unconscious conflicts that patients with neurotic syndromes and character pathology experience led Freud to successive formulations regarding the ultimate drives, culminating in the dual drive theory of libido and the death drive. The practical implication of these proposed two major motivational systems is that, as mentioned before, at the bottom, all unconscious conflicts involve conflicts between love and aggression at some level of development. This, I believe, makes eminent sense clinically and so does Freud's careful warning that the only thing we know about these two drives is their expression in mental representations and affects.

Here begins the problem: Freud had postponed linking psychological functions and structures with underlying neurobiological developments because of the primitive nature of the neurobiology of his time. He expressed the hope, however, that, eventually, more specific relationships between psychological functions and neurobiological developments might become clearer. From today's developments in neurobiological science and advances in our knowledge about instinctive behavior and its organization in mammals, particularly primates, it emerges that the primary motivational systems consist of affects of a positive and negative kind. Affects are primary motivational systems in the sense that their activation, under certain circumstances, by mechanisms of the limbic brain, initiates strong motivation to movement towards other objects or away from them. The entire series of libidinal affects: joyous encounter, euphoria, sensual gratification, and erotic arousal are all directed toward early libidinal objects, while the negative affects of rage, anger, disgust, anxiety, and, later, envy and hatred motivate us to withdraw from dangerous objects or attempt to control or eliminate them (Panksepp 1998). All affects are embedded in mental representations, that is, a cognitive organization of the context in which affects emerge, an emerging definition of the desired objects, as well as of the feared and hated ones, and wishful fantasies toward erotic objects as well as about the elimination of threatening objects. The very fantasies that reflect unconscious conflicts between love and hatred are always representations embedded in respective positive or negative affects.

In the study of patients with severe psychopathology, the borderline conditions, at the Personality Disorders Institute at the Weill Cornell Medical College, we have been able to confirm that borderline patients, who suffer from inordinate aggressive impulses and lack of impulse control—in other words, a strong predominance of negative affects and impulsivity—regularly show hyperactivity of the amygdala, a limbic structure related to the activation of negative affect. They also show a primary inhibition of the dorsolateral prefrontal cortex that is related to cognitive framing of affects and the establishment of priorities of focus, attention, and action following such affective activation (Silbersweig et al. 2007). These and other related findings have been confirmed also in various other centers, so that we are at the beginning of establishing a more direct relationship between neurobiological function and affect activation. But what does all of this say to the theory of drives?

The psychoanalytic community is struggling nowadays with the problem of whether drives should continue to be considered as the primary motivational systems or whether they should be replaced by the consideration of affects as primary motivational systems (Kernberg 2004a). The absence of any biological evidence for the original, primary nature of drives, the abundant evidence for the primary motivational function of affects, and the fact that affects always imply representations at the same time raise the question whether affective representations are the building blocks of more complex human motivational developments, thus replacing the concept of drives. Against such a radical assumption lies the fact that, clinically, the replacement of drive theory by affect theory does not do justice to the stable organization of unconscious conflicts. The multiplicity of affects and the shifting affective relationship to objects and their representations do not lend themselves to meaningful conceptualization of the organization of those conflicts. On the other hand, a pure drive theory that does not consider the specific vicissitudes of affects tends to acquire overgeneralized and rigidly dogmatic aspects that also run counter to clinical experience: to explain unconscious conflict as simple struggles between libido and aggressive drives does not do justice to the complexity of clinical experience.

As I pointed out in Chapter 8, I have proposed, years ago, and am no longer alone in this view, that affects constitute the primary motivational system and that they are integrated into supraordinate positive and negative drives, namely, libido and aggression. The drives, in turn, manifest themselves as activation of their constituent affects with varying intensity, along the line of libidinal and aggressive investments. In short, I believe that affects are the primary motivators. They organize into hierarchically supraordinate motivations, or the Freudian drives, and the drives, in turn, become activated in the form of their component affectively valenced representations manifest as unconscious fantasies (Kernberg 1992).

Within the context of these formulations, I shall propose, in the present chapter, that the concept of the death drive as a designation for the dominant unconscious motivation toward self-destructiveness is warranted in severe cases of psychopathology. I shall question, however, whether severe self-destructive aggression is a primary tendency and propose that the unconscious function of self-destructiveness is not simply to destroy the self but to destroy significant others as well.

It will be noticed that, earlier in this chapter, I have talked about aggression and then aggressive drive rather than the death drive per se. That our patients suffer from conflicts involving love and aggression from their ambivalence toward those they love and need and who gratify and frustrate them, who can never satisfy all desires and sometimes dramatically withhold the gratification of basic psychological needs, seems reasonable enough. We are talking here about aggression secondary to frustration, which conforms with the type of aggression delineated by Freud as arising from the conflict between the pleasure principle and the reality principle.

And the basis of such aggression, mingling with our deepest needs for closeness and love, naturally may be related to the biological disposition to aggression, as inborn as that to love and eroticism, and which we encounter as a common property of all mammals. I am referring to the aggressive dispositions that are a normal mechanism in the defense of the newly born mammal and its early development that requires parental protection; the aggression at the service of territoriality that protects the sources of nutrition; and the aggressive disposition involved in the competition of males for the possession of females. These biologically anchored instincts have the correspondent instinctive dispositions in human beings as well and explain the mechanism of aggression secondary to danger or frustration. But Freud discovered clinical phenomena in which aggression could not be accounted for by mere frustration of the pleasure principle and became an overriding, self-destructive motivation that proved to offer enormous resistances to its modification in psychoanalytic treatment. The clinical experience accumulated, throughout time, on the basis of psychoanalytic practice has added new evidence in support of the prevalence of severely self-destructive psychopathological constellations, indirectly supporting the theory of a death drive.

The phenomena that led Freud to the establishment and, later, to the reinforcement of the hypothesis of the death drive as opposed to a simple aggressive drive include (Freud 1920/1955, 1921/1955, 1923/1961, 1924/1961, 1930/1957):

1. Repetition compulsion;
2. Sadism and masochism;
3. Negative therapeutic reaction;
4. Suicide in severe depression (and in nondepressive characterological structures);
5. Destructive and self-destructive developments in group processes and their social implications.

Let us examine them. First, regarding repetition compulsion, the main clinical constellation referred to by Freud in his original proposal: As the name implies, the patient engages in an endless repetition of the same, usually destructive behavior that resists the interpretation of assumed, and very often well-documented, unconscious conflicts involved. Originally described as a "resistance of the id," a somewhat mysterious force from the dynamic unconscious, clinical experience has demonstrated that repetition compulsion may have multiple functions that have different prognostic implications. Sometimes it is simply the repetitive working through of a conflict that demands patience and gradual elaboration; at other times, it represents the unconscious repetition of a traumatic relationship with a frustrating or traumatizing object, with the hidden hope that "this time" the other will gratify the needs and wishes of the patient, thus being transformed, at last, into the much needed good object. Many unconscious fixations to traumatic situations have this origin, although sometimes they may reflect more primitive neurobiological processes. These primitive processes deal with the incessant rekindling of a very early behavioral chain deeply engrained in the limbic structures and their neural connections with the prefrontal and preorbital cortex. In many cases of posttraumatic stress disorder, we find that repetition compulsion is an effort to come to terms with an originally overwhelming situation. If such a repetition compulsion is tolerated and facilitated in the context of a safe and protective environment, gradual resolution may obtain.

In other cases, however, particularly when posttraumatic stress syndrome is no longer an active syndrome but operates as an etiological factor behind severe characterological distortions, the repetition compulsion may reflect an effort to overcome the traumatic situation by an unconscious identification with the source of the trauma. Here the patient identifies with the perpetrator of the trauma, while projecting on somebody else the function of victim. It is as if the world had become exclusively a relationship between perpetrators and victims, and the patient, unconsciously, repeats the traumatic situation in an effort to reverse the roles and place somebody else in the role of victim (Kernberg 1992, 2004b). The unconscious triumph that such a reversal may provide the patient then maintains repetition compulsion endlessly. There are still more malignant cases of repetition compulsion, such as the unconscious effort to destroy a potentially helpful relationship out of an unconscious sense of triumph over the person who tries to help, who is envied for not having suffered what the patient, in his or her mind, has suffered. It is an unconscious triumph, which, at the same time, coincides, of course, with the defeat of the patient himself or herself.

André Green, a leading contributor to the exploration of severe psychopathologies, has described the unconscious identification with a "dead mother," that is, a severely depressed mother who had chronically frustrated the needs for love and dependency of her infant and child. At the same time, such a mother, desperately needed, cannot be abandoned. The patient, in unconscious identification with a fantasied "dead mother," denies the existence of all live relationships in reality as if the patient him- or herself were dead to the world (Green 1993a, 1993b).

In patients with severe narcissistic pathology, repetition compulsion may have the function of an active destruction of the passage of time, as an expression of denial of aging and death, combined with the triumphant destruction of the work of the envied therapist (see also Chapter 6). That denial, on the surface, reassures the patient and protects against anxiety over his or her self-destructive avoidance of life tasks, including the analytic work. It is a manifestation of what Kleinian authors describe as a destructive narcissistic organization (R. Steiner 2009). Repetition compulsion, in short, provides clinical support to the theory of a relentless self-destructive motivation, one of the sources of the concept of the death drive.

Severe manifestations of sexual sadism and masochism are a second type of a fundamental drive to self-destruct. Cases of sexual perversion, that is, a significant restriction of sexual behavior to a specific interaction that becomes an indispensable condition for sexual excitement and orgasm, may be linked to a dangerously sadistic or masochistic behavior, reflected in severe self-injurious or self-mutilating behavior as a precondition for sexual enjoyment. Inordinate cruelty toward others and inordinate cruelty toward the self often are combined in the most severe cases. Patients with borderline psychopathology often show severe self-mutilation, cutting, burning, and, in the most severe cases, self-mutilation leading to the loss of limbs as a relentless drive, which, at times, causes all therapeutic efforts to fail. The frequent syndrome of anorexia nervosa, particularly in its most severe manifestations, also may correspond to such relentless, irreducible self-destructiveness. The unconscious conflicts of anorectic patients cover a broad spectrum of dynamics: from oedipal rivalry and rebellious protest against mother and unconscious guilt over a girl's developing sexuality to primitive hatred of the patient's own body identified with an extremely sadistic maternal image and the enactment of a self-destructive unconscious omnipotence (Kernberg 2004d).

One clinical syndrome that is particularly difficult to handle is that of perversity (not sexual perversion). Perversity involves the recruitment of love at the service of aggression, the effort to seduce another person toward love or helpfulness as a trap that will end with the destruction, symbolic or real, in a social and sometimes even in a physical sense of the person so seduced (Kernberg 1992). In normal love relationships, small doses of aggression intensify erotic pleasure. However, under pathological conditions, perversity may destroy erotic pleasure and even more so its object. The mildest cases of all these sadomasochistic developments are found in those patients who, because of unconscious guilt, usually related to profoundly forbidden oedipal urges or unconscious aggression to an early object of their dependency needs, destroy what they received. These developments are easier to understand and to treat; here self-destructiveness has the function of the "price" that must be paid in order to permit a gratifying relationship to develop and does not have the primary function of destruction of a potentially good relationship.

This brings us to the third type of manifestation of severe self-directed aggression, namely, the negative therapeutic reaction. Freud described one type of negative therapeutic reaction in his clinical observation of patients who appeared to get worse under conditions when they experienced a helpful intervention by the analyst, as an expression of unconscious guilt over being helped (Freud 1923/1961). Negative therapeutic reaction out of unconscious guilt is, in effect, the mildest form of this reaction. A much more frequent and more severe, although eminently treatable, form is the negative therapeutic reaction out of unconscious envy of the therapist, particularly characteristic of narcissistic patients. It is an expression of the humiliating envy on the part of the narcissistic patient of the therapist's capacity to help him or her and of the analyst's creativity in efforts to help the patient.

There is still an even more severe form of negative therapeutic reaction, and this one has the unmistakable signs of a highly motivated self-destructiveness, namely, an unconscious identification with an extremely sadistic object, so that it is as if the patient felt that the only real relationship he or she may have is with somebody who destroys him or her. This dynamic constellation is prevalent in the case of patients presenting severe self-mutilating behavior. One patient successively cut off segments of fingers of her hands and severed major nerves in one arm: she presented the syndrome of malignant narcissism, and her psychoanalytic psychotherapy was carried out, in part, during extended hospitalizations. She was not psychotic at any point. In the transference, the identification with an extreme aggressive and incestuous paternal image was a dominant element. It is difficult to understand this development from a position of ordinary common sense, but there are patients who relentlessly provoke the analyst until the analyst succumbs to an uncontainable negative countertransference reaction. The analyst, maneuvered into a countertransference enactment, manifests some negative behavior to which the patient triumphantly responds with further escalation of provocative self-destructive behavior. Very often these treatments end precipitously, leaving the therapist with a sense of impotence, frustration, and guilt feelings.

These patients represent severe borderline conditions and what I have described as the syndrome of malignant narcissism; that is, patients with severe narcissistic features, paranoid tendencies, ego-syntonic aggression against self and others, and antisocial behavior. These patients may utilize the treatment as a perversely gratifying form of self-destruction because they draw others into their deadly self-attacks. One of our patients presenting this syndrome repeatedly consumed rat poison, which interferes with blood clotting, to the extent of provoking severe internal hemorrhages, while she smilingly denied to her therapist and to the staff that she had done so. Even hospitalized, and with the prothrombin time extending by the day, and careful searches by the nursing staff, we were not able to control the self-mutilating behavior and the pleasurable nature with which this patient expressed it, to the extent that, finally, she was transferred for custodial care to another institution.

A fourth type of severe self-destructive impulse is reflected in suicidal urges and behavior. Freud considered suicidal tendencies in melancholia as another expression of the death drive. He described the essential mechanism of this development as the introjection of an ambivalently loved and lost object that then would draw the aggression toward that object into the ego, which is now identified with the lost object. Although Freud (1917 [1915]/1957) had originally explained suicide in melancholia as a result of turning hatred of the lost object inward, after the formulation of his dual drive theory (1920/1955), he revised his view in *The Ego and the Id* (1923/1961, p. 53), stating about melancholia: "What is now holding sway in the super-ego is, as it were, a pure culture of the death instinct, and in fact it often enough succeeds in driving the ego into death, if the latter does not fend off its tyrant in time by the change round into mania."

The work of Melanie Klein showed that such ambivalence is a normal aspect of all love relationships (Klein 1940, 1957). She described the task of the depressive position in overcoming the split between positive, idealized internalized relations with the object and aggressively invested and projected relations with the object of a persecutory type. She described, in short, the normal integration between split-off idealized and paranoid relationships as part of normal development, the depressive position, in contrast to the earlier, splitting dominated paranoid schizoid position. This integration, Melanie Klein proposed convincingly, constitutes a normal early developmental phase, repeated in all later mourning processes, so that in all losses there is not only the loss of an external object, and the working through of that loss by its internalization, but also a reactivation of the depressive position with the working through of ambivalences toward all earlier object losses. In short, normal ambivalence is an unavoidable aspect of all mourning reactions.

It is only under conditions of severe aggressive, particularly unconsciously aggressive, impulses towards the lost object when the pathology of the depressive position evolves in the form of relentless self-attacks now derived from the internalization of aggressive aspects of the object into the superego and an attack on the self from the superego and the simultaneous identification of the object with the ego or the self. This combination leads to potentially severely dangerous and very often actualized suicidal tendencies. But we do find such self-destructive suicidal behavior also in patients who are not depressed, precisely in severe narcissistic personalities. Here a sense of defeat, failure, humiliation, and, in essence, the loss of their grandiosity may bring about not only feelings of extremely devastating shameful defeat and inferiority but also a compensatory sense of triumph over reality by taking their own life, thus demonstrating to themselves and to the world that they are not afraid of pain and death. To the contrary, death emerges as an even elegant abandonment of a depreciated, worthless world (Kernberg 2007; Chapter 5 in this volume).

We have seen that severe self-destructive psychopathology warrants the clinical assumption of powerful, sometimes uncontrollable self-destructive impulses reflected in the phenomena of repetition compulsion, sadism and masochism, negative therapeutic reaction, and suicide, both in severe depression and in other forms of psychopathology. But, in addition, Freud described severe self-destructiveness as a social phenomenon in the behavior of large social group processes, in human masses as ideologically united conglomerates, in mutual identification with a grandiose and aggressive leader (Freud 1921/1955). In this process, the group projects their individual superego functions onto the group leader, with the consequence of group-sanctioned expression of primitive, ordinarily suppressed impulses, particularly of an aggressive type. A mass movement may coalesce around a drive to search and destroy enemy formations, the sense of power derived from their liberated, now focused aggression; their sense of protected dependency by their allegiance to the leader; and the regression to the most primitive dissociation of object relations into idealized and persecutory ones. This development represented for Freud the activation of severe destructiveness at a social level. The projection of the superego onto the leader, the mutual identification of all participants with him or her, as well as the sanctioned expression of aggression are the fundamental explanation for the aggressive behavior of mass movements and large social structures, applying even to international conflict. But the aggression activated in regressive group processes may also be channeled onto the group itself, guided by a grandiose, self-destructive leader, ending in a religiously or ideologically rationalized mass suicide.

Freud's theory of mass psychology, dramatically demonstrated in a thousand forms in the mass psychology of the fundamentalist movements of the last century, has been complemented by Bion's (1961) work with small groups of ten to fifteen individuals and Pierre Turquet's (1975) and Didier Anzieu's (1981) work with large groups of 100–150 individuals. I do not have space here to describe in detail all these findings (for a fuller discussion, see Chapter 16) but would summarize them by stating that when small or large groups are unstructured, that is, without a clear task and its corresponding structure relating that group constructively to its environment, and when, in contrast, the only task of such groups is meeting to study their own reactions for, say, an hour and a half during a sequence of several days or a few weeks, they present striking and similar phenomena. They show the immediate activation of intense anxiety and an effort to escape that anxiety by some soothing ad hoc philosophy expounded by a friendly, mediocre, grandfatherly leader who calms down the group's anxiety with clichés. When this effort fails, they show a tendency to the development of intense violence, the search for a paranoid leader, and the division of the group itself or its perception of the surrounding social environment into an idealized and a persecutory one, with active aggression directed against what is perceived as the hostile segment of the world in order to protect the perfection and the security of the ideal group.

Vamik Volkan (2004), who has applied psychoanalytic theory to the study of intergroup and international conflicts, has expanded these observations by systematically studying the nature of the ideal world of fundamentalist groups, the reason for their need to search for and destroy enemies, their strivings to preserve rigid boundaries and the purity of their group, and the obvious connection between these categories and fundamentalist political, racial, and religious movements. In conclusion of this point, there is impressive clinical and sociological evidence for a universal potential for violence in human beings that can be triggered too easily under certain conditions of group regression and corresponding leadership and that, from the perspective of survival of human societies, may be considered as fundamentally self-destructive.

These are the leading clinical arguments in support of Freud's theory of the death drive. Freud also attempted to link it to biological disposition to self-destruction, tracing a parallel of the psychological attraction of the "nirvana principle" with the physiological mechanisms of self-destruction in biology. In effect, the biological function of apoptosis, the controlled orders for self-destruction of certain cells, may be seen as one illustration of such a biological mechanism. While it may be tempting to explain psychological functions by analogical ones from biology, this runs the risk of reductionism by relating complex phenomena at widely different structural levels to each other. What we do have is the powerful clinical evidence for severe, relentless self-destructiveness in many cases of psychopathology. If anything, the experience with severe types of character pathology and the borderline conditions in the last thirty years has given even further evidence to the fundamental nature of deep self-destructive tendencies in human beings that clinically would support the concept of a death drive.

If we accept that severe self-destructiveness functions as a major motivational system, we may explore, from this perspective, the concept of the death drive. In my view, one solution to this theoretical challenge is a combination of several conclusions. First, if death drive is a designation for the dominant unconscious motivation toward self-destructiveness in severe cases of psychopathology, this concept is, undoubtedly, warranted. Second, severe self-destructive aggression, however, is not a primary tendency, as far as we can tell, but a particularly grave, organized motivational system that is not simply "secondary to trauma," although it may be influenced and stimulated by traumatic experience. Third, the unconscious functions of self-destructiveness are not simply to destroy the self but, very essentially, to destroy significant others as well, be it out of guilt, revenge, envy, or triumph.

Exploring jointly the clinical constellations that reflect most clearly the dominance of self-destructive impulses, they all reveal intrapsychic struggles between internalized sadistic representations of objects and masochistically submitting representations of self. Internalized sadistic object representations may represent both projected and reintrojected aggressive impulses and realistic traumatic experiences, while masochistic self-representation may represent a combination of erotization of painful, traumatic experiences and unconscious guilt-induced expiational suffering. In the case of repetition compulsion, I have referred to the unconscious identification with perpetrator and victim of a traumatic past, the unconscious identification with a "dead mother," and the triumph over a potentially helpful yet envied object by destruction of the self. In the cases of sadomasochistic pathology, the strong predominance of aggressive conflicts may turn the internalized relation with a sadistic object into overwhelming self-destructiveness. In the case of negative therapeutic reaction, the spectrum of self-directed aggression may vary from the superego-induced attacks on the self in better integrated patients to the primitive intrapsychic relationship with a battering object of dependency. Freud and Melanie Klein's clarification of the psychopathology of suicidal depression first pointed to the self-destructive consequence of a sadistic superego. So that what is sought in self-destructive motivation is not simply "nirvana" but active destruction of significant libidinal relationships with significant others.

In short, aggression as a major motivational system is always present in the mind, based on the integration of primary negative affects, but I propose that it deserves the designation of death drive only when such aggression becomes dominant, when it recruits libidinal impulses such as in the syndrome of perversity, and when its main objective is, to use André Green's (1993a) terms, the achievement of "de-objectalization," the elimination of the representations of all significant others and, in that context, the elimination of the self as well. The death drive, I propose, is not a primary drive but represents a significant complication of aggression as a major motivational system, is central in the therapeutic work with severe psychopathology, and as such is eminently useful as a concept in the clinical realm.

What determines whether aggression will be predominantly structured into internalized object relations that direct it externally or against the individual's own body or mind? Under what circumstances will self-directed aggression become the dominant unconscious motivational system? I believe we have only partial answers to these questions at this time. There is evidence for genetically determined and constitutionally given dominance of negative affect activation and for inadequate cognitive contextualization of affect, expressed in temperamental dispositions that influence the internalization of early object relations. Insecure attachment may significantly contribute to a disposition for predominantly negative affect activation. Traumatic experiences in infancy and childhood and severely disorganized family structures are clearly related to severe personality disorders with self-destructive tendencies (J. Paris, "Childhood Adversities and Borderline Personality Disorder," unpublished manuscript, 2009). But some patients with severe self-destructive tendencies do not evince such a background. Clinically, however, in those latter cases, as well as in the most severe cases of major self-destructiveness, we typically find narcissistic personality disorders—the apparently milder, self-assured, grandiose kind and the most regressed, aggression-infiltrated, pathological grandiose self of the syndrome of malignant narcissism (Kernberg 1992), the cases that Kleinian authors describe as destructive narcissism (Britton 2003; R. Steiner 2009) or pathological organization (J. Steiner 1993) and Green as negative narcissism (1983) and de-objectalization (1993a). In short, a combination of intensity of aggressive affect and the particular structuralization of internalized object relations of narcissistic personalities emerge as leading aspects of the malignant transformation of aggression into a dominant motivation for self-destruction.

The self-destructiveness of melancholia, its superego-determined suicidal tendencies, constitutes a special case, again illustrating the influence of both genetically and environmentally determined hyperreactivity of depressive affect activation and the importance of a particular structuralization of internalized object relations, namely, the pathological superego of these patients (Panksepp 1998).

This brings us, of course, to the question of the therapeutic implications of this conceptualization: where do we stand, and what has psychoanalysis achieved in this regard? Under the influence of contemporary object relations theory, psychoanalytic structural theory has evolved into the analysis of the building blocks of ego, superego, and id; namely, their constituent internalized relationships with significant others that are integrated in the form of primitive, affectively determined representations of self and significant others or objects (Kernberg 2004c). I have proposed that dyadic representations of self and others, under the dominance of a particular affective valence, are internalized as a parallel series of positive and negative internalized object relations. They consolidate according to their specific function into superego structures when they have a commanding or prohibitive quality, into ego structures when they correspond to potentially conscious and preconscious identifications and the organization of character formations, and into id structures when such internalized object relations correspond to primitive, aggressive or erotic, fantasied, desired, and feared relations with objects that cannot be tolerated in consciousness.

The importance of this reformulation of the psychic structures in terms of the internalization of object relations resides in the fact that in the most primitive types of structures that we find in severe psychopathologies, such early split idealized and persecutory object relations dominate the transferential field rather than the manifestations of mature ego and superego functions, and the treatment has to be centered in the analysis of each of these dyadic units as they emerge in the transference. Regarding our understanding of these psychopathologies, perhaps the greatest advance in recent years has been in the treatment of severe character pathologies, particularly narcissistic and the borderline conditions.

In typical cases of predominantly self-destructive efforts in the transference, behind what appears to be a disdainful rejection and ruthless tearing apart of the analyst's interpretative interventions, the problem is not a simple manifestation of the death drive but its reflection in an internalized object relation between a sadistic, murderous object representation and a submissive, paralyzed representation of self that enters into collusion with the aggressor. It is the collusive aspect of the self that, at first, becomes evident in the patient's manifest ignoring of the analyst's interventions and the lack of concern for himself or herself. The unconscious pleasure in the defeat of the analyst, out of hate or envy, emerges more slowly in the transference situation. The analyst's tolerance of such regressive transferences is the key to their eventual resolution.

Our application of psychoanalytic principles to the descriptive and structural characteristics of these patients has permitted a clearer indication of differential treatments based on a psychoanalytic modality.

It is important to diagnose early syndromes in which severe self-destructive aggression may dominate. These include particularly the syndrome of the "dead mother" that I referred to and the syndrome of malignant narcissism; severe ego-syntonic aggression manifests in arrogance, perversity, and identification with a sadistic superego, as well as self-destructive behavior that affects patients' survival in their social environment (Kernberg 1992, 2004b, 2007). With these cases, it would seem essential to analyze the developments of such self-aggressive tendencies in the transference from the very beginning of the treatment, with particular attention paid to tendencies to destroy what is provided by the analyst and to whatever hope the patient may have for the survival of the therapist in spite of the patient's aggression. It may become important to structure the treatment, in the sense of assuring the stability of its boundaries. We have learned how to prevent severe, physical acting out of aggression that would threaten the treatment boundaries by careful initial contract setting and to analyze any countertransferential deviation from technical neutrality, that is, from the normal attitude of concerned objectivity of the analyst as a result of intensively hostile transferences.

It may become particularly important to explore the pleasure in the patient's aggression against the self and others. In this regard, we might say that the death drive is not inconsistent with the pleasure principle, as evidenced by the triumphant pleasure these patients get in defeating all efforts to help them. I have suggested in earlier work (Kernberg 1992) that it is important to transform psychopathic transferences, in which the patient manifests dishonesty or dangerous withholding, and perverse transferences, in which the patient tries to recruit the benign efforts of the therapist for malignant purposes. We have to transform these psychopathic transferences into paranoid ones, that is, to analyze why the patient has to behave in a deceptive way to avoid deep fear and suspiciousness of the analyst, onto whom such aggressive impulses are projected. Full development of paranoid transferences is the first step to a gradual recognition of the projection, the acknowledgment of the origin of aggression in oneself, and the development of depressive transferences, that is, transferences in which, under the influence of the development of guilt feelings related to the recognition of his or her own aggression, the patient may be able to integrate and elaborate his or her aggressive tendencies.

In some cases, one needs to be alert to both absence of affects and absence of representations in what may appear to be "pure" affects, so that both affect storms, on the one hand, and apparent total absence of affect have to be explored systematically to unveil the underlying activated object relations. Some cases with extended therapeutic stalemates in reality are deadly repetitions of self-destructive efforts to escape conflicts and to deny the passage of time. There are times when, under the influence of extreme aggressive impulses and their projection, the reality testing of the patient decreases. The patient may develop micropsychotic episodes in the sessions, and it may become important for the analyst to spell out the existence of incompatible realities in which patient and analyst live, how to understand them, and how to resolve them.

In short, an object relations perspective on the predominance of severely self-destructive transferences has provided analytic tools to treat such patients and, we might say, has become a major front on the struggle to apply psychoanalytic principles to this area of most challenging and prognostically reserved cases. Whether the growing psychoanalytic understanding of aggressive and self-aggressive behavior of large groups and its relation to regressive processes in the social realm will lead to a contribution of their prevention and management remains to be seen. In conclusion, Freud's dramatic concept of the death drive may not reflect an inborn disposition as such but is eminently relevant in clinical practice.

References

Anzieu D: Le Groupe et l' Inconscient: l' Imaginaire groupal. Paris, Dunod, 1981

Bion WR: Experiences in Groups. New York, Basic Books, 1961

Britton R: Sex, Death, and the Superego. London, Karnac Books, 2003

Freud S: Three essays on the theory of sexuality, I: the sexual aberrations (1905), in The Standard Edition of the Complete Psychological Works of Sigmund Freud, Vol 7. Translated and edited by Strachey J. London, Hogarth Press, 1953, pp 135–172

Freud S: Mourning and melancholia (1917[1915]), in The Standard Edition of the Complete Psychological Works of Sigmund Freud, Vol 14. Translated and edited by Strachey J. London, Hogarth Press, 1957, pp 237–260

Freud S: Beyond the pleasure principle (1920), in The Standard Edition of the Complete Psychological Works of Sigmund Freud, Vol 18. Translated and edited by Strachey J. London, Hogarth Press, 1955, pp 1–64

Freud S: Group psychology and the analysis of the ego (1921), in The Standard Edition of the Complete Psychological Works of Sigmund Freud, Vol 18. Translated and edited by Strachey J. London, Hogarth Press, 1955, pp 65–143

Freud S: The ego and the id (1923), in The Standard Edition of the Complete Psychological Works of Sigmund Freud, Vol 19. Translated and edited by Strachey J. London, Hogarth Press, 1961, pp 12–66

Freud S: The economic problem of masochism (1924), in The Standard Edition of the Complete Psychological Works of Sigmund Freud, Vol 19. Translated and edited by Strachey J. London, Hogarth Press, 1961, pp 155–170

Freud S: Civilization and its discontents (1930), in The Standard Edition of the Complete Psychological Works of Sigmund Freud, Vol 21. Translated and edited by Strachey J. London, Hogarth Press, 1957, pp 57–145

Green A: Narcissism de vie, narcissism de mort. Paris, Les Editions de Minuit, 1983

Green A: Le travail du négatif. Paris, Les Editions de Minuit, 1993a

Green A: On Private Madness. Madison, CT, International Universities Press, 1993b

Kernberg OF: Aggression in Personality Disorders and Perversion. New Haven, CT, Yale University Press, 1992

Kernberg OF: Recent developments in the technical approaches of English-language psychoanalytic schools. Psychoanal Q 70:519–547, 2001

Kernberg OF: Sanctioned social violence: a psychoanalytic view, part I. Int J Psychoanal 84:683–698, 2003a

Kernberg OF: Sanctioned social violence: a psychoanalytic view, part II. Int J Psychoanal 84:953–968, 2003b

Kernberg OF: The concept of drive in the light of contemporary psychoanalytic theorizing, in Contemporary Controversies in Psychoanalytic Theory, Technique, and Their Applications. New Haven, CT, Yale University Press, 2004a, pp 48–59

Kernberg OF: Hatred as a core affect of aggression, in Aggressivity, Narcissism, and Self-Destructiveness in the Psychoanalytic Process: New Developments in the Psychopathology and Psychotherapy of Severe Personality Disorders. New Haven, CT, Yale University Press, 2004b, pp 27–44

Kernberg OF: Psychoanalytic object relations theory, in Contemporary Controversies in Psychoanalytic Theory, Techniques, and Their Applications. New Haven, CT, Yale University Press, 2004c, pp 26–47

Kernberg OF: A technical approach to eating disorders in patients with borderline personality organization, in Aggressivity, Narcissism, and Self-Destructiveness in the Psychoanalytic Process: New Developments in the Psychopathology and Psychotherapy of Severe Personality Disorders. New Haven, CT, Yale University Press, 2004d, pp 205–219

Kernberg OF: The almost untreatable narcissistic patient. J Am Psychoanal Assoc 55:503–539, 2007

Klein M: Mourning and it relation to manic-depressive states, in Contributions to Psycho-Analysis, 1921–1945. London, Hogarth Press, 1940, pp 311–338

Klein M: Envy and Gratitude. New York, Basic Books, 1957

Panksepp J: Affective Neuroscience: The Foundations of Human and Animal Emotions. New York, Oxford University Press, 1998

Silbersweig D, Clarkin JF, Goldstein M, et al: Failure of frontolimbic inhibitory function in the context of negative emotion in borderline personality disorder. Am J Psychiatry 164:1832–1841, 2007

Steiner J: Psychic Retreats: Pathological Organization in Psychotic, Neurotic, and Borderline Patients. London, Routledge, 1993

Steiner R: On narcissism: the Kleinian approach. Psychiatr Clin North Am 12:741–770, 2009

Turquet P: Threats to identity in the large group, in The Large Group: Dynamics and Therapy. Edited by Kreeger L. London, Constable, 1975, pp 87–144

Volkan V: Blind Trust: Large Groups and Their Leaders in Times of Crisis and Terror. Charlottesville, VA, Pitchstone Publishers, 2004

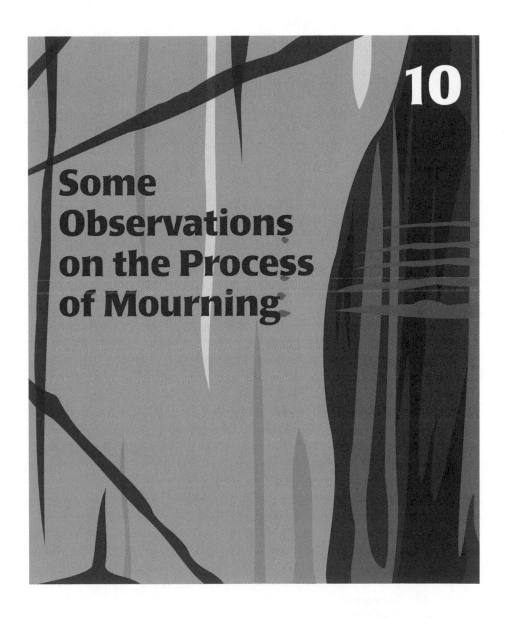

Some Observations on the Process of Mourning

10

This chapter was reprinted from Kernberg OF: "Some Observations on the Process of Mourning." *International Journal of Psychoanalysis* 91:601–619, 2010. Used with permission. Copyright 2010 John Wiley and Sons.

In this chapter, I explore the dynamics of the normal mourning process; that is, grieving for the loss of an intimately loved person, a life companion over many years, in persons who do not suffer from a psychiatric illness, particularly a form of clinically diagnosable depression. On the basis of clinical experience and the extended, in-depth interviews of persons with these characteristics and experience, I describe normal mourning as a permanent, not a transitional, process that leads to structural psychic changes manifest in typical conscious experiences and behaviors. This conclusion runs counter to the present psychoanalytic view of normal mourning and considers mourning as an ongoing psychological process that fosters emotional growth and increases the capacity for commitment to new love relationships.

Background

The origin of this chapter was a personal, painful, extended experience of mourning that gradually raised serious questions in my mind about some generally assumed characteristics of grief and mourning. Is it really a time-limited experience that is completed with a process of identification with a lost object (Freud 1917 [1915]/1957)? Is the work of mourning completed with a reworking of the depressive position and the reinstatement of the good internal object, as well as with the process of identification mentioned before? What is involved in the processes of reparation that are so central in the mourning process (Klein 1940)? Are there aspects of mourning that have not been given sufficient attention in our understanding of the experience? I have tentatively reached the conclusion that perhaps mourning processes do not simply end but, rather, evolve into more lasting or permanent aspects of psychic structures that have not been explicated fully in the corresponding literature.

In the light of these questions, I reviewed my past analytic experiences, particularly the treatment of patients who had undergone significant mourning processes in the course of their analysis. My attention was drawn particularly to a patient who, after many years of a happy marriage, had lost his spouse as a consequence of an automobile accident. His analysis, originally started because of his severe obsessive-compulsive personality features, became marked by a mourning process that overshadowed the last four years of his treatment. Although this analysis took place a number of years ago, I had, at the time, recorded very detailed process notes of sessions, and the abundance of the material of that case permitted me to review that analysis, under the impact, it must be said, of my own mourning experience, the loss of my spouse.

In what follows, I shall briefly describe the relevant developments in the treatment of this patient, including my interpretive approach then, and point to issues that now draw my attention and that I would now see as more important and requiring a broader frame for their understanding than what determined my interventions at that time. I shall then explore certain mourning experiences in a sample of persons who had undergone severe mournings and where, I believe, new evidence emerged regarding the viewpoints I developed in the course of these explorations.

A Mourning Process Triggered During an Analysis

The patient was a 51-year-old man who had started analysis three years earlier because of a rigid, obsessive-compulsive personality structure that had caused serious problems for him in his business relations, with colleagues, superiors, and subordinates, and had gradually improved throughout his analysis. He was the son of a domineering, successful businessman, whose rage attacks had successfully controlled his wife and children. The patient had a submissive and fearful attitude toward his father that, in the course of the years, gradually had shifted into an open rebelliousness. It was the anxiety he experienced when confronted with what he interpreted as the authoritarian attitudes of his business superiors that had brought my patient into treatment originally. My patient's mother was a woman who, while being submissive to her husband, was rather indulgent with their children—three daughters and one son, the patient—and in chronic conflict with her husband around the degree to which she supposedly failed to discipline them. Mother was also withdrawn and somewhat aloof, and, other than the general submissive attitude toward father expected from them, the children were left to themselves much of the time. Only when my patient was ill would mother be concerned about him, as she was, apparently, quite hypochondriacal about any physical symptoms affecting herself or the children. She also had a closer relationship to her daughters—the patient was the youngest in the family, and during the treatment it emerged that he felt quite lonely and isolated in what he perceived was mostly a "women's home."

The patient had been married for twenty-eight years, and, while he felt that he loved his wife deeply, they had frequent conflicts around his obsessive insistence on rigid schedules and plans and his overinvolvement in his work, as she saw it. She complained that he did not really seem interested in her life, while he felt that she was chronically attempting to make him feel guilty. Yet, all in all, they both felt assured of their mutual love, and, throughout the years, their relationship had remarkably deepened, which was furthered along during the treatment.

At the time of the treatment to be examined, the patient's obsessive concern with time, precision, and placement of objects and the inhibition in his work had significantly improved. At this point, however, after their son and their daughter had left home to pursue their lives in other cities in connection with their respective professions, his wife died because of the consequences of a severe automobile accident. Now the analysis shifted radically into the analytic work with his mourning process.

He experienced a severe depression of several months that gradually evolved into what might be described as more normal grief that, however, persisted throughout the next three years of treatment. In my view at that time, it was not yet completely resolved by the time we jointly decided that it was reasonable to end his analysis. During the sessions, he still expressed intense guilt feelings for not having paid sufficient attention to the needs of his wife. He remembered, again and again, the many circumstances in which she had been expressing her love and he had been taking it for granted, and he spent endless hours in internal dialogues with her and with intense grief over her loss. He repeatedly went through her belongings, letters, and photographs and over a period of months sought out the priest of his church for spiritual consolation. He struggled with persistent, repetitive feelings that his wife must still, somehow, exist in outer reality and became concerned with the question of life after death. He had not been active in the church but now experienced a deep sense of longing for faith in the possibility of an eventual reunion of his and his wife's souls.

This patient had presented much more limited periods of mourning after the death of both of his parents, which occurred during the early years of his marriage, and his present mourning experience brought to the surface the incomplete mourning of these earlier losses, particularly the death of his mother. I interpreted his present deep and protracted mourning reaction over many months. This work focused on his inordinate feelings of guilt and his desperate wish for an opportunity to redeem himself, both regarding his wife and in connection with old conflicts with his mother, the sense of chronic loneliness in his early childhood, and the repression of his anger for what he experienced as his mother's preference for his sisters. A reworking of the mourning over the death of his mother became part of the present analytic work. However, the patient persisted in the elaboration of an internal relationship with his wife over the entire four-year period of the analysis that followed her death, without showing, after approximately two years, any sign of a depression or even of a mourning reaction as far as his daily life was concerned. However, in his fantasy life, both during and outside of our sessions, he continued an intense dialogue with her. He felt that he owed it to her to dedicate whatever was left of his life to repair and compensate the limitations of his expression of his love for her while they lived their life together. This moral obligation, as he experienced it, became a source of consolation: he felt it was a way to enrich his life and to maintain contact with his wife.

In the last year before the end of his analysis, he established a new relationship with a woman from the same cultural background as his dead wife. He fell in love with her, and this relationship culminated in their marriage a few months before the termination of his analysis. He loved his new wife, but this new relationship consistently reactivated memories of his first marriage, with a pressing urge to modify and correct the limitations that he now felt he had evinced with his first wife, in a wish to change and repair old problematic behavior in the new relationship.

At the time of the termination of his analysis, I wondered whether I had been missing the analysis in sufficient depth of unconscious guilt and aggression regarding his own mother. While the patient seemed to be functioning well in his life with his new wife, and had changed significantly in his relationships at work and in his social life, I felt puzzled about what seemed like the relentless presence of his first wife and her impressive influence on his present life. It was as if the mourning process had evolved into significant characterological changes, as well as the maintenance of an internal relationship with his wife, rather than being completed, after a reasonable time, by a process of identification and "letting go."

Now, retrospectively, after a deep personal mourning experience, the review of other cases with similar experiences to those I had with this patient, and the exploratory interviewing of a selected number of persons who had experienced a loss of a spouse after many years of a happy relationship, I would approach the final stages of this analysis somewhat differently. While retracing the present mourning process to its antecedents in the patient's infantile development—and, eventually, his reaction to the forthcoming end of the analysis, I think now I would be more attentive to the ongoing mourning process related to the loss of his wife, his ongoing internal relationship with her, and the influence of this relationship on the restructuring of his superego. At the same time, I would be more attentive to the transference function of reinstating and maintaining that internalized relationship with her, while bringing it to life in the relationship with the analyst. This double function of the mourning process—superego restructuring and maintaining the relationship—I now believe deserves further exploration.

I am tentatively suggesting some new ways of conceptualizing the psychodynamics of normal mourning. Regarding the utilization of diagnostic interviews of persons whom I have not seen in analysis, the question could be raised whether the corresponding findings really may reinforce psychoanalytic hypotheses. This is a limitation of what follows, but, I submit, the similarity of certain reactions in all of these cases reinforces the merit of further psychoanalytic exploration of these proposals.

Some Phenomenological Observations

What follows are the experiences gathered in interviewing persons known to me personally and who were willing to be interviewed, all of whom having had the experience of the loss of a spouse after many years of a happy relationship. Obviously, these are not psychoanalytic observations per se, although these interviews were based on a psychoanalytic perspective. Also, I had already observed clinical features in other patients undergoing mourning processes that replicated surprisingly the features of extended mourning without clinical depression of the case I have reported before. And the conscious and preconscious manifestations that could be observed in these interviews, I believe, strengthen the hypotheses regarding the unconscious processes that, I am suggesting, may be common features of normal mourning. Also, in exploring the mourning processes of other patients who had lost significant others in the course of their treatment, I had become particularly concerned with the nature of mourning and the grieving process. In the interviews, my focus was on the different components of the mourning process, their duration, and their influence on the life of the affected persons. As a personal experience of my own had been the initial stimulus for this exploration, I was particularly concerned with avoiding, as much as possible, the influence of my own experiences on the evaluation of the information that I was receiving.

To begin, practically all of the persons I interviewed related the experience of shock following the death of a beloved one and the intense emotional conviction that the person was still there, in some unreal world, which for deeply religious persons was consonant with a rational conviction following their particular religious belief. One woman told me: "I know that his soul is somewhere. I have spent much time thinking how our love on the earth will come together with the love of God in an eventual redemption of the souls, and what will happen to the negative feelings that are so painful in one's memories…will jealousy and envy still exist?" Various persons quoted Joan Didion's autobiographical book *The Year of Magical Thinking* (2005) and C.S. Lewis's *A Grief Observed* (1961), the latter as the basis for the movie *Shadowlands*. In fact, several had not only seen the film but also remembered it in surprising detail after many years. One deeply religious person, a leader of a major educational psychological center, speaking about a beloved deceased person, said with deep conviction, "I know that we shall meet again." Others, without religious convictions, stated very clearly that the person they lost in reality continued to exist in their mind and in the mind of those who knew and loved the deceased. Talking about the lost love object with these others evoked the comforting presence of the loved one, who lived on in their minds. This experience would not decrease its intensity over many years.

But that experience, in turn, seemed only a reproduction of an ongoing process of internal relating to the person who had died, with intense longing, painfully missing the reality of a life lived together, and with the reactivation of the sense of regret over not having used the time together more completely, more intensively. That regret reflected feelings of guilt that, remarkably, was more intense, the more fundamentally satisfactory and loving the relationship had been. Persons with a chronic ambivalent relationship and who, one might assume, had good reasons to feel guilty showed much less tendencies in this regard.

One woman, describing the sudden death of her husband of twenty-two years, with whom she had had a very fulfilling relationship in terms of their sexual life, their mutual expectations and interactions in daily life, and their orientation toward values, social life, and intellectual and ideological aspirations, described the sense of concern after his unexpected death following shortly after a routine medical examination in which he had been given a clean bill of health. Had she been contributing to causing his death from a heart attack because she had been too demanding, originating stress in his life? Over many months, this concern pained her and continued in spite of repeated reassurances by professionals, including the physicians who had examined the husband for various reasons and at different times.

While loss related to sudden death tends to trigger intense feelings of guilt and regret in the survivor, death following a lengthy and painful illness may cause intense pain recalling the suffering of the deceased person, a painful re-creation and elaboration of the weeks and months of decaying health and the cycles of hope and despair that usually characterize those terrible times. During the struggle for survival, the immediate tasks, keeping hope alive for the dying person and the person who loves him or her, leave little time or mental space for mourning. The working through of these experiences comes later with long-term grieving.

One man was reviewing in his mind the experiences of a forty-year marriage to a woman he had loved deeply and who died after an extended struggle with metastatic breast cancer. Innumerable moments of their lives together kept emerging in his mind, such as invitations on her part to spend time together in travels that his work had kept him from and his lack of sufficient support, as he now saw it, of her career and education. A consistent reaction to these painful feelings that persisted over many years was his effort to re-create, in his mind, the hopes, expectations, and plans that his deceased wife could not achieve, her desires that remained unfulfilled, and her projects that remained interrupted, with efforts to actively carry out what she would have wanted to achieve or would have wanted him to do.

Another woman, who had been very dependent on her now deceased husband who would take care of all their problems of daily life, felt that it was his wish that she now become more independent and capable of relying on herself. She felt a sense of strength and satisfaction in fulfilling his wishes, a redemption from her feelings of guilt over her excessive passivity with him by changing her behavior in the direction that he would have wished her to go.

The death of a beloved person is, of course, a well-known stimulus for an effort to carry out a social function in memory and in the name of the deceased. One wife established a professional fellowship in the field in which her husband was an expert, and one man made enormous efforts to the effect that the artistic production of his wife be acknowledged and appreciated after her death.

Psychologically, what seemed important to me listening to these persons was their sense of a relationship to the lost person that actively continued, by virtue of reparative endeavors which the mourners felt were expressions of love and regret for lost time and opportunities that would be appreciated by the lost partner. One man said that thirty years after her death, he still consulted with his wife whenever it came to important decisions regarding the relationship to their children.

At the same time, several persons noted that they acquired attitudes that were similar to those of the person who had died. One man felt that something in him had died as well and that there was a split between one part of himself that felt alive and one that felt as if he had crossed over into a different world to be with his lost wife. Another man commented thoughtfully over the strange combination of having changed, as if he had taken his lost wife into himself, while yet maintaining an ongoing relationship with her in his mind, and wondered, half jokingly, "Is that schizophrenia?"

What I wish to stress is the combination of the—well-known—identification with a lost object in the sense of a modification of the self-representation, on the one hand, and the persistence of an internal object relation with the lost person. The process of identification really involves the transformation of the self-representation under the influence of the representation of the significant other—as Freud and Jacobson had pointed out—and, at the same time, the persistence of the internalized relation between self and other as a stable psychological structure. I am using advisedly the term *structure* to refer to the permanence and the functional quality of this mental dyadic relation between self- and object representation.

I mentioned earlier the emotional conviction that the person that has been lost is still there in some form in external reality: even in nonreligious persons, this may take very concrete forms through hallucinatory experiences. For example, one man felt that he was being touched in a caressing way by his deceased wife during the first month after her death, and he had difficulty to explain to me, years later, whether that was an experience in reality or whether he was dreaming. A woman mentioned, somewhat embarrassed, that she would write letters to her deceased husband with a strong conviction that he would be able to obtain the content and the meaning of these letters because of her action. She put them away, with the fantasy that, eventually, she would be able to show them to him. While these acute experiences and behaviors tend to subside over time, the internal conversation and interaction with the loved and lost person continue, as I mentioned before, over many years.

The pain of mourning gradually decreases but may be reactivated with full intensity even after years, such as during the interviews that I carried out. In fact, it was impressive how intensively most people reacted to my tactful efforts, over a time span of two to three hours, to raise questions about the persistence of a mourning process and how, before my eyes, the intense pain over the loss of the person would reemerge, with particular characteristics: first, the simple pain over the loss of somebody deeply loved, the regret over the final nature of it; second, the pain over the interruption of the life project of the other person, of what the deceased person, if alive, would want to achieve; and third, the pain over the responsibility to carry on alone a world built together, with a sad awareness that with their own future death, that world would finally disappear. It was as if the exploration of this pain would bring alive the words of Goethe: "We die twice: first, when we die, and then when those who knew us and loved us die" (Goethe 1809/1972). And fourth, the pain over the loss of a deep dependency on the loved person has clearly parental, perhaps mostly maternal features. This signifies, if one explores it further, the reactivation of all mourning processes that the individual has experienced before the traumatic loss of the beloved person and points to the underlying reactivation of the depressive position.

An efficient, apparently self-assured businessman referred to the fact that whenever an unexpected crisis developed, a momentary sense of anxiety and despair would overcome him that, in his experience, could be controlled by his calling his wife, who now had died four years ago. Under conditions of such critical moments, he would feel as if he were an abandoned child, and an intense longing for her with an upsurge of deep sadness would follow.

As an illustration of the pain over the fact that the lost person would miss out on something that was so dear to her, a usually controlled mental health professional, whose wife had died five years ago, attended the graduation from elementary school of a granddaughter whom his wife had been very close to. Suddenly, in the middle of the ceremony, his feeling of pleasure shifted into sadness and a barely controlled outburst of tears as he thought how happy his wife would have been if she were present at this moment.

The pain over the abrupt ending of the life project of the lost person also is illustrated by the grieving reaction of a widower when he faced the paintings of a certain expressionist painter whose life his wife had been exploring in the context of solving the riddle of certain symbolic objects that repeated themselves in many of his paintings. He felt knowledgeable about what she was after but incompetent to be able to follow it through, and while he was attracted to the work of this painter, it was a joy mixed with pain every time he saw one of his works.

One woman expressed the concern over the loss of a shared world upon her own death: she said, "One of the things I am most sad about when I think of him is that, when I die, all I knew about his world in the old country, his childhood, his struggle for independence, will be lost." The internally felt need to transmit to a future generation the knowledge about the life of the person whom one has lost is a powerful incentive for biographical writing.

Thus, the pain over the loss of a beloved person is composed of several currents and maintains its influence on the personality over many years. The identification with the lost person, particularly with traits that one admired and missed, is a source of strength and, indeed, fosters the experience of a sense of overcoming the mourning process. In this regard, Freud's observation that the mourning process is completed with a process of identification is confirmed in everyday experience. At the same time, however, the presence in one's mind of the relation with the lost object goes on, and the sense of guilt over the loss that Freud ascribed mostly to pathological mourning but that Melanie Klein proposed as a fundamental aspect of all mourning processes in their reactivation of the depressive position clearly seems confirmed by the consistent observation of guilt feelings, perhaps particularly in persons who had the least reason for feeling guilty.

As mentioned before, persons with severe, chronic conflicts with the person they lost and who were conscious of rather than denying their own ambivalence seem to show fewer feelings of guilt, in contrast to cases where a profound repression of the aggression against the lost person would emerge as the syndrome of pathological mourning, an expression of unconscious guilt. In my study of borderline patients, mourning processes most frequently were accompanied by intense rage and resentment at the lost person for having abandoned the surviving partner—a regression to paranoid-schizoid mechanisms, and, in the case of narcissistic pathology, the absence of any mourning process is a typical characteristic development (Kernberg 1984). Narcissistic personalities who, instead of grieving, develop an intense paranoid reaction against those they feel able to blame for the death of the lost partner, spouse, child, or parent thus are protected from the painful mourning process that patients with more normal internalized object relations have to confront.

Regarding the reactivation of past mourning processes, one man who lost his spouse remembered with strong feelings the agony of his father following the death of the patient's mother. He wished he could have been aware, at that point, of what he now had become aware of and helped his father, while, at the same time, if his father were alive now, they could console each other. One woman, because of the serious conflicts and mutual alienation she had experienced with her mother, remembered a rather ambivalent, and retrospectively, superficial mourning experience at her death. Following, however, the mourning process over the death of her husband years ago, she felt a surge of longing for her mother, spent much time reflecting on her mother's feelings and motivation, and experienced fully a double mourning process for her husband and her mother. This belated working through of a previously repressed mourning process in the light of a later one is not infrequent.

The Psychodynamics of Mourning

The psychoanalytic literature on mourning processes is mostly concerned with pathological mourning, mourning as part of depression, both neurotic and melancholia (Akhtar 2000; Coyne 1985; Fiorini 2007; Frankiel 1994; Grinberg 1992; Kogan 2007; Pollack 1975). Beyond the classical contributions of Freud (1917 [1915]/1957), Melanie Klein (1940), and Edith Jacobson (1971), there is little reference to normal mourning processes. The present study is focused on the phenomenological and structural aspects of the normal mourning process, on mourning that is not part of a clinical depression.

What follows is undoubtedly influenced by a recent personal experience of mourning and at risk for missing, therefore, the necessary objectivity of an adequately distant exploration. As mentioned before, I have tried to gain some objectivity about the questions triggered by my own experience by interviewing a number of persons who had undergone a significant loss of a spouse within the past ten to twenty years, with the explicit purpose of studying their mourning experiences, and who had given me ample evidence that they did not suffer from a significant personality disorder. Naturally, my experiences with patients in analysis and psychoanalytic psychotherapy provide the general background to this presentation.

My observations regarding the process of "normal" mourning stem from a psychoanalytic viewpoint of the processes of severe mourning experienced by persons who, both in their general personality functioning and from the descriptive aspects of their mourning processes, would not be considered cases of "pathological mourning." The latter is reflected in the characteristic clinical aspects of excessively severe or prolonged mourning, clinical depression, irrational guilt feelings, the development of regressive features of personality functioning, or other symptoms linked to that process. The main proposals derived from my observations are the following:

Mourning, in contrast to Freud's (1917 [1915]/1957) initial assumption, but recognized by him in later years (1929/1960), is not a time-limited process. Freud concluded that mourning is completed through a process of unconscious identification with a lost object and by the compensatory gratitude for being alive, in contrast to the beloved person who has died. Melanie Klein (1940) proposed that an adequate resolution of the reawakened processes of the depressive position and its elaboration completes the work of normal mourning. This is a fundamental contribution to the understanding of normal as well as pathological mourning. While Freud clarified the dynamics of melancholia, Melanie Klein clarified commonalities of normal and pathological mourning, as well as their differences in terms of the normal reactivation of the dynamics of the depressive position or the failure of this process with the dominance of regressive manic or paranoid-schizoid processes. I believe it is the process of unconscious identification with the lost object that needs to be reexamined and the extent to which the reality of an object loss determines new processes within the depressive position.

To begin, the process of identification refers to the modification of the representation of self under the influence of the representation of a significant other (Jacobson 1964). But this may not be all in the case of relatively normal persons who have suffered a signifi-

cant loss, particularly that of a spouse with whom they had an optimal relationship over many years. In fact, the traumatic loss of a
spouse under such circumstances is relatively underemphasized in
the literature on mourning, in which the mourning of parental figures or of one's children and the losses that children experience
upon the death of parents are focused upon much more frequently.
Yet clinical observations indicate the enormously traumatic aspects
of the mourning of a life partner of many years.

From my interviews, as well as my own experience, I propose
that what is also involved in this process of identification is the setting up of a permanent relationship between the representation of
self and the representation of the lost object, the combination of an
intrapsychic presence of that object, and the awareness of its objective permanent absence. From a different perspective, Gaines
(1997) proposed that the two tasks of mourning include detachment from the lost object as well as maintaining continuity in the
connection with that object. It is the dynamics and structural implications of that permanent aspect of the mourning process that
I wish to focus upon. I propose that this objective absence in the
presence of an intense subjective experience of the permanent relation between self and the lost other is at the center of the painful
experience of loss and the compensatory processes this situation
engenders. This intrapsychic duality acquires the characteristics
described by Freud and Melanie Klein, namely, an idealization of
the lost object and the reactivation of significant previous mourning
processes linked to the reactivation of the depressive position. Clinically speaking, past mourning processes are reactivated with their
elements of guilt feelings and reparative efforts. As Melanie Klein
has stressed, the more ambivalent the relation with the lost object
had been, the greater the guilt feelings over the real and fantasized
aggression toward the lost object. And, insofar as ambivalence is a
universal character of human relationships, this process also may
be observed consistently. But not only conflicts over aggression are
involved here.

Regarding the working through of the depressive position, the
reality of guilt over opportunities lost, over failure to appreciate
what one had until it was gone, cannot be retraced totally to past
internal aggressive impulses now integrated with loving ones toward the lost object. Exaggerated guilt over past experiences also
illuminates the limitations that daily reality imposes throughout
time. Daily reality militates against the full appreciation of a loving
relationship, and only retrospectively exists the possibility of a per-

spective that fully illuminates the potential implications of every moment lived together. The paradox of the capacity to only appreciate fully what one had after having lost it, a profoundly human paradox, cannot be resolved by communicating this experience to others. It is an internal learning process fostered by the painful, yet creative aspect of mourning.

There is now no possibility of correcting past shortcomings and failures, no possibility for redressing realistic grievances, and no opportunity to make up and try to be a better mate. Objectively, there is now no more forgiveness or repair. Working through of the limitations and failures stemming from the past cannot be carried out now in an objective relation to the lost object.

But reparative processes are possible by other mechanisms that deserve further attention. The desires, aspirations, and ambitions of the person who has died, particularly the wishes for his or her own life and future, as well as for the life and future of the person who mourns and for other persons who were central in the love and concern of the lost person, may be experienced by the person in mourning as a mandate, a command, a moral obligation to fulfill the wishes and hopes of the deceased. They become part of the mourner's superego, not as an impersonal aspect of superego demands and prohibitions, but, rather, preserved as highly personalized relations with the lost object.

Guilt, remorse, and reparation: these are intimately related, but not equivalent or necessarily linked aspects of the mourning process. Unconscious guilt, massive and overwhelming, as the basis of severe depression is related to unconscious aggression to the ambivalently loved, lost object, consciously represented by overvalued or even delusional self-depreciation and devaluation, if not even more disguised by a wide array of typical depressive delusions involving the self and the external world (Jacobson 1971).

But conscious guilt, whether normal or neurotic, is usually associated with remorse; that is, conscious regret for aggressive behavior toward the lost love object, whether through actions, neglect, or abandonment. Remorse is the foundational impetus for reparation, the impulse to undo the aggression in an attempt to compensate or atone for the real or imagined damage done to the lost object. But, beyond atonement, there may be a growing impulse to redeem oneself by means of personal change, constructive action, and striving to be a "better person" in ongoing and new relationships. Remorse and guilt are, as Melanie Klein suggested, the origin of the reparative drive. But remorse is not always followed

by the urge to reparation: in cases of narcissistic personality structure, remorse may be subverted to the "suffering" of the survivor, a
self-limited response that does not lead to reparative action. Guilt
feelings that don't lead to reparation or its equivalent changes in
behavior are a defensive neutralization of the very guilt sometimes
indicative of significant superego pathology.

In the course of normal mourning, however, grief creates a
powerful reparative impulse, strengthening the internalized object
relation with the lost object as an aspect of preconscious experience, and fosters the development of new value systems, a part of
superego, and particularly ego ideal structures. There is a growth
of the motivation and capacity to relate daily life with ethical aspirations and meanings. The regret over opportunities lost and over
the loss of the finite relationship in reality and the full illumination
of the value of the relationship with the lost object are the driving
motivation for this development. As part of this ego and superego
development, at any point of the remaining life of the mourning
subject, the mourning process may be reinstated: perhaps particularly at those moments of quiet reflection when the past reemerges
as part of the growing sense of continuity of the time experience as
part of the maturation throughout the life cycle.

Another aspect of this experience is the strengthening of the
normal development of a subjective, personal past world shared
with the lost object that differentiates itself from the experience of
present daily reality: a normal, delicately evolving, life-enriching
yet subtly sad experience of the historical dimension and transient
nature of life. It is a normal, subliminal but lasting mourning experience that is punctured by the acute experience of loss of the past
when a present event evokes it. It may well be that both types of
mourning experience reinforce each other.

The objective manifestations of mourning, such as a persistent,
low-toned sadness; a potential for intense episodic sadness activated
under the many circumstances that bring into sharp focus the memory of the lost person; the occasional intense pain as memories related to the lost person emerge in present interchanges with others;
and a certain degree of internal withdrawal under circumstances
that evoke past experiences shared with the lost person, may all
have subsided after a year or two as manifest symptoms. And yet,
over many years, and I am proposing that this becomes a permanent
trait of the personality that evolves in the context of such a mourning
process, the poignant memory of the lost person remains fully and
intensively present, together with moments of an acute sense of pain

and sadness. This reaction can be triggered at any time and often catches the mourning person by surprise.

There are well-known circumstances that activate this permanent, internalized relationship: first, the individual's experience of new, beautiful, emotionally intense moments that one knows would have been appreciated intensively by the person who is lost, a sadness that he or she cannot be here to enjoy an experience so related to what was so important to him or her. Second, there are moments in which a rapid, instantaneous understanding of the meaning of an event transcends the practical reality of the immediate situation and condenses many memories, understandings, and convictions, in one single instance, one idea: now the person with whom that awareness could be shared, the only one who would immediately comprehend all the elements involved, is absent. At the bottom of such experiences lies a common world, constructed with the lost person over many years, that now remains only in memory, its presence felt in absence. Third, there is the fulfillment of aspirations that the deceased did not live to see, for example, the growth of a child or grandchild. And, of course, above all, the simple longing for the person who has been lost, the yearning for the recovery of a shared mutual dependency with all its loving and regressive implications of safety and familiarity, exists, and the underlying longing for the reunion with beloved parental figures on whom one depended is a powerful context for the emergence of those other triggers of an ever renewed sense of mourning and longing. And then, there are the dreams in which the dead person is alive, interacting with the dreamer, at times reassuring the dreamer as part of the manifest content of the dream that this is not an illusion... followed by the painful awakening to reality.

Happily, the enduring nature of these experiences in the normal course of grieving does not imply a libidinal fixation on the past that permanently limits the capacity for new investments. Libidinal investments are not a zero sum capacity. To the contrary, the expansion of moral values and ethical commitments related to the mandates that reflect the desires and aspirations of the person who died, whose life project was interrupted, is frequently a powerful stimulus to reparative action of the survivor, providing a sense of purpose. They become, as mentioned before, ethical commands and aspired-for ideals. Reparative processes, in short, expand into spiritual demands.

The reparative impulses stimulate psychological growth, the capacity to learn from experience, and the capacity to enrich new love relationships with the lessons derived from the loss of the past one. The capacity to love anew increases with the tolerance and elaboration of mourning as a permanent process. In fact, the capacity to love again may become enriched by this perennial mourning process that combines the gratitude for a new relationship with the gratitude for a new opportunity to fulfill the mandate of the lost object. Normal mourning, I propose, enhances the capacity for loving. This experience of a new opportunity to love must necessarily include the belief that the lost loved ones would want us to find new happiness and go on with our lives, perpetuating the feeling of their presence in their absence. And the loving understanding on the part of the new object of the elaboration of a past loss may enrich the new relationship. Needless to say, all of this may go terribly wrong under pathological circumstances, and we know more about those situations from our clinical work.

To mourn a lost loved object and yet to be able to love again… without abandoning the love for the lost object or truncating the mourning process itself is an important and yet neglected aspect of normal mourning. It runs counter to the traditional assumption of a mechanical flow of "libidinal energy" that is withdrawn from the object and redirected but remains essentially constant. Chasseguet-Smirgel (1985) has pointed out that falling in love is not a matter of directing narcissistic libido toward an object and thus reducing the narcissistic investment but that both object-invested libido and self-invested libido increase at the same time. I propose that, similarly, the reaffirmation of investment of love for the lost object that is part of the normal mourning process or, rather, the full liberation of love for the lost object previously dampened or obscured by the daily process of living together facilitates the increase of love toward a new object. At this point, the understanding and tolerance of the new love object of the mourning partner's attachment to the lost object may enrich their relationship and facilitate further the growth of a new love.

Mourning interminable may become part of the increased capability for love and appreciation of life. In contrast to Freud's (1917 [1915]/1957) assumption that the pleasure with one's own being alive compensates for the loss of the beloved one in the overcoming of mourning, the pleasure of being alive is enriched by the moral responsibilities derived from the integration of the internal mandate proceeding from the person who has been lost.

The activation of the depressive position is reflected in the resurgence of the mourning process regarding earlier losses. In the case of the loss of a spouse or child, the typical reactivated experiences involve parental figures, which then tend to become transformed and more fully mourned by virtue of the current grief. Here the highly individualized nature of the relationship to earlier life experiences involving fully developed or avoided mourning reactions makes generalization difficult. The most important feature of those experiences, however, is the deepening of the understanding and of the internal relationship to a lost parent. Under optimal circumstances, that internal relationship may help to mitigate the pain and bring with it a sense of consolation to the new mourning experience. But, at times, the sense of loss of a love object reinforces the feelings of abandonment by the previously lost parental object.

The denial of the disappearance of the loved one, the emotional conviction that the soul of the lost other continues existing in a virtual world, an article of faith held by major religions, is beautifully illustrated in its intensity and as a central aspect of the mourning process in C.S. Lewis's book *A Grief Observed* (1961) and in Joan Didion's book *The Year of Magical Thinking* (2005). While these, of course, are not psychoanalytic studies, the profound introspection of these authors merits psychoanalytic reflection. Both authors clearly describe their difficulty in tolerating the discrepancy between the overwhelming internal presence of the lost object and the external reality of its absence. The ardent wish for a reencounter in that dark world of the unknown may take many forms and is a major source of the suicidal ideation and suicidal attempts that follow the death of a beloved one. Here the wish for one's own death is the hope for the reencounter. Also, that wish and the profound experience of the permanence of the lost object are profound sources of religious feelings.

The function of gravestones, memorial monuments, pictures and photographs, and works of art symbolically representing the lost person derive their consoling function from the assurance that the dead person is still out there, somewhere, in the external world. Burial sites further serve as "points of contact," gathering places where the soul of the departed, now in a different and mysterious world, can renew contact with the mourning person. This may function normally as painful yet reassuring symbols of the reencounter with the lost object. This normal process, however, may evolve into pathological idealization of such memorial places, or their symbolic equivalents, constituting now "linking objects" (Volkan 1972) that acquire an almost delusional function in the life of the mourner. The religious function of such symbols is a major source of communion with the deity: the presence of the host in a church and a chapel with the image of the Virgin Mary thus become places of solace, of reassuring closeness to the deity.

The profound emotional conviction about the continued existence, in another realm of reality, of the soul or the spirit of the person who has died, of the immortality of the soul, in short, is an essential component of the mourning process. It dovetails with religious assumptions of resurrection of the soul and of the body and of reencounter with the love object as an aspect of the final encounter with God. C.S. Lewis has movingly described this psychological process in its interaction with religious conviction. It raises numerous questions that involve theological and scientific issues but also, very predominantly, psychological ones. This emotional conviction of the continued presence of the lost object points to an important psychological root of the religious impulse as a basic aspect of the human psyche.

Martin Bergmann (personal communication, 2006) has suggested that religion, in this regard, affirming the survival of the soul, protects the mourner from hallucination and delusion—and hallucinatory experiences of being in touch with the lost object are, indeed, quite prevalent. But, by the same token, religious convictions also raise the question of what relationship might emerge in a world of the souls, with old and new lost objects simultaneously present. C.S. Lewis, again, proposed the reunion of all love objects in the context of the reunion with God. Different Western religions formulate alternative hypotheses about this puzzle, but what matters is the power of the emotional reality reflected in this aspect of the mourning process. In short, there is a setting up of a permanent internalized relation with the lost object that becomes, in the words of Sara Zac de Filc (personal communication, 2010), an "absent presence."

From this need also derives the therapeutic function of the capacity to share the internal presence of the lost person with others who share a loving past with the lost person and, of course, to share the person with the analyst who becomes the external depositary of this internal world. I believe I had missed the important transferential function, in the case of the patient I referred to initially, of the re-creation of the image of his dead wife in the sessions with me, re-creating her again and again in the transitional space of our relationship. And again, in these painful, yet so desired reencounters in fantasy, the earlier mentioned aspects of the mourning process are reactivated: the regret for opportunities missed, the sense of a mandate to be fulfilled in a virtual continuation of the relationship with the deceased, and the pain over the always premature disruption of the life plan of the other are essential aspects of the communicatively shared internal relationship with the lost one. The irresistible urge for reunion, the fantasy and concern over life after death, and the expanding moral universe related to the mandate all combine in the expression of powerful religious impulses, whether they take the form of adherence to an established religious belief system or are constructed individually as a painful yet indispensable aspect of spiritual existence and survival.

Mourning, of course, always implies a traumatic loss. When the trauma is compounded by violence, such as for loved ones killed in the Holocaust or assassinated by ordinary criminals, terrorists, or the repressive machinery of a totalitarian state, intense hostility mingles with the pain of mourning. Pathological mourning, on the other hand, may involve the search for culprits to project unconscious aggression toward the ambivalently loved lost object. Relatives of patients who have committed suicide often look for culprits in the mental health system, particularly in the context of a family member's chronically bad relationship with the suicidal patient.

In cases when the loss is the result of violence, paranoid and aggressive reactions color the mourning process and may temporarily or over a long time overshadow it, protecting the mourner from the full impact of the grief. Collective mourning over the death of a beloved leader may take the form of unmitigated grief, without paranoid reactions, thus acquiring an intensively painful yet mature form of mourning—as, for example, the national mourning process over the death of John F. Kennedy. Collective mourning over the victims of the Holocaust also usually takes the characteristics of a normal mourning process. Or else, paranoid features may predominate, such as in the collective memory of the disastrous battle of Kosovo, a 600-year-old Serbian trauma reactivated, as Vamik Volkan (2007) has described, within a regressive large group mourning process in which the paranoid elements predisposed the large group psychology to sadistic revenge on present-day real and imagined enemies. Here the persistence of the mourning process throughout generations clearly carries with it pathological, paranoid-schizoid features within the group identity, paralleling paranoid-schizoid features in the intolerance of the depressive position of the individual. In this regard, in contrast, the permanent features of the normal mourning process described carry important reparative features without terminating the mourning process itself.

Some General Conclusions

Perhaps the most impressive aspect of the mourning process is the previously mentioned moral or ethical injunction to carry on the aspirations of the now deceased person. It is as if the most effective way to deal with the pain of loss were the commitment to carry out that mandate, a commitment that has an ethical quality. The achievement of this mandate reinforces the moral values and moral strength of the surviving person as well as being a source of positive, loving, and creative gestures that affect others as well. Here the ethical component, the strengthening of advanced superego functions, transcends the reparative function of reestablishing the internal object of the depressive position.

From a religious perspective, Rabbi Moshe Berger (personal communication, June 2006) has formulated this development, stating that all human love relationships are finite, while the absence that necessarily follows the death of one of a couple is infinite. The paradox, he goes on, is that only at the time of infinite absence can the time of finite presence be fully appreciated in all its potential luminosity, and it is absolutely unavoidable that, in that light, feelings of regret and sadness over lost opportunities color the memory of the relationship. Those regrets, whether they take the form of guilt feelings or not, cannot be compensated; there is no repair and no forgiveness, because the person to whom reparation would be directed is irretrievably gone. Here is where the sense of the mandate emerging from the lost person becomes part of one's moral guidance system, and in carrying out this mandate evolves the creation of moral values. Rabbi Berger links this development with the fundamental religious demand of "Tikun Olam" (to improve the world), implying a moral mandate to try to improve and bring happiness, as much as we can, within the circle of one's daily life. In this regard, the desperate desire for an existence beyond death, the longing for and faith in such a spiritual world, on the one hand, and the adherence to an internalized set of transcendental principles in fulfilling a moral mandate combine to increase the religious aspect of psychological functioning. Objectively, this may be reflected in more maturity, in a more loving and concerned relationship to others, that, in turn, may elicit growth processes in others, such as the children of a person in mourning. This may be one of the sources of moral growth and development that, in the long run, may have broader impact at a social community level, counteracting the powerful regressive group processes that operate in an opposite direction.

From the perspective of contemporary object relations theory, the persistence of the internal relation with the lost object is a significant confirmation of the power of the world of internalized object relations and of the dyadic nature of identification processes. Freud described identification in his classical essay on "Mourning and Melancholia" (1917 [1915]/1957), and Edith Jacobson's *The Self and the Object World* (1964), as mentioned before, defined identification as the modification of the self-representation under the impact of the corresponding object representation. We may now conclude that identification is a complex process that includes, at least, the internalization of a relationship with the significant other, the modification of the self-representation as influenced by the object representation, and the maintenance of that internalized object relation, with a potential for its reactivation both in a direct form, the search for an object similar to or replacing the one that has been lost, and as a reactivation with role reversal, in the sense of re-creating the relationship while identifying with the object representation and projecting the self-representation on somebody else. Freud (1914/1957) describes this latter relationship in some cases of male homosexuality, but it probably is a much more generally valid process. In short, the persistence of the internal relationship in the process of mourning, with the combined presence of the representation of the other in relation to the self, the incorporation of the corresponding value systems into the ego ideal, and the identification of the self with the lost object, constitute complementary processes in the identification with a lost object. Adult mourning processes after the loss of a beloved other of many years of life together not only reactivate the infantile depressive position but also constitute a psychological experience that triggers specific mechanisms of grieving and compensation that foster new structural development. It may be that, at this point, the internalized world of object relations, under the impact of the mourning process, generates the experience of a world of ethical values, of what may be considered a spiritual realm that has general human validity, that is, a transcendental value system. Similar transformations may occur in the realm of the relation to art and erotic love and in the religious experience. An intrapsychic, consistent, silent dialogue with the lost object represents the subjective side of this structural development in the case of mourning.

References

Akhtar S: From mental pain through manic defense to mourning, in Three Faces of Mourning—Melancholy, Manic Defense, and Moving On. Edited by Akhtar S. Northvale, NJ, Jason Aronson, 2000, pp 95–113

Chasseguet-Smirgel J: The Ego Ideal: A Psychoanalytic Essay on the Malady of the Ideal. New York, WW Norton, 1985

Coyne JC (ed): Essential Papers on Depression. New York, New York University Press, 1985

Didion J: The Year of Magical Thinking. New York, Knopf, 2005

Fiorini LG (ed): On Freud's "Mourning and Melancholia." London, International Psychoanalytical Association, 2007

Frankiel RV (ed): Essential Papers on Object Loss. New York, New York University Press, 1994

Freud S: On narcissism: an introduction (1914), in The Standard Edition of the Complete Psychological Works of Sigmund Freud, Vol 14. Translated and edited by Strachey J. London, Hogarth Press, 1957, pp 67–102

Freud S: Mourning and melancholia (1917[1915]), in The Standard Edition of the Complete Psychological Works of Sigmund Freud, Vol 14. Translated and edited by Strachey J. London, Hogarth Press, 1957, pp 237–260

Freud S: Letter to Binswanger, Letter 239 (1929), in The Letters of Sigmund Freud. Edited by Freud EL. New York, Basic Books, 1960

Gaines R: Detachment and continuity: the two tasks of mourning. Contemp Psychoanal 33:549–571, 1997

Goethe JW: Die Wahlverwandtschaften (1809). München, Germany, Winkler Verlag, 1972

Grinberg L: Guilt and Depression. London, Karnac Books, 1992

Jacobson E: The Self and the Object World. New York, International Universities Press, 1964

Jacobson E: Depression: Comparative Studies of Normal, Neurotic, and Psychotic Conditions. New York, International Universities Press, 1971

Kernberg OF: Severe Personality Disorders: Psychotherapeutic Strategies. New Haven, CT, Yale University Press, 1984

Klein M: Mourning and its relation to manic-depressive states, in Contributions to Psycho-Analysis, 1921–1945. London, Hogarth Press, 1940, pp 311–338

Kogan I: The Struggle Against Mourning. New York, Jason Aronson, 2007

Lewis CS: A Grief Observed. San Francisco, CA, HarperCollins, 1961

Pollock G: On mourning, immortality, and utopia. J Am Psychoanal Assoc 23:334–362, 1975

Volkan VD: The "linking object" of pathological mourners. Arch Gen Psychiatry 27:215–221, 1972

Volkan VD: Not letting go: from individual perennial mourners to societies with entitlement ideologies, in On Freud's "Mourning and Melancholia." Edited by Fiorini LG, Lewkowicz S, Bokanowski T. London, International Psychoanalytic Association, 2007, pp 90–109

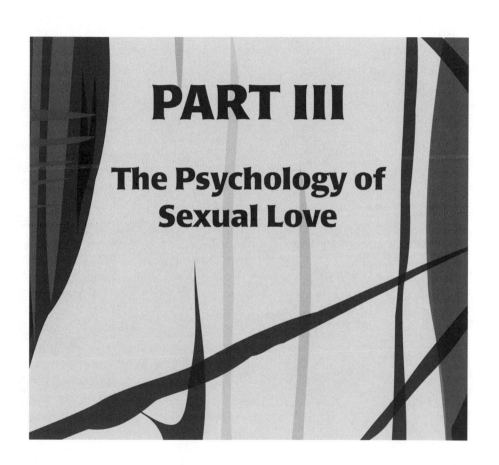

PART III

The Psychology of Sexual Love

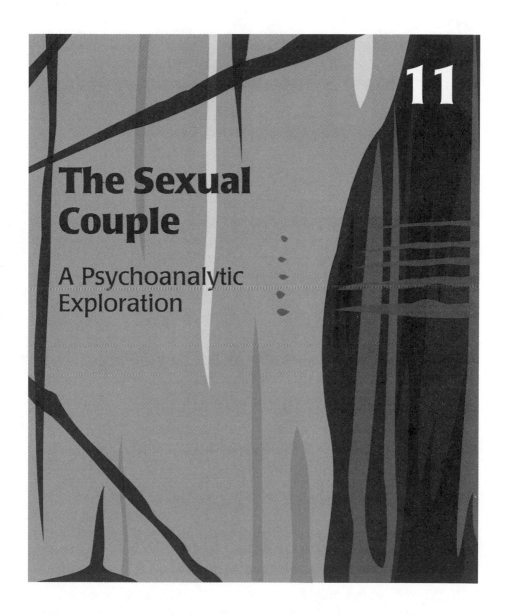

The Sexual Couple

A Psychoanalytic Exploration

Updated Sigmund Freud Lecture, originally delivered at a combined meeting
of the Sigmund Freud Institute and the Department of Psychology, University
of Frankfurt, Frankfurt, West Germany, October 21, 1988. This chapter was
reprinted from Kernberg OF: "The Sexual Couple: A Psychoanalytic Exploration." *Psychoanalytic Review* 98: 217-245, 2011. Used with permission.

In this chapter, I explore the development of the capacity for mature sexual love, starting from the neurobiology of sexual excitement, attachment, and selective attraction and exploring the transformation of the behavioral expression of these basic neurobiological systems into the complex subject experiences of erotic desire and passionate love. In this context, the integration of sexual excitement as an affect into erotic desire as an object relations–derived intrapsychic structure, reflected by specific unconscious and conscious fantasies, provides a key to the understanding of the multiple dimensions of affectionate and sexual relationships that culminate in the capacity to establish a stable love relationship. In this light, I explore what keeps a couple together and what threatens its survival, including here also the group pressures and conventional ideologies that impinge upon the love life of the couple.

What follows is a synthesis and update of my previous contributions to the psychology of mature love relationships as well as the salient forms of psychopathology of sexual love, in an effort to outline the developmental and structural preconditions for a mature love life (Kernberg 1995). The very nature of what may be considered "mature love," of course, is open to discussion (Kernberg 1997). This overview focuses on the unconscious, conflict-derived structures that underlie the conscious and preconscious disposition and capacity to fall in love and establish a love relationship in depth. The actual clinical aspects of limitations in this capacity are the subject of the chapter that follows the present one. Implicitly, in the present chapter, I also explore the affective and symbolic components of what constitutes "libido" as a drive. It represents a transition from the exploration of general psychoanalytic theory to the focus on clinical reality.

Biological Fundamentals

In the early stages of its development, the mammalian embryo has the potential to be male or female. Undifferentiated gonads differentiate into either testes or ovaries, depending on the genetic code represented by the different characteristics of the 46,XY chromosome pattern for males and the 46,XX pattern for females. Primitive gonads in the human may be detected from about the sixth week of gestation, when, under the influence of the genetic code, testicular hormones are secreted in males: the Müllerian duct inhibiting hormone (MIH), which has a defeminizing effect on the gonadal structure, and testosterone, which promotes the growth of internal and external masculine organs, particularly the bilateral Wolffian ducts. If a female genetic code is present, ovarian differentiation begins at the twelfth gestational week.

Differentiation always occurs in the female direction, regardless of genetic programming, unless an adequate level of testosterone is present. In other words, even if the genetic code is masculine, an inadequate amount of testosterone will result in the development of female sexual characteristics. The principle of feminization takes priority over masculinization. During normal female differentiation, the primitive Müllerian duct system develops into the uterus, the fallopian tubes, and the inner third of the vagina. In males, the Müllerian duct system regresses, and the Wolffian duct system develops, becoming the vasa deferentia, seminal vesicles, and ejaculatory ducts.

Whereas the internal precursors of both male and female sexual organs are thus present for potential development, the precursors for the external genitals are unitypic, that is, the same precursors may develop into either masculine or feminine external sexual organs. Without the presence of adequate levels of androgens (testosterone and dehydrotestosterone) during the critical period of differentiation, beginning with the eight-week fetus, a clitoris, vulva, and vagina will develop. But with the presence of adequate levels of androgen stimulation, the penis, including its glands, and the scrotal sac will form, and the testes will develop as organs within the abdomen. They normally migrate into their scrotal position during the eighth or ninth month of gestation.

Under the influences of circulating fetal hormones, a dimorphic development of certain areas of the brain takes place following the differentiation of internal and external genitals. The brain is ambitypic, and in it the development of female characteristics also prevails unless there is an adequate level of circulating androgens. Specific hypothalamic and pituitary functions that will be differentiated into the cyclic in women and noncyclic in men are determined by this differentiation.

The secondary sexual characteristics, which emerge during puberty—distribution of body fat and hair, change of voice, development of breasts, and significant growth of the genitals—are triggered by central nervous system factors and controlled by a significant increase of circulating androgens or estrogens, as are the specific female functions of menstruation, gestation, and lactation.

Androgens appear to influence the intensity of sexual desire in human males and females but within the context of a clear predominance of psychosocial determinants for sexual arousal. Although in low-order mammals such as rodents sexual behavior is controlled largely by hormones, in primates such control is somewhat modified by psychosocial stimuli.

The intensity of sexual arousal, the focused attention on sexual stimuli, the physiological responses of sexual excitement—increased blood flow, tumescence, and lubrication of sexual organs—are all under hormonal influence. Presently developing knowledge regarding the neurobiological mechanisms involved in the activation of sexual desire and behavior centers on the activation of a cascade of specific neurotransmitters, partly under the control of sex hormones—particularly testosterone—and largely influenced by the confluence of several neurobiological systems in addition to complex psychological mechanisms.

Oxytocin and vasopressin circuits have a central function in the activation of female and male sexual arousal and behavior. Oxytocin and arginine-vasopressin circuits also are key components of maternal nurturance and social bonding disposition, and this system, as well as the attachment-panic system, are involved as well in the complex development of the capacity for eroticism and sexual love. From a broader perspective, several basic neurobiological systems are involved in the infrastructure of human sexuality. They include the sexual-erotic system in a narrow sense, the attachment-panic system, and the social bonding–play system; all of them represented by corresponding integration of hormones, neuroamine transmitters and neuropeptides, and their related brain structures. These systems are characterized by specific activation of some of their component features for each of them and by overlapping features that reflect the overall systemic network function of the brain (Panksepp 1998).

Recent research findings regarding the neurobiology of sexual love, particularly functional magnetic resonance imaging (fMRI) brain studies of subjects, have helped to clarify this field. They have provided evidence for the combination of activation of specific hypothalamic, thalamic, and hippocampal activity, together with general activation of dopaminergic prefrontal cortical and anterior cingulate areas of subjects when presented with visual erotic stimuli, as well as love objects and nonsexual relations. Other research has provided evidence for androgen release under such conditions. Quite specifically, the evocation of images of passionate love objects activated the ventral tegmental area, nucleus accumbens, and vasopressin- and oxytocin-rich areas of the brain, together with prefrontal cortical, anterior cingulate, and hippocampal areas, reflecting activation common to both sexual-erotic and attachment-related brain structures. Images of close friendships activated related areas, but these could be clearly differentiated from those related to passionate love. Maternal love, explored with this same methodology, also activated areas related to passionate love, particularly the oxytocin- and vasopressin-related structures of, respectively, the nucleus accumbens and the ventral pallidum, but, in addition, revealed a specific activation of the lateral orbitofrontal cortex and the periaqueductal gray (Aron et al. 2005; Bartels and Zeki 2000, 2004; Fisher 1998, 2000).

Fisher (2006), based on her own research and a general review of neurobiological findings, has proposed an anthropological approach to the brain systems involved in sexual behavior: she proposes to differentiate 1) the sexual drive proper (represented by sexual arousal and search for achieving sexual relationships); 2) "selective attraction," which she equates to passionate love; and 3) attachment, analogous to what other authors (Hatfield and Rapson 1993) call "companionate" love, a combination of attachment, commitment, and intimacy. In this connection, the differentiation between two types of love, "passionate" and "companionate," first proposed by Berscheid and Hatfield (1969), corresponds to the widely accepted view that the initial intensity of erotic desire and passion in couple relationships is normatively replaced, throughout time, by a more tranquil but deeper emotional relationship, with a decrease of sexual interest, and early idealization is replaced by a sense of comradeship (Mitchell 2002). However, there is research evolving in this field that questions that assumption (B.A. Acevedo and A. Aron, "Does a Long-term Relationship Kill Romantic Love? A Review of Theory and Research," unpublished manuscript, 2008; Cuber and Haroff 1965; Hatfield et al. 1984; Tennov 1979; Wallerstein and Blakeslee 1995). A recent report by Acevedo (2008) has provided fMRI evidence of specific activation in long-time couples, when presented with pictures and evocation of their loved ones, of the same brain areas activated in individuals newly fallen in love. In addition, other brain areas related to concern and commitment are activated but can be differentiated from the reactions evoked by stimuli representing close, nonsexual friendships.

From a clinical standpoint, the capacity for passionate sexual love of long-term loving couples is quite evident, as is the failure in this regard on the part of many couples in serious chronic conflict. Of relevance here is the neurobiological basis for the assumption that several basic neurobiological and corresponding behavioral systems are involved in the development of the capacity for mature sexual love. It needs to be stressed, however, that empirically based clinical evaluation of the sexual life of adults cannot be equated simply to the behavioral expressions of basic neurobiological systems per se, for example, attachment. The "companionate" relationship of a couple in love obviously is a much more complex psychological organization than an infant's attachment behavior to mother, and the idealization of a love object is obviously more complex than "selective attraction" observed in animal behavior. There is a risk of reductionism involved, it seems to me, in relating neurobiological systems and their behavioral expression directly to complex human behavior, such as sexual love, and corresponding temptations may be found within the neurobiological and evolutionary psychology fields and within the behavioral and psychodynamic psychology fields as well.

It seems reasonable to assume that several major neurobiological systems are involved in the development of the capacity for mature sexual love: sexual excitement, attachment, selective attraction, playful bonding, and also, we should add, aggressive competiveness with sexual rivals; but our understanding of the complexities involved in adult sexual love by means of a psychodynamic exploration of the symbolic intrapsychic features of human experience is essential to give us a full picture of the complexities of the human mind in love. In what follows, I shall attempt to summarize the present approach of psychoanalytic object relations theory, as a general method of analysis and integration of the psychological development of the biological dispositions to sexual excitement, attachment, and erotic attraction, in addition to the idealization and passion that form part of the psychology of mature sexual love. To begin, we have to explore the contribution of contemporary affect theory. In summary, various basic motivational systems of the brain converge in the physiological substrate of erotic desire (Panksepp 1998). These systems operate through respectively dominant, positive and negative affect activation, so that, from a psychophysiological standpoint, affects are the signal expression of neurobiological systems, but they are influenced as well, in their behavioral and subjective expression, by the early interaction of the infant with his or her caregiving world.

Affective Development

In earlier work, I have proposed that affects are the primary motivational systems of psychic life, so that both positive, rewarding affects and negative, aversive affects are, respectively, the building blocks of the hierarchically supraordinate drives: libido and aggression. The drives, thus conceived, constitute integrated organization of the respective affects and are manifest in the activation of internalized object relations linked by the affective valence in which they are embedded (Kernberg 1992).

In my view, affects are the primary motivational system in that they are at the center of each of the infinite number of gratifying and frustrating concrete experiences the infant has with his or her environment. Affects link the series of undifferentiated self-/object representations so that gradually a complex world of internalized object relations, some pleasurably tinged, others unpleasurably tinged, is constructed. But even while affects are linking internalized object relations in two parallel series of gratifying and frustrating experiences, "good" and "bad" internalized object relations are themselves being transformed. The predominant affect of love or hate of the two series of internalized object relations is enriched and modulated and becomes increasingly complex. In contrast to primary affects as direct expression of neurobiological motivating systems, complex secondary affects—such as envy and hatred, highly individualized erotic desire and tender love, compassion and mourning—are highly influenced and determined by the individual development of internalized object relations. The advanced forms of intrapsychic motivations imply various fusions and combinations of primary neurological motivational systems.

Eventually, the internal relationship of the infant to the mother under the affect of "love" is more than the sum of a finite number of concrete, sensual, sexual, dependent, and idealized loving affect states. The same holds true for hate. Love and hate thus become stable intrapsychic structures in the sense of two dynamically determined, internally consistent, stable frames for organizing psychic experience and behavioral control in psychogenetic continuity through various developmental stages. By that very continuity, they consolidate into libido and aggression as hierarchically supraordinate motivational systems or drives, expressed in a multitude of differentiated affect dispositions under different circumstances. Affects are the building blocks, or constituents, of drives; they eventually acquire a signal function for the activation of drives.

It needs to be stressed that drives are manifest not simply by affects but by the activation of a specific self/other dyad that includes an affect and in which the drive is represented by a specific desire or wish. Unconscious fantasy, the most important being oedipal in nature, includes a specific wish directed toward an object. The wish derives from the drive and is more precise than the affect state—an additional reason for rejecting a concept that would make affects rather than drives the hierarchically supraordinate motivational system. Here we shall explore the specific unconscious fantasies that transform the biological function of sexual excitement into object-related erotic desire.

Erotic Desire

What are the clinical characteristics of erotic desire as uncovered by psychoanalytic exploration? A first characteristic of erotic desire is a search for pleasure always oriented to another person, an object to be penetrated or invaded or to be penetrated or invaded by. It is a longing for closeness, fusion, and intermingling that has a quality both of a forceful crossing of a barrier and of becoming one with the other person. The concrete sexual fantasies refer to invasion, penetration, or appropriation and include, at the level of conscious or unconscious fantasy, the relations between bodily protrusions and bodily openings: penis, nipple, tongue, finger, feces on the penetrating or invasive site and vagina, mouth, anus on the receptive or encompassing site. The rhythmic stimulation of these bodily zones promises erotic gratification, but that gratification loses its gratifying quality when it does not serve the broader function of intermingling with an object. "Container" and "contained" are not to be confused with masculine and feminine, active and passive; we find fantasy of active incorporation and passively being penetrated together with active penetration and passively being incorporated. Psychological bisexuality in the sense of the identification with both self and object in the specific sexual interaction is universal for men and women. One might say that bisexuality is first of all a function of identification with both participants of a sexual relationship or with all three in the triangulation of sexual experience.

A second characteristic of erotic desire is the gratification from identification with another's sexuality, more precisely, with the sexual excitement and orgasm of the sexual partner, with a condensation of two complementary experiences of fusion. The first element here is the pleasure derived from the desire of the other, the love expressed in the other's response to the sexual desire of the self, and the associated experience of fusion in ecstasy. Together with this may be the sense of becoming both genders at the same time, of

overcoming temporarily that ordinarily unbreachable barrier separating the sexes, with a sense of completion and enjoyment of the
penetrating and encompassing, penetrated and enclosed aspect of
sexual invasion.

A third characteristic of erotic desire is a sense of transgression; of overcoming the prohibitions implied in all sexual encounters, a prohibition derived from the oedipal structuring of sexual
life. This sense of transgression takes many forms; the simplest and
most universal is the transgression against conventional morality,
the ordinary social constraints that protect the intimacy of body
surfaces as well as the intimacy of sexual excitement from public
display.

In a deeper sense, transgression includes transgressing oedipal
prohibitions against sexual intimacy with the oedipal object, the
positive or negative oedipal object according to the predominantly
heterosexual or homosexual object choice. The wishful fantasy of
taking possession of that object constitutes a defiance of as well as
a triumph over the oedipal rival. But transgression also includes
transgression against the sexual object itself experienced as seductively teasing and withholding. Sexual excitement involves a sense
that the object is both offering and withholding itself, and sexual
penetration or engulfing of the object is a violation of the latter's
boundaries. In this sense, transgression involves aggression against
the object as well, aggression that is exciting in its pleasurable gratification, reverberating with the capacity to experience pleasure
in pain and the projection of that capacity onto the object. The aggression is also pleasurable because it is being contained by a loving relationship. And so we have the incorporation of aggression
into love and the assurances of safety in the face of unavoidable
ambivalence.

The ecstatic and aggressive aspects of the search for loss of
boundaries of the self represent a related deep and complex aspect
of erotic desire. Sexual excitement and orgasm facilitate an experience of fusion with the other that provides an ultimate sense of
fulfillment, of transcending the limits of the self (Stein 2008). They
also facilitate, in one stroke, a sense of oneness with the biological
aspects of personal experience. To induce pain in the other, and to
identify with the erotic pleasure in pain of the other, is the counterpart of erotic masochism. Sexual excitement, in this regard, also includes an element of surrender, of accepting a state of enslavement
to the other as well as being master of the other's fate. The extent to
which this aggressive fusion will be contained by love is impor-

tantly mediated by the superego, the guardian of the frame of love containing aggression. In short, both in pleasure and in pain there is a search for a peak affect experience that, temporarily, erases the boundaries of the self, a peak affect experience that gives a fundamental meaning to life, a transcendence that links sexual engagement with religious ecstasy and the experience of freedom beyond the boundary control of daily existence.

The idealization of the body of the other or the objects that symbolically represent that body is an essential aspect of erotic desire. Meltzer and Williams (1988) have proposed the existence of an early "aesthetic conflict" linked to the infant's attitude to mother's body. The infant's love for mother, in this view, is expressed in the idealization of the surface of her body and, by introjection of the mother's love expressed in the idealization of the infant's body, in the identification with her in this self-idealization. This idealization would give rise to the earliest sense of aesthetic value, of beauty.

Following Meltzer and Williams, the split-off aggression toward mother would, in contrast, be directed mainly toward the inside of her body and, by projection, in experiencing the inside of mother's body as dangerous. From this viewpoint, the desire and fantasy of violent invasion of mother's body is an expression of aggression, of envy of her outside beauty as well as her capacity to give life and love; and the idealization of mother's bodily surfaces, a defense against the dangerous aggression lurking under that surface. Mother's physical ministrations of the infant activate the erotic awareness of his or her own body surfaces and, by projection, the erotic awareness of the body surfaces of mother. Love received in the form of erotic stimulation of body surfaces becomes the stimulus for erotic desire as a vehicle for the expression of love and gratitude.

The lack of activation or the extinction of body-surface eroticism when intense aggression and a parallel lack of pleasurable body-surface stimulation combine in such a way as to interfere with the development of early idealization processes as part of erotic stimulation determines a primary sexual inhibition. The secondary repression of sexual excitement linked to later superego functioning and later oedipal prohibitions is much less severe and has a much better prognosis in treatment.

The wish for teasing and for being teased is another central aspect of erotic desire. This wish cannot be completely separated from the excitement stemming from overcoming the barrier of something forbidden and hence experienced as "sinful" or "amoral." The sexual object is always, in a profound sense, a forbidden oedipal object and the sexual act a symbolic repetition and overcoming of the primal scene. But here I am stressing the object's self-withholding, teasing as a combination of promise and withholding, of seductiveness and frustration.

Sexual teasing is typically though not exclusively linked to exhibitionistic teasing and illustrates the intimate connection between exhibitionism and sadism. By the same token, voyeurism is the simplest response to exhibitionistic teasing and implies a sadistic penetration of an object that withholds itself (Kernberg 1991b). As with the other perversions, it is characteristic that voyeuristic perversion is a typical sexual deviation of men, whereas exhibitionistic behavior is much more frequently interwoven with the character style of women. Psychoanalytic interpretations of female exhibitionism as a reaction formation to penis envy need to be amended to incorporate our more recent awareness of the complex step the little girl undertakes in shifting her object choice from mother to father: exhibitionism is a plea for sexual affirmation at a distance. Father's love and acceptance of his little girl and her vaginal genitality reconfirm her feminine identity and self-acceptance (Paulina Kernberg, personal communication, August 2005).

The experience of women's sexuality as both exhibitionistic and withholding, that is, as teasing, is a most powerful stimulus to erotic desire in heterosexual men. And it is also a source of aggression, a motive for the aggressive implication of the invasion of a woman's body, a basis for the voyeuristic aspects of the sexual relation that contain the wish to dominate, expose, and encounter and overcome barriers of true and false shamefulness in the woman who is loved. Parallel developments in homosexual men's reaction to father experienced as teasingly loving determine similar aggressive implications of the erotic desires to explore, dominate, and invade male bodies.

The voyeuristic impulse to observe a couple in sexual intercourse—at a symbolic level, to violently penetrate the primal scene—is a condensation of the wish to penetrate the privacy and the secrecy of the oedipal couple and to take revenge against the teasing object. Voyeurism is an important component of sexual excitement in the sense that every sexual intimacy implies an element of privacy and secrecy and, as such, identification with the oedipal couple and a potential triumph over it.

This leads us to one more aspect of erotic desire, namely, the oscillation between the search for secrecy, intimacy, and exclusiveness in the relationship, on the one hand, and the search for a radical discontinuity, for shifting away from sexual intimacy, on the other. The conventional cliché of our society at this time is that it is women who want to maintain intimacy and continuity in love relationships beyond their sexual implication and that men dissociate themselves from intimacy following sexual gratification and orgasm. This assumption does not take into consideration the differences in development in male and female sexuality and confuses the early stages of male development with mature development in both sexes. In clinical practice, we see as many husbands whose dependent longings are frustrated by their perception of their wife's affectionate dedication to their infants and small children as we see women complaining about their husband's failure to maintain sexual interest in them.

Braunschweig and Fain (1971; Braunschweig and Michel 1975) have developed an appealing theory of the characteristics of erotic desire in terms of the early development of the infant's and small child's relationship to mother. To summarize their viewpoint: the early relationship of the infant of both sexes with mother influences fundamentally the child's later capacity for sexual excitement and erotic desire.

Braunschweig and Fain attribute a crucial role to the mother's psychological turning away from the infant; they contrast mother's erotic stimulation of her male infant with the discontinuity established by her withdrawing her erotic interest from him and returning it to her husband. It is at this moment that the infant identifies himself with the frustrating yet stimulating mother, with her erotic stimulation and with the erotic stimulation of the sexual couple, that is, father as mother's object. This identification of the infant with the two members of the oedipal couple would provide the basic frame for a psychic bisexuality and consolidate the triangular situation in the child's unconscious fantasy.

The male infant's acknowledgment of this frustration and of the implicit censorship of his erotic desire for mother would then shift his erotic stimulation into masturbatory fantasy and activity, including the desire to replace father and, in primitive symbolic fantasy, to become the father's penis and the object of mother's desire.

In the case of the little girl, mother's subtle and unconscious rejection of the sexual excitement that she would freely experience in relation to the little boy gradually inhibits the little girl's direct awareness of the original vaginal genitality; she would therefore gradually become less aware of her own genital impulses while being less directly frustrated by the discontinuity in the relationship with mother. The identification with mother's eroticism would take more subtle forms, derived from mother's tolerance and fostering of the little girl's identification with her in other areas. With a tacit understanding of the "underground" nature of her own genitality, the little girl's deepening identification with mother would also strengthen her longing for father and her identification with both members of the oedipal couple.

The little girl's change of object from mother to father determines her capability for developing an object relation in depth with the loved and admired and yet distant father and the secret hope of eventually being accepted by him and of becoming free once more in the expression of her genital sexuality. This development fosters the little girl's capacity to commit herself emotionally to an object relationship that determines the woman's greater capacity for such a commitment in her sexual life, from early on, than is the case with men.

The explanation resides in the early exercise of trust, in the little girl's turning from mother to father, in his love and affirmation of her femininity "from a distance," in her capacity to transfer her dependency needs to an object physically less available than mother, and also, by the same change of object, the escape from preoedipal conflicts and ambivalence toward mother. Men, whose continuity of the relationship from mother to later female objects signifies potential perpetuation of both preoedipal and oedipal conflicts with mother, have greater difficulties in dealing with ambivalence toward women and evince a slower development than women in their capacity to integrate their genital with their tender needs.

Unconscious Object Relations

From this point on, I shall focus exclusively on the development of the love relationships between men and women. My experience with sexual conflicts of homosexual couples is too limited to integrate the corresponding literature meaningfully with my own psychoanalytic observations. The capacity to fall in love is a basic pillar of the relationship of the couple (Kernberg 1976). It implies the capacity to link idealization with eroticism and, implicitly, the potential for establishing an object relationship in depth. A man and a woman who discover their attraction and longing for each other, who are able to establish a full sexual relationship that carries with it emotional intimacy and a sense of fulfillment of their ideals in the closeness with the loved other, are expressing their capacity not only to link unconsciously eroticism and tenderness, sexuality and the ego ideal, but also to recruit aggression in the service of love; a couple in a fulfilling love relationship defies the ever-present envy and resentment of the excluded others and the distrustfully regulating agencies of the conventional culture in which they live (Kernberg 1988). The romantic myth of the lovers who find each other in a hostile crowd expresses in mythological form an unconscious reality for both partners. Some cultures may highlight romanticism, and others may rigorously attempt to deny it, but as an emotional reality, it is revealed in the erotic art and literature throughout historical times (Bergmann 1987).

The unconscious dynamics underlying the couple's defiance include overcoming oedipal prohibitions against sexual involvement with a loved and idealized object of the other sex. Behind this oedipal father, a woman's lover represents the preoedipal mother as well, satisfying her dependency needs while expressing tolerance of sexual intimacy with a symbolic oedipal object. For both man and woman, the love relationship represents daring to identify with the oedipal couple and overcoming it at the same time (Kernberg 1976).

Love and the Stable Couple

With sexual intimacy comes further emotional intimacy, and with emotional intimacy, the unavoidable ambivalence of oedipal and preoedipal relations. Granted the frequency of severe unconscious oedipal guilt and of narcissistic defenses derived from both oedipal and preoedipal sources, the question is, what factors are responsible for creating and maintaining a successful relationship between a man and a woman?

From a psychoanalytic viewpoint, the longing to become a couple and so fulfill the deep unconscious needs for a loving identification with paternity and maternity in a sexual relationship is as important as the aggressive forces that tend to undermine the couple; and what destroys passionate attachment and may appear to be a sense of imprisonment and "sexual boredom" is actually the activation of aggression, which threatens the delicate equilibrium between sadomasochism and love in a couple's sexual and emotional relationship.

But more specific dynamics come into play as emotional intimacy develops. The unconscious wish to repair the dominant pathogenic relationships from the past and the temptation to repeat them in terms of unfulfilled aggressive and revengeful needs determine their reenactment with the loved partner. By means of projective identification, each partner tends to induce in the other the characteristics of the past oedipal and/or preoedipal object with whom he or she experienced conflicts around aggression (Dicks 1967). If such conflicts were severe, this includes the erotic possibility of reenacting primitive, fantastically combined mother-father images that carry little resemblance to the actual characteristics of the parental objects (Kernberg 1991a).

Unconsciously, an equilibrium is established by means of which the partners complement each other's dominant pathogenic object relation from the past, and this tends to cement the relationship in new, unpredictable ways. Descriptively, we find that couples in their intimacy interact in many small, "crazy" ways. From an observer's position, the couple enact a strange scenario, completely different from their ordinary interactions, a scenario that, however, has been enacted repeatedly in the past. This "union in madness" ordinarily tends to be disrupted by the more normal and gratifying aspects of the couple's relationship in the sexual, emotional, intellectual, and cultural realms. In fact, a normal capacity for discontinuity in their relationship plays a central role in maintaining it.

Discontinuities

This capacity for discontinuity, described by Braunschweig and Fain (1971; Braunschweig and Michel 1975), has its ultimate roots in the discontinuity of the relationship between mother and infant.

The capacity for discontinuity is played out by men in their relationships with women: separating from women after sexual gratification reflects an assertion of autonomy (basically, a normal narcissistic reaction to mother's withdrawal) and is typically misinterpreted in the—mostly female—cultural cliché that men have less capacity than women for establishing a dependent relationship. In women, this discontinuity is normally activated in the interaction with their infants, including the erotic dimension of that interaction, which leads to the man's frequent sense of being abandoned: once again, in the cultural cliché—this time a male one—of the incompatibility of maternal functions and heterosexual eroticism in women.

The differences in capacity for tolerating discontinuities in men and women also show in their discontinuities regarding love relationships, as Alberoni (1987) has pointed out: women usually discontinue their sexual relationships with a man they no longer love and establish a radical discontinuity between an old love relationship and a new one. Men are usually able to maintain a sexual relationship with a woman even if their emotional commitment has been invested elsewhere; that is, they have a greater capacity for tolerating discontinuity between emotional investments in a woman, in reality and in fantasy, over many years even in the absence of an ongoing relationship in reality with her.

Men's discontinuity between erotic and tender attitudes toward women is reflected in the "Madonna-prostitute" dissociation, their most typical oedipal defense against the unconsciously never abandoned, forbidden, and desired sexual relationship with mother. But beyond that dissociation, profound preoedipal conflicts with mother tend to reemerge in undiluted ways in men's relationships with women, interfering with their capacity to commit themselves in depth to a woman. For women, having already shifted their commitment from mother to father in early childhood, their problem is not the incapacity to commit themselves in depth to a dependent relationship with a man but to tolerate their own sexual freedom in that relationship. In contrast to men's assertion of their phallic genitality from early childhood on, in the context of the unconscious erotization of the mother-infant relationship, women have to rediscover their original vaginal sexuality, unconsciously inhibited in the mother-daughter relationship. Throughout time, one might say that men and women have to learn what the other comes prepared with, in establishing the love relationship: for men, to achieve a commitment in depth and for women, sexual freedom. Obviously, there are significant exceptions to this rule, such as narcissistic pathology in women and severe types of castration anxiety of any origin in men.

Throughout many years of living together, a couple's intimacy may be either strengthened or destroyed by enacting certain types of unconscious scenarios. I am referring to unconscious scenarios enacted throughout time that differ from the periodic enactment of ordinary, dissociated past unconscious object relations. I am referring here, above all, to the enactment of oedipal scenarios linked to the invasion of the couple by excluded third parties as a major disruptive force and to various imaginary twinship relations enacted by the couple as a destructive centripetal or estranging force. Let us first explore these latter relations.

Narcissistic conflicts manifest themselves not only in unconscious envy, devaluation, spoiling, and separation but also in the unconscious desire to complete oneself by means of the loved partner, who is treated as an imaginary twin. Didier Anzieu (1986), in developing Bion's (1967) work, has described the unconscious selection of the love object as a homosexual and/or heterosexual completion of the self: a homosexual completion in the sense that the heterosexual partner is treated as a mirror image of the self. Anything in the partner that does not correspond to that complementing schema is not tolerated. If the intolerance includes the other's sexuality, it may lead to severe sexual inhibition. Behind the intolerance of the other's sexuality lay the narcissistic envy of the other sex. In contrast, when the selection of the other is as heterosexual twin, the unconscious fantasy of completion by being both sexes in one may act as a powerful cement. Bela Grunberger (1979) first pointed to the unconscious narcissistic fantasies of being both sexes in one.

It is a frequent observation that after many years of living together, partners begin to resemble each other, and one marvels at how two such similar persons found each other. The narcissistic gratification in this twinship relationship, the wedding, we might say, of object love and narcissistic gratification, protects the couple against the activation of destructive aggression. Under less ideal circumstances, such twinship relationships may evolve into what Anzieu (1986) has called a "skin" to the couple's relationship, a demand for complete and continuous intimacy that first seems an intimacy of love but eventually becomes an intimacy of hatred. "Do you still love me?" as a constantly repeated question that reflects the need for maintaining the couple's common skin is the counterpart of the assertion, "You always treat me like that!" signaling the shift of the quality of the relationship under the skin from love to persecution.

Triangulations

Direct and reverse triangulations, which I have described in earlier work (Kernberg 1988), constitute the most frequent and typical of unconscious scenarios, which may at worst destroy the couple or at best reinforce their intimacy and stability. Direct triangulation refers to the unconscious fantasy of an excluded third party, an idealized member of the subject's sex—the dreaded rival replicating the oedipal rival. Every man and every woman unconsciously or consciously fears the presence of somebody who would be more satisfactory to his or her sexual partner, and this dreaded third party is the origin of emotional insecurity in sexual intimacy and of jealousy as an alarm signal protecting the couple's integrity.

Reverse triangulation refers to the compensating, revengeful fantasy of involvement with a person other than one's partner, an idealized member of the other sex who stands for the desired oedipal object, thus establishing a triangular relationship in which the subject is courted by two members of the other sex for the idealized oedipal object of the other sex. I propose that, given these two universal fantasies, there are potentially, in fantasy, always six persons in bed together: the couple, their respective unconscious oedipal rivals, and their respective unconscious oedipal ideals.

One form that aggression related to oedipal conflicts frequently takes in clinical practice and in daily life is the unconscious collusion of both partners to find, in reality, a third person who represents a condensed ideal of one and rival of the other. The implication is that marital infidelity, short-term and long-term triangular relationships, more often than not reflects unconscious collusions between the couple, the temptation to enact what is most dreaded and desired. Fantasies about excluded third parties are typical components of normal sexual relationships. The counterpart of sexual intimacy that permits the enjoyment of polymorphous perverse sexuality is the enjoyment of secret sexual fantasies that express, in a sublimated fashion, aggression toward the loved object. Sexual intimacy thus presents us with one more discontinuity: discontinuity between sexual encounters in which both partners are completely absorbed in and identified with each other and sexual encounters in which secret fantasied scenarios are enacted, thus carrying into their relationship the unresolved ambivalences of the oedipal situation.

The perennial questions—What do women want? What do men want?—may be answered by saying that men want a woman in multiple roles—as mother, as a little baby girl, as a twin sister, and, above all, as an adult sexual woman. Women, because of their fateful shift from the primary object, want men in fatherly roles but also in motherly roles, a little baby boy, a twin brother, and an adult sexual man. And at a different level, both men and women may wish to enact a homosexual relationship or to reverse the sex roles in an ultimate search for overcoming the boundaries between the sexes that unavoidably limit narcissistic gratification in sexual intimacy: both long for a complete fusion with the loved object with oedipal and preoedipal implications that can never be fulfilled.

Superego Features

I propose that superego integration and maturation, expressed in the transformation of primitive prohibitions and guilt feelings over aggression into concern for the other—and the self—protect the object relation of the couple: the mature superego fosters love and commitment to the loved object. But, by the same token, because the superego always includes prohibitions against the remnants of oedipal conflicts, it may threaten the capacity for sexual love by prohibition directed against genital impulses and against the integration of sexual and tender feelings. Thus, the superego may guarantee the lasting capacity for sexual passion, or it may destroy it. When primitive superego pathology dominates, sadistic superego precursors are enacted and projected by the partners in the form of primitive dissociated object relations activated in their relationship (Kernberg 1993). In extreme cases, what amounts to a practical "absence" of normal superego functions may be the crucial factor that destroys the couple.

The setting up of the ego ideal as a crucial substructure of the superego is a fundamental precondition for the capacity to fall in love. The ego ideal reflects the capacity for the development of idealization beyond the self. The idealization of the loved other reflects the projection onto the other of aspects of one's own ego ideal. It is a projection that coincides with the profound attachment to this projected ideal, the sense that the loved other represents the coming alive in external reality of a desirable, profoundly longed for ideal. In this regard, the relationship in reality with the loved other implies an experience of transcendence beyond the limits of one's own psychic boundaries, an ecstatic experience that enters into a dialectical contrast to the ordinary world of daily reality and provides a transcendent meaning to life.

Superego functions become actualized at several levels of a couple's relationship. The first level is the enactment of superego functions in each of the partners, reflected, under normal circumstances, in the capacity for a sense of responsibility for the other and for the couple, of concern for their relationship, and of protection of the relationship against the consequences of the unavoidable activation of aggression as part of normal ambivalence in intimate relationships.

At a second level of superego activation, the projection of repressed aspects of the infantile superego onto the partner makes each of the partners particularly susceptible to criticism from the other. Those we love most can not only hurt us most but also, particularly, make us feel most guilty. A halo of projected primitive superego features reinforces the aggressive quality of objective criticism from the other. By the same token, however, by "rebelling" against the partner's criticism and guilt-raising behavior, one's own infantile superego is "counterattacked" and temporarily overcome. Cycles of projection of superego functions onto the other and the "rebellion" against these projected superego functions may contribute to the psychological equilibrium of the couple.

There is still a third level of activation of superego functions of the couple, a more subtle and intangible but extremely important one. Here, it is the healthy aspects of the ego ideal of both of them that combine to create a joint structure of desirable and aspired values reflecting an ego ideal function for the couple, as well as of undesirable and forbidden values that reflect prohibitive superego functions shared by both of them. At this level, a preconsciously adhered to value system of the couple is gradually mapped out, elaborated, and modified throughout the years and provides a boundary function for the couple in terms of their joint value systems.

It is at this third level where the couple's conscious aspirations for what their joint life should be are mapped out, their ideal aspirations for their relationship as a couple per se, and for their integration into—and autonomy from—the surrounding culture. And it is in appealing to this joint system of values that a couple can creatively contribute to solving their conflicts at all levels. It is at this level where, in the middle of a couple's conflicts, an unexpected gesture of love, of remorse, of forgiveness, of the creative gift, of the subtle reminder, and of humorous appreciation may keep aggression within bounds. It is also at this level where tolerance for shortcomings and the acceptance of limitations in the other, as well as in the self, are silently integrated into the relationship.

Conflicts at Relatively Mild Degrees of Superego Pathology

In essence, the problem here is a well-integrated but excessively severe and restrictive superego in one or both partners, jointly shared or unconsciously imposed upon the relationship. In this case, there is a mutual reinforcement of a rigid idealization of the conscious expectation of marriage, brought about by the confluence of the couple's identification with the cultural values and ideology of a specific social group and their similar conscious role expectations of themselves and their partner in a marital relationship. Their mutually projected and rigidly adhered to ego ideal may provide stability for the couple but also drown their sexual needs. The unconscious mutual projection of prohibitions against oedipal sexuality and against the integration of tender and erotic feelings facilitates the unconscious mutual activation of their corresponding oedipal relationship; their current interactions show a growing similarity to their dominant past relationships with the oedipal figures.

Conflicts at Severe Degrees of Superego Pathology

Here, a lack of overall superego integration predominates sufficiently to foster the inordinate reprojection of superego nuclei onto the partner and for one or both partners to tolerate his or her chronic enactment of contradictory character patterns.

Mutual reprojection of superego functions dominates, with consecutive attribution of blaming, critical, and derogatory attitudes to the partner, and, by means of projective identification, an unconscious induction of such behaviors in the partner. These mutual projections may be reflected, in the simplest cases, in a defensive emotional distancing that evolves over a period of months or years between the partners. Sometimes, the couple may simply "freeze" in a distancing position that becomes reinforced throughout time and leads to the eventual destruction or breakdown of the love relationship (Dicks 1967).

The most frequent expression of severe, chronic, mutual superego projection is one partner's experience of the other as a relentless persecutor, a moralistic authority who sadistically enjoys making the other feel guilty and crushed, while that second partner experiences the first as unreliable, deceitful, irresponsible, and treacherous and feels enraged because the other is attempting to "get away with it." These roles are often interchangeable. Chronic sadomasochistic relationships without any interventions of "excluded third parties" are probably the most frequent manifestation of superego pathology at this level of severity. These relationships may include satisfactory sexual relationships, but, in the long run, the vicious sadomasochistic interactions secondarily affect the couple's sexual functioning as well.

An important aspect of the enactment of superego conflicts in the relationship of the couple may be the development of deceptiveness in their relationship. Deceptiveness may serve the purpose of protection against real or fantasied aggression from the other and of hiding or keeping under control one's own aggression against the other. Deceptiveness in itself, of course, is a form of aggression. It may be a reaction against feared attacks from the other that, in turn, may be realistic or reflect the projection of superego features. Deceptiveness may also attempt to protect the other from pain, narcissistic lesion, jealousy, and disappointment because of the dishonest, aggressive, potentially unacceptable behavior of the self. Sometimes "absolute honesty" is simply a rationalized aggression.

Even in good relationships, there are discrete cycles of what might be called 1) deceptive, 2) paranoid or mutually suspicious, and 3) depressive or guilt-determined behaviors in the interaction that express as well as defend against the direct affective communication of the couple. From the viewpoint of the unconscious dynamics involved, deceptiveness is a defense against underlying paranoid fears and paranoid behavior in turn a defense against deeper depressive features, but self-blame may also be a defense against paranoid tendencies.

The capacity to forgive usually reflects a mature superego. The mature capacity to forgive others stems from having been able to recognize aggression and ambivalence in oneself and from the related capacity to accept the unavoidable nature of the mixture of love and hatred in intimate relationships. Authentic forgiveness is an expression of a mature sense of morality, an acceptance of the pain that comes with the loss of illusions about self and other, faith in the possibility of recovery of trust, and the possibility that love will be re-created and maintained alive in spite of and beyond its aggressive components. In contrast, forgiveness based on naiveté or narcissistic grandiosity has much less value in reconstructing the life of a couple based on a new consolidation of their shared concern for each other and for their life together.

There are cultures that may be considered "paternalistic," where a double morality prevails, and the main sexual taboos are directed against male homosexuality and against female marital infidelity. In contrast, in "maternalistic" cultures, the main sexual taboos are directed against male infidelity and father-daughter incest (Alberoni 1987). These taboos correspond, respectively, to the dominant insecurities and fears of men and women: for men, the threat to their sexual identity and the abandonment by mother; for women, the betrayal by father and the rupture of the oedipal prohibitions against the sexual involvement with him.

Group Processes

In earlier work (Kernberg 1980), I suggested that the couple in love represents both an ideal of and a threat to the large group, the fulfillment of each individual's fantasies. Each member of the group longs to break away from the anonymity of the large group and to become a partner in the private, secret, and symbolically forbidden new couple (the symbolic oedipal couple). At the same time, the group also experiences an intense envy of the couple that has managed to escape from the anonymous nature of the group and to accomplish what each of the isolated individuals in the large group fears cannot be accomplished.

The wishes to destroy the couple, derived from deep preoedipal sources of envy that tend to be activated under the conditions of large group processes and from direct oedipal rivalry and competition as well, resonate with the internal sources of aggression within the couple, referred to before, the ambivalence of their emotional relationship, and the temptation to set up direct and reverse triangular relationships. The couple needs the group to disperse in it aggression that otherwise might destroy it in isolation. The triumph of the couple that maintains itself within the threatening conditions of the large group reinforces its bonds. Couples and large groups need each other and threaten each other, especially when groups are unstructured, such as in informal community meetings, political rallies, congresses, public celebrations and recreational events, and large informal parties. The couples' ordinary social life reduces the manifestations of these group processes but maintains the tension between the boundaries of each couple and the threat to these boundaries derived from the activation of direct and reverse triangulation. In fact, the sexual tensions generated within the network of couples are a major cohesive force of social life as well as a threat to individual couples.

The relationships to the leader of the horde, described by Freud (1921/1955), are transformed, under ordinary social circumstances, by the relation of a community to the common boundaries of conventional morality expressed in the laws regulating, among other issues, sexual relationships. Such laws, as illustrated in the Judeo-Christian tradition in the Ten Commandments (and the expanded version of them in Leviticus 18, 19, and 20 of the Old Testament), are basically directed against incest and parricide and geared to protecting the boundaries of sexes and generations against massive invasion by regressive polymorphous perverse sexuality under the dominance of primitive aggression. Chasse-guet-Smirgel (1984) has detailed these functions of institutional-ized morality in opposition to dangerous regression to primitive group processes that would tend to deny the prohibition against in-cest and parricide together with the exclusive nature of the oedipal couple and of the autonomous adult couple as its derivative.

I would add that the collective projection of infantile superego features upon the abstract systems of laws and moral authority that regulate public behavior within informal human communities cannot but transform rational moral law into a derivative form of morality heavily influenced by infantile prohibitions against sexu-ality. This distortion takes the form of a conventionalized tolerance of sexuality that affirms the sacred nature of the autonomous cou-ple but suppresses the recognition of all elements of polymorphous perverse infantile sexuality, together with an attendant ritualiza-tion of sexual behavior to reduce the private freedom of the couple.

These developments generate an unresolvable contradiction between public and private morality, a hidden contradiction be-tween the couple's striving for sexual freedom and the public re-striction of sexuality to conventional social norms.

Paradoxically but not surprisingly, group rebellion against such conventional morality destroys both the conventional suppression of polymorphous perverse sexuality and the protection of the couple's sexual love. The protective functions of the superego are brushed aside together with its sexually restrictive ones. Group processes that illustrate this phenomenon are seen in boys' latency groups wherein sex is talked about freely but with derisory and largely anal terminology and in adolescent groups that, in the case of boys, also permit free communication about mechanical sexuality devoid of emotional value and, in the case of girls, romanticize but de-enitalize the idealization of popular stars (Braunschweig and Fain 1971). Similar devaluation of the integration of erotic and tender love of sexual passion of the couple can be observed in the cultural atmosphere of "old boys' clubs" and the corresponding female equivalents.

From a historical perspective, repeated cultural oscillations between "puritanical" periods in which love relationships become de-eroticized and eroticism goes underground and "libertine" peri-ods in which free sensual sexuality deteriorates into emotionally degraded group sex can be observed. In my view, such oscillations reflect the long-term equilibrium between the dynamics of the social need for destroying, protecting, and controlling the couple and the couple's aspirations to break out of conventional constrictions of sexual morality, a freedom that, in extremes, becomes self-destructive.

References

Acevedo BP: The neural basis of long-term romantic love. Doctoral dissertation, State University of New York at Stony Brook, 2008

Alberoni R: L'Erotisme. Paris, Ramsay, 1987

Anzieu D: La scéne de ménage: l'amour de la haine. Nouvelle Revue de Psychanalyse 33:201–209, 1986

Aron A, Fisher H, Strong G: Romantic love, in The Cambridge Handbook of Personal Relationships. Edited by Vangelisti A, Perlman D. New York, Cambridge University Press, 2005, pp 595–614

Bartels A, Zeki S: The neural basis of romantic love. Neuroreport 11:3829–3834, 2000

Bartels A, Zeki S: The neural correlates of maternal and romantic love. Neuroimage 21:1155–1166, 2004

Bergmann MS: The Anatomy of Loving. New York, Columbia University Press, 1987

Berscheid E, Hatfield E: Interpersonal Attraction. New York, Addison-Wesley, 1969

Bion WR: The imaginary twin, in Second Thoughts: Selected Papers on Psycho-Analysis. Northvale, NJ, Jason Aronson, 1967, pp 3–22

Braunschweig D, Fain M: Eros et Anteros. Paris, Payot, 1971

Braunschweig D, Michel F: La Nuit, Le Jour: Essai psychanalytique sur le fonctionnement mental. Paris, Presses Universitaires de France, 1975

Chasseguet-Smirgel J: Creativity and Perversion. New York, WW Norton, 1984

Cuber JF, Haroff PB: The Significant Americans. New York, Appleton-Century, 1965

Dicks HV: Marital Tensions. New York, Basic Books, 1967

Fisher HE: Lust, attraction, and attachment in mammalian reproduction. Human Nature 9:23–52, 1998

Fisher HE: Lust attraction, attachment: biology and evolution of the three primary emotion systems for mating, reproduction, and parenting. J Sex Educ Therapy 25:96–104, 2000

Fisher HE: The drive to love, in The New Psychology of Love. Edited by Sternberg R, Weis K. New Haven, CT, Yale University Press, 2006, pp 87–115

Freud S: Group psychology and the analysis of the ego (1921), in The Standard Edition of the Complete Psychological Works of Sigmund Freud, Vol 18. Translated and edited by Strachey J. London, Hogarth Press, 1955, pp 65–143

Grunberger B: Narcissism: Psychoanalytic Essays. New York, International University Press, 1979

Hatfield E, Rapson RL: Historical and cross-cultural perspectives on "passionate love" "compassionate" love and sexual desire. Annu Rev Sex Res 4:67–98, 1993

Hatfield E, Traupmann J, Sprecher S: Older women's perceptions of their intimate relationships. J Soc Clin Psychol 2:108–124, 1984

Kernberg OF: Object Relations Theory and Clinical Psychoanalysis. New York, Jason Aronson, 1976

Kernberg OF: Love, the couple and the group: a psychoanalytic frame. Psychoanal Q 49:78–108, 1980

Kernberg OF: Between conventionality and aggression: the boundaries of passion, in Passionate Attachments: Thinking About Love. Edited by Gaylin W, Person E. New York, Free Press, 1988, pp 63–83

Kernberg OF: Aggression and love in the relationship of the couple. J Am Psychoanal Assoc 39:45–70, 1991a

Kernberg OF: Sadomasochism, sexual excitement, and perversion. J Am Psychoanal Assoc 39:333–362, 1991b

Kernberg OF: Aggression in Personality Disorders and Perversions. New Haven, CT, Yale University Press, 1992

Kernberg OF: The couple's constructive and destructive superego functions. J Am Psychoanal Assoc 41:653–677, 1993

Kernberg OF: Love Relations: Normality and Pathology. New Haven, CT, Yale University Press, 1995

Kernberg OF: Perversion, perversity, and normality: diagnostic and therapeutic consideration. Journal of the Psychoanalytic Institute of the Postgraduate Center for Mental Health 14(suppl):19–40, 1997

Meltzer D, Williams MD: The Apprehension of Beauty: The Role of Aesthetic Conflict in Development, Art, and Violence. Perthshire, Scotland, Clunie Press, 1988

Mitchell SA: Can Love Last? The Fate of Romance Over Time. New York, WW Norton, 2002

Panksepp J: Affective Neuroscience. New York, Oxford University Press, 1998

Stein R: The otherness of sexuality: excess. J Am Psychoanal Assoc 56:43–71, 2008

Tennov D: Love and Limerence: The Experience of Being in Love. New York, Stein & Day, 1979

Wallerstein JS, Blakeslee S: The Good Marriage. Boston, MA, Houghton Mifflin, 1995

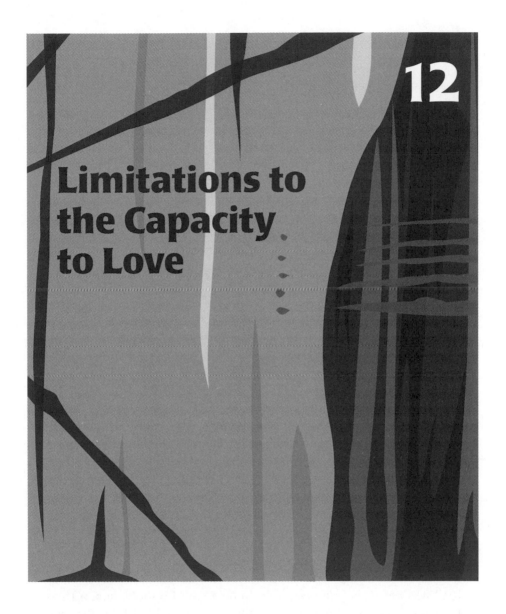

12

Limitations to the Capacity to Love

In this chapter, I describe limitations in the capacity for mature sexual love as reflecting various psychopathological conditions. These limitations include a variety of psychological restrictions determined most frequently by masochistic, narcissistic, and paranoid personality features. Clinical case material illustrates both mature and disturbed capability for love relationships. The developmental features of the capacity for mature love relationships explored in Chapter 11 are the underlying dispositions to what clinically can be explored as fully functional or dysfunctional expressions of this capacity, and I describe typical symptoms of the limitations to love that reflect the pathology in the realm of these dispositions.

Interferences to the Capacity to Love

What I have attempted in this chapter is to spell out the manifestations of passionate love that we usually take for granted and leave to poets to describe in detail. It is a meditation on the potential for and problems of establishing and maintaining loving and passionate relationships, drawn from a lifetime of struggling with these issues in the course of doing analysis. The methodology followed in this chapter is to describe the capacities involved in love relationships on the basis of their noticeable absence under various pathological conditions and to use psychoanalytic observations of their interference or absence to construct a composite frame of the corresponding assumed mature functions. Such a structural frame should facilitate an early diagnosis of the main features of pathology of love relationships in individual cases. Clinical vignettes will suggest characterological features that compromise the corresponding functions. I am aware of the risk that what follows may be misunderstood as a "prescriptive" set of characteristics of "normality." It is not. It is intended only to be a set of dimensions, a theoretical frame with the diagnostic potential to highlight, by contrast, major areas of difficulty or pathology in the capacity to love. This exploration also is a complement to earlier work analyzing the psychodynamic preconditions underlying the capacity for sexual love (Kernberg 1995).

Because the large majority of cases I have been able to analyze have been heterosexual patients, I limit my discussion to the dynamics of heterosexual love: clearly, a parallel study of homosexual love relationships remains to be done.

Falling in Love

Obviously, in the state of "falling in love," we expect to see a degree of idealization of the other person, an enchantment with the partner's physical, sexual, and personality features; an interest in and respect for the other person's value systems; and an intense longing for sexual intimacy, emotional closeness, and a meeting of the minds regarding joint ways to experience the world and relate to it (Chasseguet-Smirgel 1973). It is a passionate experience. This is in sharp contrast to narcissistic patients' typical "market analysis" of the pros and cons of potential partners' attributes, to masochistic patients' anxious idealization of their love object with the fantasy that rejection would mean a major devaluation of themselves, and to paranoid patients' fearful attention to not being treated badly or being cheated. The lack of the capacity to fall in love is a charac teristic symptom of severely narcissistic personalities; the incapacity to fall in love is an important diagnostic marker.

Necessarily, the initial idealization of falling in love will shift into the awareness of some shortcomings in the other and in the relationship of new aspects of their interaction that have to be incorporated into the image of the other, both good and bad. The accumulation of gratifying experiences, intense moments of life together that enrich the relationship in the sexual, emotional, and value systems realms, while fostering a deep feeling of gratitude for love received and responded to, generates a sense of personal value and emotional wealth derived from the relationship and leads to the transforming of falling in love into being in love, that is, a stable love relationship (Dicks 1967). The nature of the idealization of the love object shifts throughout time. Again, narcissistic patients, given their difficulties in establishing object relations in depth, often evince a tendency to repeatedly evolving, transient falling in love or "infatuations." They have great difficulty in maintaining a stable love relationship. The unconscious envy of the sexual partner, defended against by a process of relentless devaluation, is a dominant dynamic of these cases (Kernberg 2004).

Interest in the Life Project of the Other

Here, a central aspect of the capacity to love will emerge, one that may require time to become fully evident, namely, an ongoing curiosity and interest in the life of the beloved person, in his or her emotional experience, personal history, ideals, and aspirations as an unending source of stimulation and growth of one's own life experience. The interest in the life and emotional development and growth of the person one loves is a source of personal enrichment and adds a dimension of depth regarding joint exploration of intellectual interests and the relation to nature, art, and human conflicts, and it further deepens love and gratitude for what the couple shares. It implies the capacity for a mature object relationship in depth. In a deeper sense, a process of identification with the beloved person takes place, an identification with the interests and values of the other that become part of one's own aspirations and commitments. This development differs sharply from narcissistic patients' lack of interest in what strongly moves their partner.

The absence of this psychological capability of curiosity and interest in one's partner is one of the most dramatic consequences of narcissistic pathology, with its tendency to take the other for granted, a boredom with the subjective experience of the other, and the experience of the relationship as more "transactional" than interpersonal, dominated as it is by concern with "who of the two is getting more from the other." And, of course, a submersion in the subjective experience of the other necessarily may become distorted by excessive projective mechanisms characteristic of paranoid character traits or by a predominantly aggressive infiltration of the relationship related to the destructive pathology of envy, both conscious and unconscious, of narcissistic personalities.

All of the patients in clinical cases mentioned in this chapter were in psychoanalytic treatment with me, four sessions per week.

One patient, suffering from a severe narcissistic personality, fell in love in the third year of his analysis. He admired the beauty, social grace, and intellectual prominence of his girlfriend and basked in the social import that his new relationship signified among the members of his family and his friends. However, he showed practically no curiosity about her inner life or her reactions to experiences they shared and only perceived acutely whatever he considered positive or critical reactions she might have toward him. Gradually, as her impact on his social life became more routine, and the admiring acceptance of her—and its reflection on him—by his social group diminished as a source of narcissistic gratification, he became bored with the relationship. More importantly, her evident success in her professional life, her being admired and appreciated in her own right rather than simply reflecting his importance, became a major source of his unconscious envy of her. Traveling abroad with her, he found less and less to talk about with her, felt bored, and experienced her presence as restrictive to his freedom.

In addition, his awareness of her enjoyment of life and of her very capacity to love him evoked intense envy and secondary devaluation of her. Enthusiastic reactions of hers to people, art, and situations made him feel uncomfortable and resentful.

This case illustrates a defensive narcissistic devaluation of unconscious envy as a major cause of the lack of curiosity and of interest and enjoyment in the mind and the life of the other. The very capacity to love and to enjoy the love of the other is severely restricted under such circumstances. To the contrary, the pleasure with the happiness of the other, resonating with the fulfillment of the other's hopes and dreams, personal and professional success, and profound gratification with the enjoyment of the other, are normal expressions and sources of further growth of a love relationship.

Basic Trust

A second characteristic of the capacity for mature love is the presence of a basic trust in the partner's empathy with oneself and the goodwill of the other. A corresponding capacity is the freedom to be open about oneself, including about one's weaknesses, conflicts, and frailties, daring to express one's needs for help and understanding, one's doubts in oneself at time of crisis or regarding conflictual aspects of the self, with the implicit trust that the other will understand and tolerate one's uncertainty and sense of frailty and that love will not be affected negatively by revealing one's vulnerabilities. At the bottom, this capacity implies the internal security in depending on a loving maternal introject, even when oedipal guilt complicates this deep sense of a secure attachment. Without it, such basic trust remains frail.

The ability to be open and honest must, of course, be reciprocal, so that both parties may feel free to reveal themselves and thus challenge each other to contribute to their growth as individuals and as a couple.

Honesty may become a major test of the love relationship. Of particular importance is the question of infidelity, always a major threat to the love relationship, indicating as it does a profound conflict in at least one of the members of the couple. Honesty about involvement with a third party poses a serious challenge to trust in the understanding, the tolerance, and the capacity for an authentic forgiveness on the part of the other. To be able to openly acknowledge behavior that hurts the other, accepting one's own responsibility in an honest communication that trusts the other's good will (although one cannot be certain of the other's understanding and forgiveness), reflecting the commitment to honesty above the certainty of preservation of the relationship, is an indication of such basic trust. It may become a major test of the survival potential of a love relationship.

> A married woman in her late thirties, in analysis for several conversion symptoms and a chronic, neurotic depression, had established, in the course of the treatment, a relationship with another man, thereby acting out negative transference developments related to a seductive and rejecting father figure and in response to a chronic conflict with her narcissistic husband. His initial idealization of her and his later apparent indifference revived her oedipal resentment toward father, powerfully activated in the transference as well, leading to this acting out and to an extended period of working through this conflict through transference analysis. At one point, having ended the extramarital relationship, she felt threatened by a third party who might reveal that relationship to her husband. A period of obsessive rumination followed about whether to preventively confess this relationship to the husband or not. She was afraid of his narcissistic reaction, his revengefully walking out on her, but also, as a consequence of analytic work, she became aware that infantile roots of her fears of being punished for "forbidden sexual behavior" projected onto her husband exacerbated her anxiety over the past affair. Also, reaching the conclusion that in effect, in spite of his characterological limitations, her husband really did love her and that she trusted him in this regard, she was able to assess more realistically his capacity to overcome such a traumatic revelation and appreciate her honesty and her wish to resolve the difficulties of their marriage. Finally, she decided that he would be able to recognize her good will and commitment to their relationship and openly discussed her now past affair with him. It was an anxious time for her and in her analyst's countertransference. She was not disappointed: her greater maturity and her husband's capacity to work through his narcissistic lesion and mourning process significantly deepened the marital relationship.

Obviously, many cases with similar difficulties end in separation and divorce. Here, particularly the masochistic amplification of the experience of betrayal by the partner and the narcissistic intolerance of having been injured are important complicating features.

Capacity for Authentic Forgiveness

The reciprocal capacity not only to ask for forgiveness but also to forgive the behavior of the other, to be able to start again after serious conflicts and temporary dominance of aggression over love in the relationship is a major test of mature love. But, such a capacity for trust has to be differentiated from the denial of aggression and mistreatment on the part of the other—in other words, from masochistic submission to an unrealistic view of the couple's relationship, in which trust is not in the other person but in a fantasized relationship that does not correspond to reality. This latter development usually coincides with an incapacity to really enjoy the personality of the other and to be truly interested in the other's experience. It may be a masochistic submission to and idealization of an aggressive or abandoning object that usually goes hand in hand with the absence of a realistic assessment in depth and with a remarkable lack of interest in the subjective experience of such a partner. Trust in the other and openness about the self imply the expectation of a mutuality of understanding that can survive conflicts. Such a trust would not, therefore, be compatible with a lack of response at the same level from the other. Naturally, when the effort to maintain the relationship by the other one is based not upon the search for reconfirmation of intimacy but upon opportunistic criteria regarding advantages of staying together, such a neutrality is not expected. That, of course, is a solution not infrequently adopted by couples in conflict, but, by the same token, it indicates the limitation of their relationship.

In this connection, in analytic treatment, there are usually many opportunities for observing a patient's capacity to raise questions when feeling misunderstood, hurt, or mistreated by a partner and expressing his or her unhappiness over the situation without attempting to induce guilt feelings in the other as another dimension of the capacity for mature love. Communicating one's feelings of being hurt without blaming the other is a subtle but essential quality of open communication that reflects trust in the other person. "I need to tell you how I feel on the basis of what happened, because I trust you are not wanting to hurt me, and you need to know that this is what I felt," reflects a very different attitude from "Look what you did to me." A chronic tendency to evoke guilt feelings in the other, a frequent manifestation of masochistic (or sadomasochistic) pathology, not only reflects efforts to deflect the attacks of a persecutory superego onto the partner but also may serve as the expression of unconscious guilt over the possibility of a happy marital relationship (Dicks 1967). All of this does not mean that there is not a place for being enraged and letting the other know that one is enraged with the other but that, in a deep love relationship, such a communication would occur in the context of the conviction that one's rage will not affect the basic love of the couple and that the other one knows it. In a deeper sense, the capacity to forgive reflects the achievement of the depressive position, the acknowledgment of one's own aggressive potential, and the confidence in repairing a traumatized relationship.

Humility and Gratitude

Mature love, in addition, it seems to me, always contains an element of humility, of deeply felt gratitude for the existence of the other person, for the love received, for the possibility of dependency on the other person, as well as the acceptance of the uncertainty derived from potential future developments in reality that may cause changes in the relationship that cannot be predicted (i.e., financial breakdowns, illness, and death). Implicit in mature love is an honest acceptance of one's essential need of the other in order to achieve full enjoyment and security in life. And yet, such humility has to be differentiated from a desperate clinging, from an unwillingness to accept the reality of the end of love if it should occur, and from an unwillingness to accept the suffering of separation as a necessary, essential alternative to maintaining a dependent relationship with somebody who is no longer responding to one's love. Humility may be considered the counterpoint of sexual passion and should be congruent with a realistic self-regard.

> A woman in her early forties, who consulted because of chronic difficulties in maintaining a love relationship, was consciously desirous of establishing a marital relationship but experienced her life as moving from one unhappy relationship to the next. She presented a combination of markedly narcissistic and masochistic characterological patterns. She could only accept successful and brilliant, good-looking men from her own cultural environment and was easily attracted to what appeared to be severely narcissistic men who were unwilling to establish a stable relationship with her on her terms. If, however, men seemed genuinely interested in her, she would rapidly devalue them: how good could they be if they seemed to need her more than she needed them? By the same token, men who seemed to be really mature and nice, and without the attitude of being special or unique, would not be taken seriously by her.

Her analysis revealed both intense unconscious envy and resentment of men as representations of a powerful and corrupt father image and unconscious guilt over the oedipal implications of all love relationships. At the same time, an unconscious search for an all-understanding and sheltering mother figure—the opposite of her own distant and aloof mother—further complicated her insatiable demands of men with whom she was involved.

What I wish to highlight here was her deep sense that without an ideal man with whom, unconsciously, she could merge, life was truly intolerable. She needed a love relationship to feel complete, to avoid a sense of emptiness, aloneness, and lack of purpose in life. She was desperately clinging to impossible men yet ending relationships with men who loved her but expected some degree of reciprocity from her on an enraged note of frustrated entitlement. She would make endless demands and seemed unable to experience a sense of gratitude for love received. She oscillated between a haughty grandiosity and a desperate sense of being abandoned. Her limitation to love was characterized by an incapacity to depend on a love object and to experience gratitude for love received, a lack of humility in the sense described, and particularly a remarkable lack of interest in the internal life of men she was involved with. She was impressed by the prominence of one man she was involved with in international artistic circles but could not tolerate his sharing with her the technical challenges of his actual work.

In the transference, these dynamics played themselves out in repetitive cycles of alternating idealizing dependency, rageful frustration, and contemptuous devaluation of the analyst. At times, I was moved by her description of the loving attention to her wishes on the part of her lover that, evidently, she had taken for granted: a painful countertransference experience. Only very slowly could these mutually split-off states be integrated, with a growing tolerance, on her part, of the ambivalence of her relationship to me and with the gradual elaboration of her unconscious relationship with the corrupt, powerful father and her regression to an ambivalent relationship to an absent mother.

At one point, she became both able to feel grateful for my not giving up on her and able to maintain an internal relationship with me even under conditions of intense rage. Her newly achieved tolerance for acknowledgment of her profound ambivalence permitted her to experience the interaction with me more realistically and to become anxiously aware of her difficulties in evaluating our interactions. Now, for the first time, she became attentive to men's realistic relationship to her rather than to simply search for reconfirmation of her grandiosity by means of their admiration. But she was still far from the capacity to establish a stable love relationship.

A Common Ego Ideal as a Joint Life Project

To be dedicated to a love relationship as a life project that infiltrates the tasks of every day is another major, perhaps the most essential, aspect of a love relationship, the counterpart to the capacity for an ongoing, enlivening, and exciting interest in the personality and the subjective experience of the other. It is an expression of the joint ego ideal established by the couple through time, the basis for ongoing work on the relationship and for the protection of its boundaries and of its survival under adversity (Kernberg 1995).

The awareness and acceptance of the unavoidability of conflicts, of aggression, and of discrepancies in daily life arrangements, in sexual experiences and expectations, in the relationship to children and family of origin, and in ideology and value systems are part of what makes the life of a couple dangerous yet exciting. Here, an ongoing assessment of one's own essential values as a fundamental, indispensable part of one's personality that must be respected by the other, and what the corresponding basic, essential values and requirements are of the other that have to be tolerated and respected and adjusted to, is another task and condition of love. The commitment to a joint life based on mature love facilitates the establishment of valuable and gratifying compromise solutions where conflicts and competing agendas arise. This involves the assessment of problems in self and the other that have to be acknowledged and dealt with honestly, with the underlying pleasure in the capacity to achieve such an understanding that strengthens the boundaries of the couple in that context.

It may sound trivial to stress the importance of communicating love for each other to each other as an ongoing communication, and it certainly may become a routine, stereotypical behavior; however, as an expression of an ongoing, always new pleasure in the daily encounter and reencounter, sharing with the other the very pleasure with the other's presence and love may be part of a consistent mutual communication of life experience. It signals the ongoing awareness of the life project of the couple. It is the counterpart of the capacity to tolerate temporary separations, not simply in terms of time or geographic distance but in terms of the unavoidable—and necessary—discontinuities of a relationship that confirm difference and individuality, independent experiences that may later be joined, and the normal acting out of the ambivalence of all love relationships.

An obsessive man in analytic treatment complained about his wife's consistent expression of unhappiness with him because he never shared his feelings with her. During one session, he pointed out to me that this was similar to his mother's chronic complaining about his behavior, attempting to make him feel guilty. He openly expressed his feelings about his wife to me, didn't he?, he asked. I acknowledged that he expressed his feelings about her openly to me, including, in recent times, his feelings of love for her....So there seemed to be a strange discrepancy between the sessions and the relationship with his wife. At that point, he realized that being "too open" about expressing his loving feeling to his wife made him feel uncomfortable about his relationship with me—now representing his jealous mother. It was an unconscious aspect of his fear to reveal his loving dependency to his wife. And would she believe that it was childish of him to love her so much?

Sharing with each other the pleasures the other one gives us in such ordinary daily experiences as watching each other in social encounters; observing spontaneous behavior of the other that has an endearing quality; sharing as a source of enjoyment a peculiar, sometimes comical, and sometimes moving gesture and reaction; and giving a sudden expression of pleasure of the other, form strong bonds in the union of the couple. Love should permit to open one's eyes to pleasure the other has experienced and has helped us to discover; love implies sharing meanings we construct on an ongoing basis of life experience and shifting life realities. It is the opposite of a couple taking each other for granted. Frequently, oedipal guilt, not daring to experience a better marital relationship than the one a patient's parent shared in reality or in the patient's fantasy, may be the source of an excessive constraint in mutual enjoyment. A frequent masochistic acting out in long-standing couples is the accusatory statement by one partner: "He (she) should have remembered this anniversary...been aware that that statement hurt me...know from experience what I want." Many patients—and not only patients—have to learn that humans are not telepathic.

Mature Dependency as Opposed to Power Dynamics

Mature dependency has to be differentiated from masochistic submission and is closely related to the ongoing sense of gratitude for love received, love not taken for granted, and love from the other acknowledged consistently as a gift from destiny or heaven. Love of the other, fused with gratitude for the love received, also implies a sense of responsibility for the other, for the achievement of the life project and the happiness of the other as an essential personal goal.

One important aspect of the experience of dependency on the other as a component of mature love is the capacity to let oneself be taken care of by the other without suffering from a sense of inferiority, shame, or guilt, particularly under conditions of illness and fear-arousing experiences. In the case of serious, life-threatening illness, or crippling life situations, to be held by the love of the other; not to lose the sense of being part of the couple's living experience; tolerance of one's own and the other's frailties under such conditions; and the natural, loving commitment to take care of the other are part of the experience of mature love (Balfour 2009). Once again, profound disturbances in this capacity are closely related to narcissistic conflicts, a sense of humiliation or inferiority when a fantasied independent superiority is challenged, and, at the bottom, the failure of a safe relationship to a loving, maternal introject.

The willingness to take over (or for the other to take over), helping the other, stepping in for the other, is expressed, in less dramatic ways, in the natural wish to share responsibilities, burdens, and tasks and to actively want to help the other as well as being able and willing to ask for help, with a sense of fairness in the distribution of tasks and responsibilities. A sense of fair distribution of tasks and responsibilities is the opposite to the concern over power distribution and power relations under conditions when aggression infiltrates the love relationship and takes the form of the need to protect oneself against real or fantasized aggression from the other. The concern with power struggles as the supposedly unavoidable conflict between men and women represents, I believe, a conventional rationalization of pathological dominance of aggression in a couple's relationship, in contrast to the normal ambivalence of all relationships that can be absorbed and utilized in the positive functions of a love relationship.

Psychoanalytic psychotherapy of couples frequently reveals mutual power struggles as dominant themes of chronic marital conflicts. Psychodynamic exploration of such conflicts typically shows dominance of projective mechanisms, in the area of both aggressive aspects of ambivalent object relations in their daily interactions and superego-derived mutual projection of infantile demands and prohibitions. Conventional clichés regarding the mis-

understandings and "wars" between the genders provide easy rationalizations of power struggles (Person 2006, 2007). Conflicts
about who was right and who was wrong, the search for culprits,
and the identification with sadistic parental images color these interactions. Naturally, a severely paranoid personality structure
maximizes the dominance of such mechanisms, but they reflect
deep-seated ambivalences, and they are a universal aspect of intimate love relationships, as Henry Dicks (1967) first observed.
Revengeful persecution of a disappointing partner for years after
the end of a relationship is a frequent development in paranoid personalities.

The Permanence of Sexual Passion

A frequent assertion in the literature dealing with love relationships, particularly in its popularized form, is that the initial intensity of sexual desire and erotic passion in the life of a couple is
normally replaced by a more tranquil but deeper emotional relationship, in which sex becomes less important and a sense of comradeship replaces early idealizations (Fonagy 2008; Mitchell 2002).
I have questioned this assumption in earlier work (Kernberg 1995)
and would only reiterate, on the basis of analytic work with individual patients and with conflicts of couples in later life years, that
passionate encounters and an intense sexual relationship are a
long-range aspect of a love relationship that does not necessarily
diminish or disappear over time. Inhibitions in the passionate nature of sexual encounters of long-lasting relationships usually reflect unconscious conflicts throughout the entire spectrum of a
couple's object relationship and may improve dramatically in the
course of treatment. Mutual superego projections and acting out of
conflicts around aggression are leading psychodynamic features of
these conflicts (Kernberg 1995, 2007). The fact that, physiologi-
cally, the frequency of desire for sexual relationships decreases in
the case of men while it maintains itself relatively stable in the case
of women does not imply the decrease of the intensity of meaningfulness of erotic engagements at any stage of life. I do not have the
space here to review in detail the corresponding literature and arguments. In essence, passionate sexual intimacy is a disruption of
the boundaries of reality, a merger into one's own bodily functions,
a penetration and being penetrated, and a fusion in abandonment
and momentary dissolution of the boundaries between self and

other (Stein 2008). For couples in a mature love relationship, passionate love is an ever-recurring, exhilarating experience, a "well-kept secret" (Hunt 1974). Both oedipal prohibitions and guilt and narcissistic dissociation between tenderness and eroticism play a central role in inhibiting the normal integration of total object relations, polymorphous infantile and genital sexuality, and the mature ego ideal of the couple, all of which play a role in facilitating sexual passion.

The present interest in the interaction of the early attachment system and sexuality tends to focus somewhat reductionally on mother-infant interaction as directly related to adult sexual behavior, neglecting in the process the complexity of intrapsychic determinants, both preoedipal and oedipal conflicts, and unconscious fantasy in general (Britton 1989, 1992, 2004; Diamond and Yeomans 2007; Widlöcher 2002).

The development of sexual boredom in a long-term, lasting relationship is a typical symptom of narcissistic pathology. This is a widespread symptom, particularly exacerbated, of course, as part of a persisting syndrome of separation of idealized desexualized love objects and devalued but sexually exciting ones, perhaps the most frequent expression of a combination of unresolved oedipal conflicts and narcissistic pathology.

> A typical manifestation of severe narcissistic pathology is represented by one patient, a man in his early fifties, married to a wife whom he treated, practically, as a slave for whose maintenance and daily satisfaction he assumed full responsibility, without feeling more than the gratitude for having somebody totally dedicated to all his wishes and needs. His sexual feelings, regarding her, were practically totally absent. He frequented a string of high-class prostitutes, with whom he experienced a fully pleasurable sexual gratification without any emotional involvement. This was a rather stable equilibrium for many years, which, however, had began to crumble under a growing sense of depression and loneliness that brought him to treatment. In the course of this analysis, it became clear that his wife represented both the hated and feared mother of his early childhood and a forbidden oedipal object in the struggles with his internalized punitive father image. In a slow development over several years, these various components of his dominant unconscious conflicts could be worked out in the transference, and gradual changes in the relationship with his wife constituted "markers" of transference elaborations. Only in his early sixties was he able, for the first time, to experience a passionate desire for and appreciation of his wife of many years.

Under conditions of a successful love relationship, a wide-ranging and flexible capacity for mutual adjustment of sexual interest and needs may take place, in contrast to the typical exacerbation of whatever discrepancy of sexual interests may become the manifest battlefield of deeper conflicts in the life of a couple.

In a mature love relationship, the idealization of the body of the other, the experience of physical beauty of the other in the light of one's love, is a permanent aspect of love and does not need to be affected by the changing aspects of the body as an effect of aging or illness. To love the other with shortcomings and problems includes the love of the other with physical imperfections, as is the capacity to honestly share with the other one's concern about physical shortcomings or imperfections in oneself. To share the intimacies of one's body is the counterpart to sharing the intimacies about one's emotional life and problems, sharing one's sexual desires and uncertainties in the same way as one's uncertainties, fears, and conflicts regarding competition, jealousy, financial uncertainties, threatening family members, and conflicts with parents and adult children. The tolerance of the manifestations of aging, in oneself and the other, without any loss of the erotic excitement with the body of the other, is a consequence of the dominance of love over aggression, of maintained idealization of the surface of the body in contrast to the unconscious projection of aggression into the body of the other, the early mechanism of the origin of the sense of beauty described by Meltzer (Meltzer and Williams 1988).

At the bottom, the real unconscious conflict is not between the tender, stable nature of emotional commitment and passionate eroticism but between love and aggression within both the tender emotional and the passionate sexual realm and within the superego structures involving the ego ideal of the couple and persecutory superego features (Kernberg 1995; Stoller 1979).

Acceptance of Loss, Jealousy, and Boundary Protection

It has been said, "If you love it, let it be free": this applies to the expression of mature love, which implies the commitment to love the other person, with the acknowledgment that the person is a free agent and that nobody can be forced to love more than is natural, not by coercion, not by raising guilt feelings. It means that in the reciprocity of a love relationship, it is reasonable to expect that love and commitment be responded to and that if the loved person is not able to respond to one's love, this has to be accepted and the mourning process over the end of the relationship be tolerated. It means, in practice, a non-guilt-raising exploration of the difficulties in the relationship—of the experience of having been hurt or attacked, neglected, or mistreated by the other, and raising it as a question for exploration and resolution—with the expectation that this will be a natural concern of the other person as well.

All of this does not imply that, under ordinary conditions, aggression should not be available to defend the boundaries of a love relationship against "intruders." The capacity for jealousy is a normal protective function, achieved as part of the entry into the dominance of oedipal conflicts. It stands in contrast to its frequent absence in severe narcissistic pathology. But lack of normal jealousy also may express the acting out of oedipal guilt over the possibility of a gratifying sexual relationship.

> One patient, a rather shy man in his early thirties, in analysis for a chronic fear of loss of bowel control, related to the analyst as a frightening, extremely severe father image to whom he felt he had to submit. A close friend of his was giving indications that he was trying to seductively approach the patient's fiancée. The denial of the competitive feelings and jealous rage toward his friend was expressed in a reaction formation of rather extreme tolerance of his friend's behavior and suppressed anger toward his fiancée. The analytic resolution of his guilt-deterring masochistic submission to the analyst finally helped him to become aware how his submission to his friend's aggressive courting of his fiancée and his contributing unconsciously to drive her into his arms expressed the same fear of asserting himself in protecting his love relationship.

The ambivalence of all relationships implies that events of mutual aggression are unavoidable in the course of a life lived together, but, by the same token, the possibility of their clarification and resolution carries with it the possibility of further strengthening and deepening the relationship. If, however, to the contrary, in that context, it emerges that one cannot really expect a loving commitment from the other, there exists the need to acknowledge and, in the end, accept that. To accept the limit or end of a relationship is part of a responsibility to oneself to expect mutuality of commitment in a mature love relationship.

If the other cannot love us as we love him or her, this must be accepted and with it, the end of the relationship. Particularly in cases of triangulations, the invasion of the couple's relationship by a third party or infidelity in the relationship, such a clarification of where the other really stands is essential. There are many reasons for such a shift in sexual and emotional interest of one or both partners to outsiders, from divergent maturational and developmental processes and changing external circumstances to severe masochistic, narcissistic, or paranoid pathology. Whatever the reason, the exploration of how and whether the love relationship will survive requires an exploration of what can be expected from the other and from the self, the possibility of resolution and forgiveness, and if not possible, resignation to the termination of the relationship. The possibility of life together under conditions of the end of love may be a psychosocially reasonable compromise but is profoundly destructive to the basic fulfillment of the aspiration of a gratifying love relationship.

In some way, every long-lasting marital relationship is really several marriages. The resolution of crises changes the nature of the relationship, for better or for worse. Ideally, the resolution of crises may foster growth in the relationship, as well as in the self-awareness of the partners. When the end of a relationship occurs under conditions of a predominance of depressive over paranoid mechanisms of interaction, that is, with a dominance of sadness and mourning over the loss rather than of hatred, frustration, and wishes for revenge, such a mature way of working through the trauma of separation may foster the capacity of a more mature relationship with a new partner.

Love and Mourning

A positive development, even under conditions of a deeply painful emotional working through, may follow the death of a beloved partner. As I have pointed out in earlier work (Kernberg 2010; Chapter 10 in this volume), the painful awareness of the full value of a lost love relationship that, in all its many valuable aspects, can only be fully appreciated after the loss may trigger the development of an increased capacity for love of a new partner by mechanisms of reparation, as well as the fulfillment of the ethical mandate derived from the recognition of one's own limitations in the lost relationship. Normal mourning reinforces the capacity for love, while, naturally, that very capacity signifies a major intensity of the mourning process that follows the loss of such a relationship.

In this connection, normal mourning after the loss of a loved one, be it through separation, abandonment, or death, would not be dominated by excessive guilt feelings, self-devaluation, or pervasive insecurity. Particularly after the end brought about by abandonment from a loved partner, the depth of mourning should be free of self-devaluation, in contrast to the characteristic self-depreciation in the case of masochistic pathology and the sense of humiliation in narcissistic pathology. One's capacity to love should function as a major reassurance of one's value. In narcissistic personalities, the unconscious envy of that very capacity in one's partner is a major source of the poisoning of love relationships.

Separations as a consequence of severe conflict, disappointments, or abandonment may provide a time for reflection and search for a new encounter. If both parties are committed to working on themselves and are then able to communicate new understandings and awareness, this separation period may be fruitful. A long-lasting stalemate in a "trial separation," without any new development, in which one or both participants engage in endless prolongation of the status quo, usually indicates loss of love on the part of one of them and bodes poorly for continuing the marriage. Uncertainty within the relationship needs to be respected, within a limit of time. When uncertainty cannot be resolved by means of a trial separation, and there is a lack of urgency to reach a decision, except under conditions of pressure from the other, this is usually an indication of the need to accept the loss and move on with one's life. Such a mature resolution contrasts sharply with masochistic submission to an impossible situation or a narcissistic denial of the possibility that one may be rejected.

One's feeling of love for the other, as well as the expectation of an equal commitment of the other as a precondition to maintaining or resuming the relationship, should permit one to find a middle road between a naiveté based on denial of the reality, on the one hand, and a paranoid attitude about the partner's motivation, on the other.

In describing specific clinical features interfering with the capacity for sexual love, I have expressed the experience that the awareness of these components of mature love relationships may facilitate the diagnosis of the subtle aspects of masochistic and narcissistic pathology that reduce the capacity for normal enjoyment of love life and are common sources of chronic conflicts of individuals and couples. I believe that the consistent awareness of these features in the mind of the analyst treating patients and couples in severe conflicts may provide a helpful frame that sharpens the focus on the expression of the pathology of love relationships.

The analyst may highlight areas of ego-syntonic freezing or limitations in a patient's love relationship that open the patient's awareness of unconscious conflicts blocking the full experience and expression of love: fear of dependency, denial of an idealization that would evoke guilt, reaction formations against envy, or jealousy. Analytic exploration may expand the depth and scope of a love relationship by highlighting and exploring such "blind spots" and resolving, in the process, what are almost universal masochistic features: unconscious, oedipally determined guilt over a happy love relationship.

References

Balfour A: Intimacy and sexuality in later life, in Sex, Attachment, and Couple Psychotherapy: Psychoanalytic Perspectives. Edited by Clulow C. London, Karnac Books, 2009, pp 217–236

Britton R: The missing link: parental sexuality in the Oedipus complex, in The Oedipus Complex Today. Edited by Britton R. London, Karnac Books, 1989, pp 83–101

Britton R: The Oedipus situation and the depressive position, in Clinical Lectures on Klein and Bion. Edited by Anderson R. London, Routledge, 1992, pp 34–45

Britton R: Subjectivity, objectivity, and triangular space. Psychoanal Q 73:47–61, 2004

Chasseguet-Smirgel J: Essai sur l'idéal du moi. París, Presses Universitaires de France, 1973

Diamond D, Yeomans F: Oedipal love and conflict in the transference/countertransference matrix: its impact on attachment security and mentalization, in Attachment and Sexuality. Edited by Diamond D, Blatt S, Lichtenberg J. New York, Analytic Press, 2007, pp 201–230

Dicks HV: Marital Tensions. New York, Basic Books, 1967

Fonagy P: A genuinely developmental theory of sexual enjoyment and its implications for psychoanalytic technique. J Am Psychoanal Assoc 56:11–36, 2008

Hunt M: Sexual Behavior in the 1970s. New York, Dell, 1974

Kernberg OF: Love Relations: Normality and Pathology. New Haven, CT, Yale University Press, 1995

Kernberg OF: Aggressivity, Narcissism, and Self-Destructiveness in the Psychotherapeutic Relationship: New Developments in the Psychopathology and Psychotherapy of Severe Personality Disorders. New Haven, CT, Yale University Press, 2004

Kernberg OF: Love relations of the heterosexual couple, in Love and Its Obstacles. Edited by Pollack R. New York, Center for the Study of Science and Religion, Columbia University, 2007

Kernberg OF: Some observations on the process of mourning. Int J Psychoanal 91:601–619, 2010

Meltzer D, Williams MD: The Apprehension of Beauty: The Role of Aesthetic Conflict in Development, Art, and Violence. Perthshire, Scotland, Clunie Press, 1988

Mitchell SA: Can Love Last? The Fate of Romance Over Time. New York,
WW Norton, 2002

Person ES: Masculinities, plural. J Am Psychoanal Assoc 54:1165–1186,
2006

Person ES: The link between love and power, in Love and Its Obstacles. Edited by Pollack R. New York, Center for the Study of Science and Religion, Columbia University, 2007, pp 7–16

Stein R: The otherness of sexuality: excess. J Am Psychoanal Assoc 56:43–
71, 2008

Stoller RJ: Sexual Excitement. New York, Pantheon, 1979

Widlöcher D: Primary love and infantile sexuality: an eternal debate, in Infantile Sexuality and Attachment. Edited by Widlöcher D. New York,
Other Press, 2002, pp 1–35

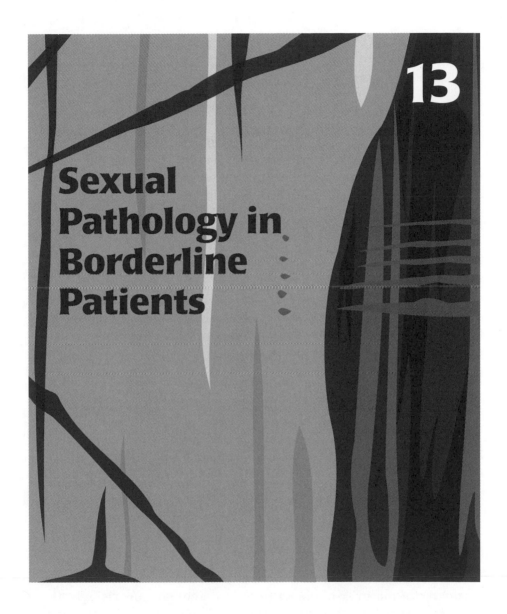

13

Sexual Pathology in Borderline Patients

This chapter was reprinted from Kernberg OF: "Sexual Pathology in Borderline Patients," in *Borderline-Störungen und Sexualität*. Edited by Dulz B, Benecke C, Richter-Appelt H. Stuttgart, Germany, Schattauer, 2009, pp. 167–174. Used with permission.

In this chapter, I continue the exploration of limitations in the capacity for mature love relationships, exploring the relationship between the degree of severity of personality disorders and the corresponding pathology in their love life. I stress the fundamental importance of exploring the love life of patients with severe personality disorders, including both their patterns of sexual activity and fantasy life and the nature of the object relations they established in the context of their sexual behavior. The relation between the severity of paraphilias or perversions, on the one hand, and that of the patient's personality disorder, on the other, provides the clinician with essential information in order to formulate an appropriate therapeutic and prognostic assessment.

What follows is an overview of the relation between the degree of severity of personality disorders and the spectrum of severity of sexual pathology that we have been able to observe in our work with these patients at the Personality Disorders Institute of the Weill Cornell Medical College. It is an overview of our clinical experience and the basis of our present development of efforts to empirically explore this relationship between severity of sexual pathology and severity of personality disorders. Preliminary empirical work (Hull et al. 1993) has indicated that HIV-positive patients with borderline personality disorders may be grossly classified into a group with most severe personality disorders who show a significant degree of overall sexual inhibition and a group with less severe personality disorders who evince a very active and, often, chaotic sexual behavior. This finding corresponds, indeed, with our overall clinical experience in the study of severe personality disorders as summarized in what follows.

The study of an individual's sexual behavior needs to include both the actual sexual activities, fantasies, and fears and the capacity to engage in a love relationship in depth with the person who is the individual's sexual partner. The capacity to fall in love and to maintain stable love relations is a fundamental expression of the degree of maturity of object relations, and, not surprisingly, the more severe the personality disorder, the more limited these emotional capabilities (Kernberg 2004a, Chapter 1). The combined analysis of the capacity for a love relation and of the nature and degree of difficulties in the realm of sexual behavior permits, in practice, differentiation of a broad spectrum of sexual pathology, ranging, at one extreme, from the sexual pathology of patients with severe antisocial behavior and antisocial personality proper to, at the other extreme, a flexible and broad sexual functioning in the context of a stable, deep love relationship with a specific partner.

Normality

It is tempting to describe the latter capacity mentioned above as "normality." Obviously, however, the concept of normality presents the problem of reflecting either the average behavior of a relatively normal population or an idealized, normative concept that, in turn, may be highly influenced by cultural values. From a clinical viewpoint, it would seem reasonable to consider the capacity for falling in love and for establishing a stable love relationship, in the context of which there evolves the capacity for sexual arousal and for sexual intercourse with a progressively increasing degree of excitement culminating in orgasm, as a reasonable characterization of normal sexual functioning in the context of emotional maturity. This combination, indeed, is quite prevalent normally and in patients without a clinically significant personality disorder.

Neurotic Personality Organization

A first, relatively minor level of sexual pathology is frequently found in patients with a "high-level" personality disorder, or neurotic personality organization, as represented by patients with hysterical, obsessive-compulsive, and depressive-masochistic personality disorders, particularly patients with hysterical personality disorder (Kernberg 1995). Patients with these disorders generally present with an integrated identity, the capacity for establishing object relations in depth, a predominance of high-level defensive operations, a capacity for mature emotional reactions, and excellent reality testing. Here the capacity for falling in love and for an intense and stable love relationship is present quite frequently in the context of some degree of sexual inhibition. This includes occasional, relatively mild degrees of impotence in the case of men and, particularly, a significant degree of sexual inhibition in the case of women, in the form of a reduction or an incapacity for achieving full sexual excitement and orgasm in intercourse.

Some degree of inhibition of the orgasmic capacity of women, particularly during the early stages of engagement in sexual intercourse, is quite frequent and may not be considered pathological. In the presence of a personality disorder at a neurotic level, one may also find, in both men and women, a typical sexual inhibition in the form of dissociation of the capacity for full sexual enjoyment with someone who is not emotionally significant to the patient, while there develops some degree of inhibition in the sexual intimacy with the person who is actually loved. This pattern presents more frequently in men than in women, particularly in men with significant hysterical or narcissistic features, who present a typical "Madonna/prostitute" dissociation: they can only enjoy sex with women they do not love, while idealizing other women with whom they may be involved emotionally but toward whom they evince no sexual interest at all. Women, in contrast, particularly those with depressive/masochistic features, quite frequently have the capacity for full sexual gratification only in the context of the development of a masochistic love relationship.

In any case, throughout this entire level of neurotic personality organization, the capacity for a full love relationship with sexual involvement, be it with some degree of inhibition in the capacity for sexual excitement and orgasm, is prevalent. From a psychodynamic viewpoint, these patients present a typical predominance of oedipal conflicts, with unconscious guilt feelings and repression of oedipal strivings, and related prohibitions against infantile genital impulses and related castration anxiety. There is relatively little infiltration of the conflicts around pregenital aggression that are so central in more severe psychopathology.

Narcissistic Pathology

A second, more severe level of pathology of love relationships corresponds to the higher level of patients with borderline personality organization, particularly the better functioning narcissistic personalities. These patients present a well-organized but pathological grandiose self and significant problems in their object relations but a relatively normal functioning in the ordinary social realm. At this level, the capacity for sexual excitement and orgasm is apparently normal, and, these patients may be involved in an intense search for frequent sexual relationships, while, to the contrary, their capacity for significant, stable love relationships seems clearly limited. Characteristically, narcissistic patients at this level have difficulty in sustaining a long-term love relationship, while manifesting frequent, transitory infatuations, falling in love with a partner who is sexually exciting to them but with whom both love and sexual excitement decrease rapidly in the course of weeks or a few months. They show repetitive cycles of idealization and devaluation of their sexual partners, with a corresponding, initially intense, sexual desire and activity, followed, soon enough, by a total loss of sexual interest and boredom with the partner in the emotional realm (Kernberg 1995).

This pattern used to be particularly prevalent in men, while corresponding narcissistic pathology in women showed different features. Narcissistic women presented generally exploitive patterns of behavior in their social and family life related to the characteristics of a paternalistic culture, with strong prohibitions against sexually promiscuous behavior of women, in contrast to cultural support of such a behavior in men. With the development of the emancipation and liberation of women in the social and economic realm, a similar pattern to that traditionally ascribed to men has emerged, so that it seems fair to say that the same pattern of sexual promiscuity has now become typical for narcissistic personalities of both genders. From a psychodynamic viewpoint, these patients present a narcissistic organization that combines defenses against preoedipal envy with anal regression from oedipal conflicts, intense envy of and rivalry with their sexual objects, and significant decrease in their capacity for object investment (Chasseguet-Smirgel 1984).

Borderline Personality Organization (Higher Level)

At the next level of severity of sexual pathology, corresponding to the broad spectrum of borderline personality organization, including patients with histrionic or infantile, borderline, and narcissistic personality disorders functioning at a borderline level, sexual functioning tends to veer into a prevalence of what may be called a polymorphous perverse infantile type of sexuality. These patients tend to combine chaotically significant sadistic, masochistic, voyeuristic, exhibitionistic, fetishistic, and bisexual features—so that chaotic heterosexual and homosexual interests may combine, in contrast to a stable heterosexual or homosexual orientation. At this level of borderline personality organization, the syndrome of identity diffusion emerges clearly as these patients lack an integrated concept of self and significant others. They show predominance of primitive defensive operations centering on splitting and related defenses, severe pathology of object relations, and significant difficulties in their work or profession and in their love life. The love lives of these patients may appear chaotic, not only because of their intense, yet unstable object relations and their multiple love objects but also because of the apparent sexual freedom to express multiple polymorphous infantile trends. A significant absence of ordinary social restraints on sexual behavior goes hand in hand with the ambivalent and chaotic nature of the object relations of the patients in this group.

The incorporation of multiple polymorphous perverse infantile features of sexuality into their fantasies and activities must be differentiated from perversions (paraphilias) proper: in these latter syndromes, a particular perverse activity has become an exclusive, repetitive, obligatory condition of their sexual activity, indispensable to achieve full sexual excitement and orgasm (Kernberg 2004a, Chapter 5). The borderline patients we are considering may impress the clinician, given their chaotic love life, as more severely ill than they actually are: their maintained capacity for an intense, pleasurable sexual interaction may shift, in the course of the treatment, into the capacity of a committed investment in a stable relationship with the object of their sexual desire, a partner in love, with whom the quality of the object relation improves in the context of this very sexual interest. Their apparent sexual promiscuity, therefore, is a prognostically favorable indicator, except when it appears in the context of a severe narcissistic personality disorder. From a psychodynamic perspective, here dominates the typical condensation of preoedipal aggression with oedipal conflicts of borderline personality organization and pervasive splitting and other primitive defensive operations rather than repression.

Borderline Personality Organization (Lower Level)

The next, and still more severe, level of sexual pathology is observable in the cases of the most severe personality disorders with borderline personality organization, particularly severely borderline, narcissistic, sadomasochistic, paranoid, and schizotypal personality disorders, in which a severe inhibition in the capacity for engaging in a stable love relationship and an incapacity for falling in love combine with a pervasive sexual inhibition, characterized by lack of sexual arousal, lack of sexual excitement and orgasm, and, in fact, a lack of sensual response to sexual stimulation of body surfaces in general. These patients sometimes show a total incomprehension regarding the very nature of sexual interest, arousal, excitement, and orgasm. Patients in the previously mentioned groups, even if they present some degree of sexual inhibition or limitation of sexual pleasure in sexual intercourse, are usually able to achieve excitement and orgasm with masturbation: in this latter group, there is usually a striking absence of masturbation and an incapacity to achieve sexual excitement and orgasm by any means.

The psychodynamic exploration of these patients' unconscious conflicts in the course of a psychoanalytic psychotherapy, such as transference-focused psychotherapy (TFP) (Clarkin et al. 2006), gradually reveals primitive erotic fantasies intimately fused with aggressive fears and impulses. As they emerge in the treatment, these fantasies convey the impression that severe early trauma and frustrations and aggressive experiences that overshadowed their early relationships with significant others had been effective in neutralizing their early capability for sensual activation and response. These patients evince a corresponding lack of development of skin eroticism and the predominance of erotic fantasies involving sexual organs and activities serving aggressive impulses, with related fears of destructive, mutual bodily invasion as the prototype of sexual intimacy.

The severe sexual inhibition of these patients interferes with the development of a fully gratifying love relationship, even after these patients recover their capacity for investment in depth in the relationships with significant others. I have found that long-term psychoanalytic psychotherapy, combined with sex therapy with a dynamically trained sex therapist, in the advanced stages of the treatment may significantly improve their sexual relationships and intimacy.

The Aggressive Antisocial Spectrum

The most extreme level of severity of personality disorders is the case of the aggressive type of antisocial personality disorder (Kernberg 2004a, Chapter 3) or, in Michael Stone's (2009) proposed terminology, at the level of the psychopath proper. This personality disorder reveals unmotivated, excessive, violent aggression directed against others, without any capacity for feelings of guilt, concern, or empathy, in which a particular pattern of sexual behavior may evolve. The patient's erotic desires are totally controlled by sadistic impulses, so that sexual encounters are at the service of brutal assault of another person's intimacy, physical well-being, or even life. Here we find an unrestricted impulsivity regarding a sexual behavior that often reflects the characteristic of a sadistic perversion, in the context of a total absence of the capacity of investment in the human relationship, let alone any capacity for loving feelings.

In patients with the syndrome of malignant narcissism, which, clinically, occupies an intermediate realm between the narcissistic personality with antisocial features, on the one hand, and the antisocial personality proper, on the other, some capacity for ambivalent investment in significant others and capacity for guilt feelings and concern may remain, but usually with total dissociation between such a limited capacity for a loving relationship and their sexual behavior. This syndrome is characterized by the combination of narcissistic personality disorder, antisocial behavior, ego-syntonic aggression, and paranoid traits.

Perversions (Paraphilias)

The correspondence between personality disorders and perversions, or paraphilias, is related to the overall spectrum of pathology of the sexual life described above (Kernberg 2004a, Chapter 5). To begin, it needs to be stressed again that the definition of perversion involves an obligatory, consistent restriction of the patient's sexual fantasy or activity to one particular component of polymorphous perverse infantile sexuality, such as voyeurism, masochism, sadism, exhibitionism, or fetishism, to refer to the most frequent types of perversion. The prognosis of the various perversions depends on particular characteristics that, in turn, are closely related to the underlying personality pathology.

At a normal level of sexual behavior, polymorphous perverse sexual fantasies, wishes, and activities are integrated into ordinary sexual fantasy, play, and activity. These components, reflecting early sexual capabilities, add excitement and intensity to the sexual relationship, and they may contribute to the intimacy of the sexual encounter. From a psychodynamic viewpoint, these early components of sexuality, similarly to the genital impulses proper, express aggressive as well as erotic impulses, a combination of predominantly tender erotic wishes for mutual penetration with the aggressively derived wishes to control, dominate the sexual partner physically or visually, and/or be controlled and dominated by the sexual partner in this way. To penetrate and to be penetrated by the other, in real and symbolic ways, is an important aspect of the wish for erotic fusion. The early superego-determined prohibitions against these manifestations of infantile sexuality determine the most frequent forms of mild sexual inhibition, quite frequent in a normal population, where these polymorphous infantile sexual impulses undergo repression.

The frequent experience of sexual couples who have undergone sex therapy, in the sense that following such therapy they experience a degree of sexual freedom, pleasure, and intensity that exceeds that which they were able to achieve "normally" before, may illustrate this point. Such a heightened sexual capability, derived from decrease of superego pressures, however, tends to again "normalize" (i.e., decrease) after a period of months, presumably because of the reassertion of unconscious superego pressures operating in the couple's relationship and overriding the decreased internalized prohibitions regarding infantile sexual impulses gained during the sex therapy.

In any case, the paradoxical relations of the capability of integrating polymorphous perverse infantile sexuality into normal sexual behavior and intercourse, on the one hand, and, on the other, the predominance of one of these tendencies with restriction of all other sexual behavior, and with an obligatory character of the enactment of this perverse behavior as a condition for achieving sexual excitement and orgasm, illustrate the contrast between the dynamics of conflictual, dissociated impulses and the sublimatory manifestations of integrated pregenital erotic and aggressive impulses.

Levels of Perverse Pathology

At the highest level of perverse pathology, the perverse activity permits the expression of unconscious aggressive fantasies in the context of a sexual encounter in a dissociated condition or scenario. Typically, perversion at the level of a neurotic personality disorder is manifest in the form of a rigid scenario activated by the patient in following a highly individualized script, with maintenance of the capacity for a normal object relation in depth with a consistently loved object. A strictly delimited perverse sexual encounter in the context of a normal love relationship and the capacity for an object relation in depth represent a perversion at that high level and usually indicate an excellent prognosis for treatment.

At a second level of pathology, again in the case of the better functioning narcissistic personalities, a stable perversion may coexist with a typical incapacity to maintain an object relation in depth and with the cycles of idealization and devaluation of a love object mentioned before. At the same time, a stable relationship with a sexual partner with whom there is no emotional relationship but a common agreement for a sexual relationship that involves that perversion may complement the structure of the patient's sexual life. Instead of one perverse partner, there may be an interchangeable series of such specialized objects of a restricted sexual perversion. In contrast to a perversion at a neurotic level, the (temporary) love relationship and the perverse relationship usually are split from each other. Here, the treatment of the perversion is dependent on the resolution of the narcissistic personality structure in the context of transference analysis. Both these narcissistic cases, as well as the cases of perversion at a neurotic level, do present an indication for psychoanalysis.

A third, more severe level of perversion may present in cases of the more severe forms of borderline personality organization, with chaotic object relations, difficulty in maintaining a love relationship in depth, and multiple infantile sexual perverse trends. In these cases, a particular perversion tends to be much less structured than in the cases mentioned before and, paradoxically, less of a therapeutic problem in itself. The overall prognosis depends on the severity of actual aggressive impulses embedded in the perverse behavior and also manifest in the patient's general object relations. At this level, the prognosis for treatment of all kinds of sexual pathology depends, on the one hand, on the general quality of object relations of the patient and, on the other, on the quality of superego functions and the direct manifestations of aggression in the patient's social as well as intimate sexual life. These patients, in our experience, tend to respond better to a psychoanalytic psychotherapy—particularly TFP—than to psychoanalysis.

This general prognostic principle also holds true for the most severe cases of perversion to be referred to in what follows, where a perversion evolves in the context of severe limitations of all object relations and they are replaced by a specific perversion. When this perversion includes health- or life-threatening aggression, the residual quality of superego functions and the remaining capacity for object relations are fundamental in determining the prognosis.

One might summarize the prognosis of all perversions that involve clearly antisocial behavior, such as pedophilia, and that enter the realm of forensic psychiatry, as dependent on the personality structure of the individual, ranging from excellent prognosis with a neurotic personality organization, to less ideal but still a favorable prognosis with borderline personality organization that does not include the narcissistic personality proper, to reserved prognosis in the case of a narcissistic personality disorder, and to probably extremely negative, "zero" prognosis in the case of an antisocial personality disorder.

Homosexuality–Heterosexuality

The foregoing formulations apply to both heterosexuals and homosexuals. The nature of homosexuality, its genetic and/or psychodynamically determined etiology, and its "normality" or "pathology" still remain controversial, particularly within the psychoanalytic approach to these conditions (Kernberg 2004b). From a clinical viewpoint, normality in the sexual realm as defined in this chapter, that is, the capacity for a loving and stable relationship with a partner, with full range of sexual expression within the relationship, applies equally to homosexuality and heterosexuality. One finds the same varying relationship between the capacity to fall in love, the integration of a love relationship and sexual behavior, their potential dissociation, and the more severe degrees of pathology of sexual relationships mentioned before in the case of homosexual as well as heterosexual patients.

There are differences regarding the sexual behavior of men and women, gender differences that, in turn, may be determined partly by genetic and, probably, mostly by cultural features. There seems to be a clear difference in terms of gender regarding bisexuality: in my experience, in men, it usually coincides with a severe type of personality disorder, while, to the contrary, bisexuality in women, particularly the late-onset homosexuality in women who originally presented a heterosexual lifestyle, frequently emerges in women with normal or neurotic personality structure. Undoubtedly, cultural bias and prejudices still interfere with the objective, scientific approach to homosexuality, but the general principle of the relation between severity of personality disorders and the spectrum of pathology of sexual behavior seems to be valid for both genders of homosexual and heterosexual patients.

Diagnostic Evaluation

In the diagnostic evaluation of patients with personality disorder, it is extremely important to evaluate the nature of their sexual functioning. Their sexual life clearly exerts profound influences on their object relations and contributes significantly to the prognosis of the treatment of their personality disorder. The patient's sexual life both reflects and influences his or her intrapsychic and interpersonal conflicts and constitutes a major dimension in the therapeutic effort to help him or her to achieve a satisfactory, intimate love life. In the Personality Disorders Institute at Cornell, we systematically explore, as part of the initial evaluation of patients, their sexual activities, fantasies, and daydreams, particularly their masturbatory activities and fantasies, and the relation between their sexual orientation in their dreams, fantasy life, and actual sexual engagements. We study their capacity (or lack of) to fall in love and to maintain love relationships and the relation between love and sexual behavior and gratification.

Sex therapy may have an important place in the treatment of certain sexual difficulties, with particularly good prognosis in the case of sexual inhibition in women limited to the phase of excitement after penetration, and orgasm, and equally positive prognosis for the treatment of milder cases of premature and retarded ejaculation in men. The diagnosis and treatment of impotence is a complex area that exceeds what can be explored in this chapter. As a general principle, it is important to evaluate organic causes of impotence, for which there are now effective treatments, and to differentiate primary, generalized types of impotence that reflect a reserved prognosis, from secondary and selective forms of impotence, which have a good prognostic implication.

Consultation including a specialized urologist or neurologist, an analytically trained psychotherapist, and a cognitive-behavioral or psychodynamically oriented sex therapist may be optimal in developing a particular strategy for individual patients. The evaluation of sexual behavior and functioning, in short, is relevant for the diagnosis, prognosis, and treatment of the personality disorder, as well as the sexual difficulties themselves, be it a task for the psychodynamic psychotherapy or for additional therapeutic interventions.

There are several principles that have helped our group both to learn about the individual dynamics underlying the sexual difficulties of borderline patients and to assess the obstacles in their psychotherapeutic treatment related to these dynamics. First, as mentioned before, it would seem essential to take a full history of the patient's sexual behavior and love relationships at the beginning of the treatment. In fact, it is not an exaggeration to say that the most important knowledge necessary before starting the psychoanalytic psychotherapy of a borderline patient is a careful and full analysis of his or her functioning at work or in a profession in relation to colleagues, superiors, and subordinates, and within his or her sexual life, history of love relationships, and sexual experiences and behavior or fears. These two major features are too often neglected in the early study of patients with severe personality disorders, where the focus seems to be mostly on the severity of symptoms and the patients' past history rather than on their present functioning in realms of love and work. To this, a third domain of assessment should be added, that of social and creative pursuits. Careful attention to the patient's capacity to make and maintain friendships, have appropriate social engagement, and become invested in creative interests will help determine overall personality organization and levels of severity of pathology.

Second, in the presence of significant difficulties in the patient's sexual life, the therapist has to be prepared to be attentive to whether and when these issues will emerge in the context of transference developments in the treatment or, as frequently happens, whether they are submerged under apparently non–sexually related conflicts or obscured by a conventionalized control in the patient's free associations: mentioning what is going on in his or her daily experiences while refraining from bringing up the fantasy life, particularly sexual fantasies and the psychological impact of ongoing sexual experiences. It may seem strange to have to stress this, but this area of exploration is frequently avoided not only by non–analytically trained therapists but also by psychoanalysts. The frequent omission of exploring fully the patient's sexual fantasy and love life and its implications for the developments in the transference may reflect, I believe, the extent to which the conventional suppression of open exploration of sexual issues is the counterpart to the provocative eroticization of the media in our culture.

Third, the general principle holds that in the case of severe sexual inhibitions, including those implicit in the structures of perversion, the major underlying conflicts have to be explored in the transference for their eventual resolution. The defenses against full expression of patients' sexual conflicts in the transference are often reinforced by countertransference difficulties and the therapist's fear of "invading" intimate areas of the patient's life or of defenses against erotic reactions in the countertransference. It helps if the therapist has a satisfactory sexual life and good personal experiences of its importance as a source of gratification, intimacy, and creativity.

References

Chasseguet-Smirgel J: Creativity and Perversion. New York, WW Norton, 1984

Clarkin JF, Yeomans FE, Kernberg OF: Psychotherapy for Borderline Personality: Focusing on Object Relations. Washington, DC, American Psychiatric Publishing, 2006

Hull JW, Clarkin JF, Yeomans F: Borderline personality disorder and impulsive sexual behavior. Hosp Community Psychiatry 44:1000–1002, 1993

Kernberg OF: Love Relations: Normality and Pathology. New Haven, CT, Yale University Press, 1995

Kernberg OF: Aggressivity, Narcissism, and Self-Destructiveness in the Psychotherapeutic Relationship: New Developments in the Psychopathology and Psychotherapy of Severe Personality Disorders. New Haven, CT, Yale University Press, 2004a

Kernberg OF: Contemporary Controversies in Psychoanalytic Theory, Technique, and Their Applications. New Haven, CT, Yale University Press, 2004b

Stone MH: The Anatomy of Evil. Amherst, NY, Prometheus Books, 2009

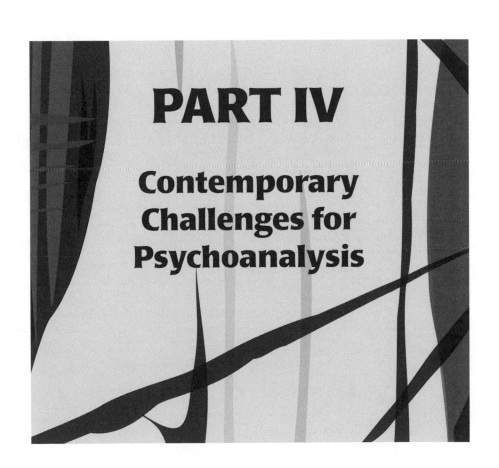

PART IV

Contemporary Challenges for Psychoanalysis

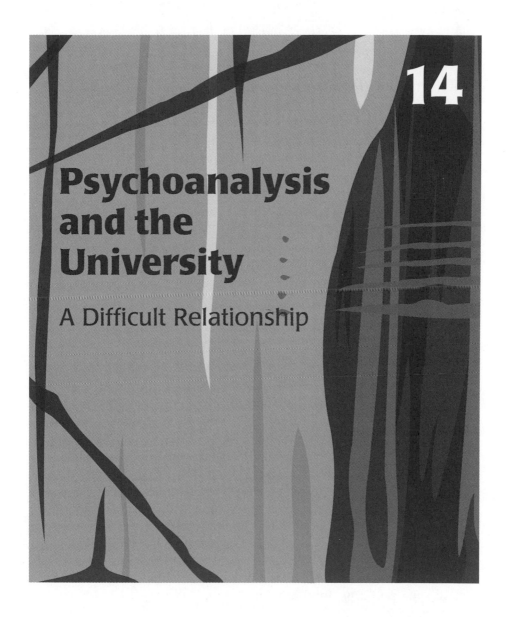

Psychoanalysis and the University

A Difficult Relationship

14

A critique of present-day isolation of psychoanalytic institutes and of their lack of emphasis on research and scientific development is followed here by concrete proposals for reorienting psychoanalytic education toward university settings, for the ultimate purpose of bringing together psychodynamic understanding of psychological development and psychopathology with the fundamental contemporary contributions of neurobiological science. Efforts that are already under way in this direction and practical recommendations for further steps to integrate psychoanalytic education and research within university settings are the main subject of this chapter. This emphasis corresponds to my fundamental conviction that these two major fields of investigation of the human psyche, neurobiology and psychoanalysis, need each other for a sophisticated progress of psychological science.

The Problem: I. External Reality

The pressing need for psychoanalysis to establish or reestablish a strong relation with universities and academic centers of higher learning has become broadly acknowledged and accepted by the psychoanalytic community in recent years—at least, in principle. Statements by leading educators and scholars of the International Psychoanalytical Association have underlined this need and have called for action in this regard (Auchincloss and Michels 2003; Cooper 1987; Ferrari 2009; Garza Guerrero 2006; C. Garza Guerrero, "Psychoanalysis—Requiescat in Pace? [A Critique From Within and a Radical Proposal]," unpublished manuscript, 2010; Glick 2007; Holzman 1976, 1985; Levy 2009; Michels 2007; Paul 2007; Wallerstein 1972, 1980, 2007, 2009). The reasons for these alliances are quite obvious: psychoanalysis has been accepted as a major contribution to the culture of the twentieth century, but its future role as a science and a profession is uncertain and is being challenged (Kernberg 2006, 2007).

Attacks from academic and cultural centers, challenging the scientific status of psychoanalysis and its effectiveness as a treatment, have become fashionable as psychopharmacology and cognitive-behavioral treatments have gained ascendancy, offering as they do short-term, less costly treatment alternatives for all manner of psychopathology once the exclusive province of psychoanalysis. From a simple economic viewpoint, the restriction of payment for extended psychotherapies on the part of insurance companies and National Health Service systems has particularly affected psychoanalysis, reinforcing its negative image within the professions of clinical psychology and psychiatry. Psychoanalytic institutes, in regions where they have long been established, have experienced significant reduction in candidates seeking psychoanalytic training and in patients seeking analysis (H. Thomä, "Remarks on the First Century of the International Psychoanalytic Association [IPA] and a Utopian Vision of Its Future," unpublished manuscript, 2010).

The fundamental contributions that psychoanalysis has made to the related fields of psychology and psychiatry have been absorbed and integrated by those disciplines but are less and less cited as scientific and professional contributions of psychoanalysis. The most recent example, perhaps, is the important development of attachment theory. Bowlby, steeped in the psychoanalytic tradition, saw attachment paradigms as intrapsychically central to development across the life span. Attachment theory is increasingly being explored from a predominantly behavioral perspective, ignoring the development of intrapsychic structures and unconscious fantasy (Polan and Hofer 1999). The descriptions of major personality disorders, such as the narcissistic, masochistic, and borderline personality disorders, that stem from psychoanalytic research are acknowledged but tend to get incorporated into classificatory systems and theories of etiology that, again, bypass the developmental history of unconscious intrapsychic structures. Psychoanalytic contributions to the understanding of early sexuality, gender-determined differentiation of psychological development, and disturbances in sexual functions equally have been absorbed and reformulated in a combination of neurobiological and cognitive-behavioral perspectives. The psychoanalytic basis of psychodynamic psychotherapies has expanded this field into a broad spectrum of autonomous psychotherapeutic institutions and applications that have become disconnected from their original psychoanalytic sources.

Also, important psychoanalytic contributions to the field of early childhood development, as well as personality studies, psychopathology, and psychotherapy, have been carried out by psychoanalysts embedded in university settings as professors of social work, psychiatry, and psychology. Many such academic positions have disappeared over the years, particularly in countries where psychoanalysis had managed to have a firm basis in the university, such as in Germany and the United States. In recent generations of psychoanalysts, we see a decreasing number of academically active, scientifically engaged professionals. In fact, a major problem posed in the development of new academic leadership in psychology and psychiatry is that it has become more and more estranged from psychoanalysis, as few psychoanalytic scholars are able to compete academically for such positions. To some extent, this process has not been as pervasive in the humanities, where interest in psychoanalysis persists in areas such as linguistics, literary analysis, and the arts, but it is painfully clear in the mental health sciences. All of this reflects the social and cultural environment that psychoanalysis is facing at this time. These challenges are compounded, unfortunately, by important internal realities affecting the psychoanalytic community.

The Problem: II. Internal Reality

A major problem is the discrepancy between the general recognition, on the part of the psychoanalytic community, that a move to approach the university and establish a closer link with it would be highly desirable, and the fact that, in practice, very little, if any, movement in that direction has taken place because the main center of educational activity and potential research interests naturally would be linked to the tasks of psychoanalytic institutes, the educational enterprise of psychoanalysis, rather than to psychoanalytic societies, the professional side of the field. Universities, of course, have as their major mission to transmit knowledge and to create new knowledge, education and research being their major, intimately linked functions.

Psychoanalytic institutes, to the contrary, are strongly focused on transmitting knowledge but reluctant to carry out research to develop new knowledge. Insofar as all research implies questioning what is known to this point, as part of the process to advance further knowledge, this challenge actually has been reacted to as a threat by the general culture of psychoanalytic institutes (Cooper 1995; Kernberg 2004).

The history of psychoanalysis may shed some light on the antagonism to psychoanalytic research within institutes: having developed outside university structures, the sense of frailty of the independently developing new science of psychoanalysis has determined, I believe, a defensive stress on the maintenance of traditional theories and approaches. Particularly, the hierarchical organization of psychoanalytic education linked to the training analysis system has been pointed to as a source of authoritarian tendencies, dogmatism regarding locally dominant approaches, and discouragement of independent thinking and original research work as part of psychoanalytic education. The regressive effects of the training analysis system carried out within an institution where candidates, training analysts, and those graduates not, or not yet, designated as training analysts live together exacerbate dynamics of idealization, submission, paranoia genesis, and rebelliousness, reinforcing the regressive features of the personal analysis and, eventually, promoting the infantilization of candidates. This contributes to reducing the curiosity and emphasis on critical evaluation and development of new knowledge (Kernberg 1986).

The scientific isolation of institutes from the development in science at the boundaries of psychoanalysis generates a further threatening, implicit insecurity regarding new knowledge and distrust of external sources of knowledge that might influence or even threaten psychoanalytic thinking. A fearful attitude regarding any challenges to traditional psychoanalytic thinking reflects the sense of isolation and implicit frailty of psychoanalytic institutes and stimulates the phobic attitude toward empirical research that still dominates large segments of the psychoanalytic educational enterprise, rationalized most frequently on the basis of the "uniqueness of each long-term psychoanalytic encounter" that defies generalizations and efforts at quantitative assessment.

The regressive effect of a personal analysis not only operates upon the student body in inducing anxiety, excessive idealizations, and paranoiagenic reactions but also affects the training analysts. Immersion in a social atmosphere of candidates whose personal intimacy they know, and over whom they wield unchallenged decision-making authority as to selection, supervision, progression, graduation, and, above all, evaluation of analytic competency, creates gratifying power for the training analyst's body, on the one hand, and distrust of an external world that may challenge this power and this entire structure, on the other. A permanent ambience of transference and countertransference reactions is reflected in the establishment of guru-like figures, on the one hand, and vehement critique of alternative theories to those that dominate within a particular institute, on the other. Add to this a basic anxiety about the firmness and stability of cherished convictions and approaches, and you have a breeding ground for conservatism, ideological monopolies, and a petrified intellectual atmosphere that runs counter to the generally growing conviction within the psychoanalytic community at large that a major rapprochement with the university is essential for the future of psychoanalysis.

In short, the basis of the major potential of transmission of knowledge and development of knowledge, of potential research on psychoanalytic theory and technique and on its application to a broad spectrum of related disciplines in the humanities and in neurobiology and medicine, as well as to psychotherapeutic approaches in general as a major contribution to the mental health professions, resides precisely in the same institutions where opposition to change and, at best, a defensive indifference to it are maximal. Thirty years ago, psychoanalytic candidates in many countries were implicitly or explicitly dissuaded within psychoanalytic institutes from following parallel careers in psychiatry and psychology and other fields. Only after the more recent decrease of candidates interested in psychoanalytic training and the aging of the profession throughout established psychoanalytic societies made it clear that we are at risk for becoming irrelevant to a younger generation has this negative attitude slowly began to change.

It would be unfair, however, to describe psychoanalytic institutes as places where no new knowledge and experimentation occur. After all, important new psychoanalytic theories and techniques have evolved, and the exploration of the psychoanalytic situation has led to significant advances in knowledge regarding early development, psychopathology, diagnosis, and treatment, as well as creative ideas regarding the application of psychoanalysis to other fields.

In all fairness, in spite of the organizational and cultural restrictions operating in the realm of psychoanalytic education, psychoanalytic institutes and societies witnessed the development of important new knowledge, innovative new theories and their applications to psychoanalytic technique, and derivative psychotherapeutic procedures. The second half of the last century witnessed the development of Kleinian and neo-Kleinian, particularly Bionian, theory and technical innovation in psychoanalysis in Great Britain; the emergence of relational psychoanalysis in the United States; the influence of Lacanian concepts on French psychoanalysis; new applications of ego psychology to a vast field of psychoanalytic psychotherapy; new knowledge regarding the psychopathology of severe personality disorders, sexual pathology, and the application of psychoanalytic psychotherapy to group, couples, and family therapy; advances in the application of psychoanalytic understanding of group processes to the study of ideology and political processes; and, more recently, progress in the understanding of the relation between neurobiology and psychodynamics of affects, with particular reference to depression. In the humanities, psychoanalytic concepts were applied to the study of linguistics and literary criticism and to the analysis of the social pathology related to totalitarian regimes.

However, the conservative and restrictive atmosphere within psychoanalytic institutes precluded research into the implications of these new developments within the institutes themselves or development of comparative studies on the differential effects of alternative new psychoanalytic formulations, indications, and limitations of the expanding modalities of psychoanalytically oriented psychotherapies. Within psychoanalytic institutes, alternative theories to the locally dominant one were initially ignored, and subsequently attacked, as occurred in the "wars" between Kleinian and ego psychological institutes and authors from the 1950s through the 1970s. More recently, in an ecumenical spirit that reflected the gradual intellectual opening of psychoanalytic institutes, alternative theories were taught and comparative discussions regarding them tolerated within many institutes themselves. But the resistance against formalized research has led to a passive acceptance of multiple, in many ways contradictory, approaches, with an implicit devaluation of the scientific importance of advancing in the knowledge of their true value. At times, theories have been treated as metaphors, contrasting them with the practicality of psychoanalytic technique itself. At the same time, however, systematization of psychoanalytic technique to a degree that would permit empirical study of the relation between alternative technical approaches and outcome has been lacking. Empirical research regarding psychoanalytic psychotherapies has been carried out within college and university settings by psychoanalytically trained researchers but not within psychoanalytic institutes proper. The theoretical work of applying psychoanalysis to the study of group and social processes, religion and philosophy, and the understanding of artistic language, for the most part, has all occurred in university settings unrelated to psychoanalytic institutes. As mentioned before, psychoanalytically based new knowledge and derived research were incorporated by other disciplines and became disconnected from the mainstream of psychoanalytic endeavors. Within the clinical realm, the development of independent institutes centered on psychoanalytic psychotherapy, competing with psychoanalytic institutes proper, has represented the clinical side of this paradoxical growth and alienation of psychoanalytically derived knowledge.

The Transformation of Psychoanalytic Institutes: Some General Preconditions

If the preceding overview of the challenges that psychoanalysis faces at this time—the internal dynamics of the training analyst system within psychoanalytic institutes, the paradoxical development of psychoanalytic knowledge, on the one hand, and a stultifying absence of scientific spirit, and educational stagnation of institutes, on the other—represents an adequate overview of the present situation, some interrelated strategies for overcoming the present crisis of the psychoanalytic profession and science seem promising. Several major contributions to a potential response required at this time have signaled the components of such an approach.

1. Psychoanalytic education has to be radically innovated. The hierarchical rigidity and its derivative deadening of intellectual curiosity need to be overcome. This requires an embrace of the knowledge explosion in boundary sciences by inviting leading faculty of related fields to become part of the teaching faculty of institutes. Structurally, the functions of seminar leaders and supervisors should be separated to recognize those who demonstrate specific capacity for supervising clinical work, on the one hand, and those who have original contributions to make to the understanding and development of the cognitive body of contemporary psychoanalysis, on the other. The personal psychoanalysis should be completely separated from the educational functions of the institute, and politically loaded appointment of training analysts should be replaced with a generally accepted method of certification in proficiency as psychoanalytic practitioner, equivalent to the specialty boards in medicine, with free selection by psychoanalytic candidates of their personal analyst within all those certified by such a generally recognized, supra-institutional specialty board. I have described elsewhere (Kernberg 2006, 2007) the advantages, preconditions, and methods of implementation proposed to abolish the training analysis

system and to replace it with a functional arrangement for a high-quality personal analysis for psychoanalytic candidates.

2. Formalized research as an essential aspect of psychoanalytic education—not with the intention of making every psychoanalyst a researcher, but of fostering and rewarding research-oriented candidates and faculty, particularly those with academic aspirations, and providing them with appropriate institutional mentoring and support, drawing on the vast clinical material available to psychoanalytic institutes—would lead to the development of new psychoanalytic knowledge. This means, at the very least, the establishment of a department of research in psychoanalytic institutes with the freedom to extend inquiry into every aspect of theory, technique, and applications that is part of the curriculum and reflecting, at all levels, a concern for critical evaluation of what is taught. Experts in research methodology should become an essential part of the leadership of the psychoanalytic institution. The academic credentials of research methodologists within the psychoanalytic institute would facilitate an alliance with the corresponding academic centers, within which collaborative research with the institute could be carried out. University faculty working within the institute would have access to its human resources as well as clinical material, while collaborative research with the university might provide the funding support that would facilitate candidates and faculty to pursue an academic career, in parallel to their analytic one. Again, such a career probably would develop for only a small proportion of psychoanalytic candidates, but the benefit of the critical input from related disciplines within the educational atmosphere of the institute would be powerfully strengthened. This development, of course, would imply overcoming the past prejudice against those candidates and analysts not dedicated exclusively to their analytic career.

3. The development of a cadre of scholars within psychoanalytic institutes has been the potentially strongest element in fostering new knowledge in the context of psychoanalytic education. Radical innovators have come from the intense involvement with psychoanalytic work and often have been able to generate an atmosphere of exciting new developments in psychoanalytic theory and technique. Total immersion in the psychoanalytic treatment of patients should be fostered and facilitated for those candidates and faculty evincing particular interests and

creativity in their clinical work and related scholarly writing. But this should not be the only path to the development of new knowledge or a rationale for discouraging all other roads to progress.

In the past, original scholars whose thinking strongly diverged from the dominant ideology of a particular institution were driven into the periphery of the educational process, leading to contentious splits within the psychoanalytic institution. Rather than merely being tolerated, originality should be actively fostered as a stimulus for intellectual productivity by inviting distinguished scholars from fields related to psychoanalysis to join the faculty, with the purpose of stimulating a mutually enriching dialogue. The participation of such distinguished scholars from other fields, as well as from the particular institution itself, requires, naturally, an adequate forum to provide a real opportunity for intellectual interchange rather than an implicit isolation of such scholars from the daily educational enterprise. All of this implies open, systematic discussion of new developments and controversial subjects, while strengthening clarity and the realistic potential for theoretical integration, as well as a scientific approach to incompatible hypotheses.

4. Last but not least, the teaching faculty of the institute should include psychoanalytic practitioners whose clinical practice has been expanded to analytically derived areas: the various forms of psychoanalytic psychotherapy, a broader psychiatric practice oriented within a psychoanalytic viewpoint, institutional work, forensic work, organizational consultation, and the arts. This development would end the widespread, painful alienation of many psychoanalytic graduates who have chosen to pursue other clinical specialties rather than focusing on specific psychoanalytic treatment and, in general, the disappointed alienation presently prevalent among graduate analysts who were interested in participating in the work of psychoanalytic institutes and who, not having been appointed as training analysts, constitute an implicitly devaluated group within the present ambience of the institute.

Here, naturally, the question may be raised whether this is not the task of psychoanalytic societies rather than psychoanalytic institutes proper. The reality, at the present, is that educational activities within the society are generally treated as a secondary type of educational activity, mostly the communication of psychoanalytic knowledge "to the uninformed" or training in psychoanalytic psychotherapy of other mental health professionals, often given to teachers as a "consolation prize" for those who have not become training analysts. Distrust and fear of the introduction of teaching psychoanalytic psychotherapies within the setting of the institute proper play an important role and contribute to the striking paradox that analytic candidates are being trained to carry out a treatment geared to only a minority of the patients they will see, while their main practice of psychoanalytic psychotherapy remains largely unaddressed and is being taught at competing institutions.

Practical Solutions Under Way

If we examine jointly the required preconditions proposed as the basis for the urgently needed change within our training institutes, the relation of psychoanalysis to academia emerges as the central pillar of the establishment of a new system of psychoanalytic education. Psychoanalysis needs the university, although it is not clearly aware of it at this time, and, I believe, in the long run failure to establish these alliances will constitute a severe threat to the future of the psychoanalytic profession and science (Cooper 1987; Garza Guerrero 2006; C. Garza Guerrero, "Psychoanalysis—Requiescat in Pace? [A Critique From Within and a Radical Proposal]," unpublished manuscript, 2010; H. Thomä, "Remarks on the First Century of the International Psychoanalytic Association [IPA] and a Utopian Vision of Its Future," unpublished manuscript, 2010). By the same token, a case can be made for the benefit to academia of psychoanalyses as a science that illuminates the impact of unconscious determinants on psychic life, in the world of the humanistic disciplines as well as in the psychosocial and the naturalistic sciences, particularly in the interface between neurobiology and the functions of the mind. But academia, of course, can very well survive without psychoanalysis, while it is questionable whether, in the long run, psychoanalysis can survive without this link (Auchincloss and Michels 2003; Michels 2007). I believe that this fact is gradually being recognized throughout the psychoanalytic community and has led to a number of attempted solutions.

First of all, an "internal" solution, totally in the hands of the psychoanalytic community itself, is a new relation between the training institute and the psychoanalytic society. There has tended to be a destructive ideological barrier between the psychoanalytic institute as the "elite" of psychoanalysis and the psychoanalytic society as a second-range body that threatens the preservation and development of psychoanalysis. Within the United States, the concept of the development of a "psychoanalytic center," that is, an integration of the educational, professional, application, and outreach functions that jointly constitute the psychoanalytic enterprise, has fostered a new organizational model on the basis of a shared and integrated direction of all of the activities of such a center (Wallerstein 2007, 2009). It facilitates the teaching of psychoanalytic psychotherapy as part of the regular educational program of the institute, using the clinical expertise as well as theoretical developments of the society members mostly engaged in some form of individual, group, or couples psychotherapy and the application of psychoanalytic approaches to psychotherapeutic as well as psychiatric consultation.

The psychoanalytic center fosters the participation of senior faculty in outreach involvements organized by the society, in the form of symposia and conferences that relate psychoanalysis to its local community. The center also facilitates the development of specialized seminars of interest to both candidates and members of the society, involving candidates early in their training in society activities, as well as in important clinical or theoretical new interests or controversies within the society life. It also facilitates the dismantling of the traditional assumption that anointed training analysts are the best seminar leaders and supervisors. If the leadership of such an integrated psychoanalytic center is constituted, at least, by the director of the institute, a representative of the faculty at large, the president of the society, a representative of the outreach division, the chairperson of the society's program committee, and a representative of the research enterprise (if and when such a specialized department has been developed), in addition to a representative of the candidates' organization, a workable cooperative and functional structure may evolve.

This model does not resolve the isolation of the center from the university but may be an important step toward greater awareness of the reality faced by the psychoanalytic practitioner in the external world in the current sociocultural environment. Exciting conferences and scientific activities carried out jointly by society members and students, clinical conferences of candidates and members, joint study groups, and supervisory experiences foster a stimulating atmosphere for the educational enterprise. Psychoanalytic institutes and societies in Philadelphia, Pennsylvania, and in San Francisco, California, have reorganized their structure to implement a center model, with various features among those outlined here.

However, as mentioned before, the model of the psychoanalytic center does not resolve the basic problem of the isolation of the psychoanalytic institution from the world of science and academia. A more direct and organizational relation with university settings may offer many more opportunities and the possibility of a qualitative transformation of psychoanalytic education and, with it, of the science and the profession as well. A close relation with university settings facilitates creation of departments of research within the psychoanalytic institute, the availability of experts on research methodology from the university, and the linkage with technical and financial resources from the university in a mutually beneficial interaction between the faculties of both institutions. The fact that models involving this rapprochement with universities have already been developed and are flourishing is an extremely encouraging and promising development of psychoanalysis (Levy 2009; Michels 2007; Wallerstein 2007, 2009).

One obvious model is that of a psychoanalytic institute that is part of a university department of psychiatry or psychology. The Columbia University Center for Psychoanalytic Training and Research is such an institution that, for many years, has been part of the Department of Psychiatry of Columbia University, with financial and space support from the Department of Psychiatry and a corresponding commitment to participate actively in the education of psychiatric residents and trainees and in the research enterprise of the department. The director of the psychoanalytic institute is appointed by the chairman of the department, on the basis of the proposal by a committee constituted of representatives from the Department of Psychiatry, the medical school, and the institute faculty. The faculty of the institute are eligible for university appointments, following the general rules and regulations for academic promotion, with heavy emphasis on the research and educational background of candidates for academic promotion. A department of research within this psychoanalytic institute stimulates and coordinates research activities including faculty and psychoanalytic candidates, as well as selected trainees within the Department of Psychiatry. Important publications in the area of research on education have been achieved, and the intellectual atmosphere of the institute is remarkably open to absorbing new theoretical formulations and technical developments within the psychoanalytic realm. The Association for Psychoanalytic Medicine, the psychoanalytic society of the Columbia psychoanalytic community, is an independent institution that has been involved, jointly with the Columbia Psychoanalytic Institute, in outreach activities including the provision of teachers within various colleges of Columbia University and interdisciplinary activities in the form of public conferences involving faculty from the psychoanalytic community as well as other university colleges.

Another variation of this model in the United States is offered by the Psychoanalytic Center of Emory University in Atlanta, Georgia (Levy 2009). This is a complex structure that includes a psychoanalytic institute within the department of psychiatry of the medical school and an autonomous center dedicated to facilitate psychoanalytically oriented education and research throughout the entire university, offering consultation and teaching to various university departments and arranging for interested students throughout the university to participate in classes of the psychoanalytic institute. All institute seminars, with the exception of the supervision of clinical cases and seminars on psychoanalytic technique, are open to all Emory students, and the center organizes specific educational activities and conferences for the university at large. This original program seems an ideal solution to the problem and challenges outlined above.

A major problem with this model is that it is difficult to replicate at this time. A psychoanalytic institute, in order to become eligible to function within or in relation to a department of psychiatry or clinical psychology of a major university, would require the availability of senior, academically productive and recognized members of the psychoanalytic community whose curricula vitae would permit them to compete successfully for faculty positions—or even chairmanships of university departments in those disciplines. The lack of a strong body of psychoanalytic academicians within a younger generation of psychoanalysts makes this a major constraint; one hopes this model might become a more generalized one in the long run, if and when academically active and recognized psychoanalytic candidates for senior faculty positions and for chairmanships again become available, as was the case for an earlier generation of psychoanalysts in countries such as Germany and the United States. A more viable variation of this model, however, is the possibility of a more loose and flexible association of an independent psychoanalytic institute with a university department of psychiatry or psychology, with teaching commitments of the psychoanalytic faculty in return for voluntary faculty positions affiliated with the university. The cooperative arrangement between the New York University Psychoanalytic Institute and the Department of Psychiatry of the New York University Medical School represents this type of the university-linked model.

An alternative model is the development of an autonomous university institute within or related to a major university setting, the psychoanalytic institute taking on the responsibility of developing a full-fledged program—say, in clinical psychology—acceptable as part of the educational and professional standards of the university, within the rules, regulations, and overall control of the university of such a program. Large psychoanalytic societies may have sufficient intellectual resources to be able to carry out such a program, and this is the model adopted by the Psychoanalytic Association of Buenos Aires (APdeBA), which has developed an Institute of Psychology granting a master's degree in clinical psychology, under the sponsorship and control of APdeBA, following the general Argentinean rules and regulations governing private universities, and in close professional interchange with the Association of Private University Institutes (Ferrari 2009). The psychoanalytic institute provides the faculty that are committed to teach all the requirements for a master's degree in psychology of the university, with a particular accent on psychoanalytic theory and its applications. The students acquire knowledge of psychoanalytic theory and its development, the epistemological questions raised by the study of the dynamic unconscious, the evidence supporting psychoanalytic theory, as well as controversial aspects of it, and a theoretical knowledge about the application of psychoanalytic theory to diagnosis and treatment of the major types of psychopathology within the realm of a psychoanalytic approach. They do not receive clinical training in psychoanalysis proper but are encouraged, if they are so interested, to undergo a personal psychoanalysis or psychoanalytic psychotherapy. The success of this program is reflected in the increasing awareness of and attention to psychoanalysis within the overall university ambiance, an increase in interdisciplinary activities, and, last but not least, an increase in students seeking their own analysis, regardless of their eventual career choices.

In Germany, a somewhat similar program has been initiated in Berlin with the creation of the International Psychoanalytic University, an independent university institute that offers a bachelor's degree in psychology and a master's degree in psychology, fulfilling all the requirements for granting these degrees by the German law governing university mandates and requirements, including the teaching of a comprehensive spectrum of psychological theories and approaches and the development of a research program and corresponding research training that satisfies the general criteria of standards of research training in German university settings (J. Körner, personal communication, 2009).

This program does not include clinical teaching of psychoanalytic techniques or psychoanalytic psychotherapy, but its graduates, hopefully, will be able to apply psychoanalytic theory to the diverse specialties they will be involved in later, and it provides an important gateway to psychoanalytic training proper for some of them. The impressive initiative of the International Psychoanalytic University in Berlin was funded by a private donor, a senior, highly respected training analyst who had for many years held the chairmanship of a department of psychology of another university in Germany.

Financial constraints remain, in general, a major factor that limits innovative programs in university settings. At the same time, however, collaborative efforts between university departments interested in research development and with access to particular sources of funding, on the one hand, and the willingness of psychoanalytic institutes to provide faculty time, patient material, and even space for joint research and educational programs, on the other, should offer realistic possibilities.

Another significant constraint may be the hostile reception of psychoanalysis in many departments of psychiatry and psychology, particularly under conditions when long-term competitive struggles between psychodynamic approaches and cognitive-behavioral approaches have characterized the mental health field. I believe it is the task of psychoanalytic institutes and societies to try to reverse the bias against psychoanalysis derived from such an intellectual background. Particularly in the United States, the historical dominance of psychoanalysis in many leading university departments of psychiatry in the 1950s and 1960s that was characterized in some cases by gross neglect of (if not outright opposition to) the parallel development of biological psychiatry led to a corresponding "revenge" once biologically oriented psychiatry gained ascendancy, while a parallel process shifted departments of clinical psychology from a psychodynamic into a cognitive-behavioral direction. Here patience and political action are required, opening up the psychoanalytic institute to influences from the university, and the institute offering faculty and space and patient material resources for joint projects with university-based disciplines.

The programs referred to in this chapter are major illustrations of viable models of integration or reintegration of contemporary psychoanalysis into university settings and academic life. The enormous resistances of psychoanalytic institutions against change and the slowness of the process throughout the international psychoanalytic community should not deter us from working in pursuit of this objective. As mentioned before, I believe the future of psychoanalysis as a science and a profession depends on it, even while the contribution of psychoanalysis as a body of knowledge to the cultural development of humanity may already be assured.

First Steps

What follows are some early developments in the creation of new relations of psychoanalytic institutes with university settings that, I believe, are open to institutes now and are realistic possibilities in many countries. To begin, it would be helpful, in the acceptance of candidates for psychoanalytic training, to foster the selection of academically interested and active applicants, such as psychiatrists and psychologists interested in academic careers in research in specialized fields at the boundary sciences of psychoanalysis, as well as distinguished scholars in the humanities and the social and natural sciences. It would be desirable to combine a selection process for candidates so as to include students interested exclusively in psychoanalysis as well as students with other creative professional interests who may wish to apply psychoanalysis to their specialty field. Naturally, the latter group of candidates needs to be supported in their efforts to apply psychoanalysis to other specialty fields.

Institute leadership should attempt to approach chairpersons of departments of psychiatry and clinical psychology of universities to explore the possibility of collaborative projects. Inviting leading scientists and scholars to teach relevant subjects at the institute, while offering institute faculty for teaching and supervision at those university departments, and holding jointly sponsored public conferences, may be confidence-generating, mutually helpful initiatives. Particularly, experts in sciences at the boundary of psychoanalytic theory and developments may enrich psychoanalytic education and create an atmosphere favorable to possible collaborative studies and research.

Sometimes the ideal area for a productive collaboration resides in the humanities: literature, cultural anthropology, linguistics, and philosophy. Interdisciplinary approaches, of course, have to be based on an honest desire for mutual learning...it cannot be a one-way street. The area of psychosomatic medicine offers an opportunity for collaboration, as both psychiatry and psychoanalysis can benefit from each other's contribution to the understanding of this issue.

Opening up courses at the psychoanalytic institute to students and faculty of a university with which the institute is engaged in some collaborative effort may be an optimal channel for interesting young academicians in a psychoanalytic career: such interest has already been actualized in some of the initiatives mentioned such as the Emory Center and the German International Psychoanalytic University (Levy 2009).

In short, opening the psychoanalytic institute to a genuine attempt at rapprochement with the university may be a viable beginning for creative and really essential new avenues for the future development of psychoanalysis as a science and a profession.

References

Auchincloss EL, Michels R: A reassessment of psychoanalytic education: controversies and changes. Int J Psychoanal 84:387–403, 2003

Cooper A: Changes in psychoanalytic ideas. J Am Psychoanal Assoc 35:77–98, 1987

Cooper A: Discussion: on empirical research, in Research in Psychoanalysis: Process, Development, Outcome. Edited by Shapiro T, Emde RN. Madison, CT, International Universities Press, 1995, pp 381–391

Ferrari H: IUSAM-APdeBA: a higher education institute for psychoanalytic training. Int J Psychoanal 90:1139–1154, 2009

Garza Guerrero C: Crisis del psicoanálisis: desafíos organizativos y educativos contemporaneos [Crisis of Psychoanalysis: Contemporary Organizational and Educational Challenges]. Mexico City, Mexico, Editores de Textos Mexicanos, 2006

Glick RA: Psychoanalytic education needs to change: what's feasible? Introduction to Wallerstein. J Am Psychoanal Assoc 55:949–952, 2007

Holzman PS: The future of psychoanalysis and its institutes. Psychoanal Q 45:250–273, 1976

Holzman PS: Psychoanalysis: is the therapy destroying the science? J Am Psychoanal Assoc 33:725–770, 1985

Kernberg OF: Institutional problems of psychoanalytic education. J Am Psychoanal Assoc 34:799–834, 1986

Kernberg OF: Resistances to research in psychoanalysis, in Contemporary Controversies in Psychoanalytic Theory, Technique, and Their Applications. New Haven, CT, Yale University Press, 2004, pp 86–93

Kernberg OF: The coming changes in psychoanalytic education: part I. Int J Psychoanal 87:1649–1673, 2006

Kernberg OF: The coming changes in psychoanalytic education: part II. Int J Psychoanal 88:183–202, 2007

Levy ST: Psychoanalytic education then and now. J Am Psychoanal Assoc 57:1295–1309, 2009

Michels R: Optimal education requires an academic context: commentary on Wallerstein. J Am Psychoanal Assoc 55:985–989, 2007

Paul RA: Optimal education requires an academic context: commentary on Wallerstein. J Am Psychoanal Assoc 55:991–997, 2007

Polan HJ, Hofer MA: Psychobiological origins of infant attachment and separation response, in Handbook of Attachment. Edited by Cassidy J, Shaver PR. New York, Guilford, 1999, pp 162–180

Wallerstein RS: The futures of psychoanalytic education. J Am Psychoanal Assoc 20:591–606, 1972

Wallerstein RS: Psychoanalysis and academic psychiatry—bridges. Psychoanal Study Child 35:419–448, 1980

Wallerstein RS: The optimal structure for psychoanalytic education today: a feasible proposal? J Am Psychoanal Assoc 55:953–984, 2007

Wallerstein RS: Psychoanalysis in the university: a full-time vision. Int J Psychoanal 90:1107–1121, 2009

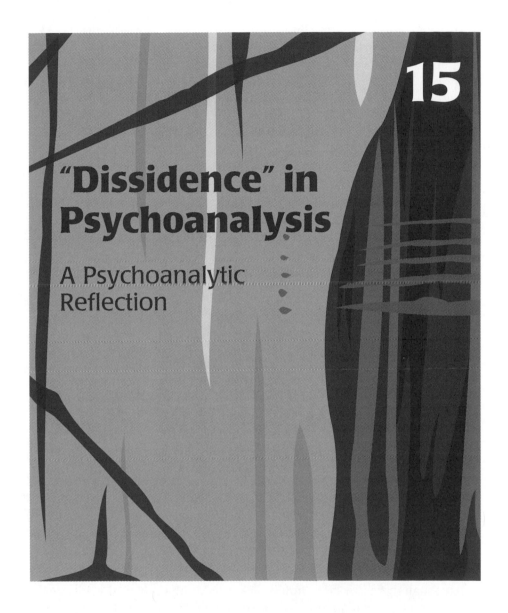

"Dissidence" in Psychoanalysis

A Psychoanalytic Reflection

This chapter was reprinted from Kernberg OF: "'Dissidence' in Psychoanalysis," in *Power of Understanding, Essays in Honour of Veikko Tälikä*. Edited by Laine A. London, Karnac, 2004, pp. 55–72. This chapter also appeared in *Understanding Dissidence and Controversy in the History of Psychoanalysis*. Edited by Bergmann MS. New York, Other Press, 2004, pp. 129–146. Used with permission.

In this chapter on the vicissitudes of psychoanalytic institutions, I focus on the ideological battles between the psychoanalytic "mainstream" and challenging "dissidents" who, for a variety of reasons, developed new theoretical formulations and technical approaches to treatment that resulted in a collision course with the "establishment." I propose that the lack of a tradition of research in psychoanalysis interfered with the possibility of finding scientific answers to such controversies and that, instead, both internal organizational dynamics and external, culturally determined ideologies influence these theoretical struggles. The optimal development of scientific contributions from psychoanalysis, I conclude, is to be open to new ideas, explore alternative approaches, carry out empirical research to resolve the corresponding controversies, and generate new knowledge in the process. The presently developing empirical research on psychodynamic psychotherapies has already signaled the viability of this way of proceeding.

The present "age of pluralism" in psychoanalytic theorizing justifies a new look at the historical aspects of dissidence and change in the development of psychoanalysis during the past century. A conference on this subject organized around a fundamental contribution to this subject by Martin Bergmann (M.S. Bergmann, "Rethinking the Problem of Dissidence and Change in the History of Psychoanalysis," unpublished manuscript, 2001) stimulated this contribution. What follows is a general reflection on dissidence in psychoanalysis.

Dissidence is defined (*Concise Oxford Dictionary*) as disagreement, especially with the religious doctrines of an established church. Dissidence within psychoanalysis thus implies an ideological or religious quality of psychoanalytic convictions and implicitly raises questions about the scientific nature of psychoanalysis. Bergmann (M.S. Bergmann, "Rethinking the Problem of Dissidence and Change in the History of Psychoanalysis," unpublished manuscript, 2001) quotes Freud as stating that disagreements regarding psychoanalytic theories should be settled with empirical evidence. Yet Freud, Bergmann goes on, also asserted that rejection of some basic psychoanalytic theories reflected psychologically motivated resistance to the truth of psychoanalysis, implying that the perfectly analyzed psychoanalyst would not present such opposition. Dissidence, according to this latter view, again has the connotation of opposing ideological or religious belief systems rather than of engaging in scientific discourse.

If one translates the question of dissidence into the question of the nature of scientific evidence in psychoanalysis, the focus shifts to the development of methods for empirical examination of controversial issues. I assume that even in the current relatively immature stage of methodology of scientific research in psychoanalysis, some issues may be approached empirically. These might include the nature of the analytic relationship, the interaction of technique and process and between process and outcome, and the effectiveness of psychoanalytic treatment, for example. But many fundamental questions must remain open and can only be resolved gradually by means of the cumulative clinical experience of the profession and the shared communication and evaluation of this clinical experience over time.

As Bergmann (M.S. Bergmann, "Rethinking the Problem of Dissidence and Change in the History of Psychoanalysis," unpublished manuscript, 2001) pointed out in his overview of the main contributions stemming from psychoanalytic dissidents, many of their theories, originally rejected by the psychoanalytic community, were eventually woven into the main fabric of psychoanalytic theory and method. Bergmann raises the fascinating question, what made some of these dissidents "dissidents," and what made some potential dissidents into "modifiers" who enriched psychoanalytic theory with their contributions? His central thesis is that, at least in the early generation of dissidents, the personal relationship with Freud played a major role. It is an open question to what extent the personal relationship to Freud's thinking continues having such a central role for the dissidents and modifiers who continued to emerge after his death. While I am in essential agreement with the major proposal of Martin Bergmann, in what follows I shall take on the role of a "modifier," building on his rich contributions while focusing on the varying influence that personal, scientific, cultural, and institutional factors have on the emergence of dissidents.

The Personal Relationship With Freud

Bergmann describes convincingly the importance of the development of personal conflicts, particularly rivalries between Freud and his early disciples, with clear implications of oedipal conflicts and sibling rivalry as major contributors to the development of dissidents. Perhaps the most striking illustration of this dynamic is the gradual sharpening of the disagreements between Freud and Adler and the eventual departure of Adler from the psychoanalytic group. But it is one among many that include Jung, Rank, Ferenczi,

Horney, and Wilhelm Reich. All of these dissidents had personal relationships with Freud, but at a certain point, when their contributions ran counter to Freud's convictions and the related boundaries of psychoanalytic formulations of the time, they met with sharp criticisms that reinforced their insistence on their particular views, finally leading to a split.

I agree with Bergmann that a personal disappointment either in their psychoanalysis or in the relationship with Freud played an important role. Obviously, behind that conflict were issues of the psychopathology of all participants, activated by the regressive effects of the personal psychoanalysis and by the institutional reinforcement of such conflicts as these resonated with the psychoanalytic movement's relation to its founder and charismatic leader. In fact, one might raise the question whether what appeared on the surface as personal conflicts with Freud might not have been unconsciously stimulated by the "innocent bystanders" of the psychoanalytic movement. By the term *innocent bystanders,* I am referring to the psychology of regressive group processes that enact profound ambivalence toward their leader, expressing the hostility by a selected opponent or subgroup, which permits the silent majority to deny their own aggression, acting as "innocent bystanders." While they admired Freud and followed him without questions, their unconscious hostility might have been enacted through fostering the conflict with Freud of a selected "representative"...or scapegoat.

Freud was open to new ideas and changed his views significantly in the course of time but was strongly assertive of them at any particular point. His efforts to integrate the thinking of his disciples when it did not correspond entirely to his own may at times have been facilitated by those closest to him. At other times, the influence of his close friends may have increased the sharp differences between Freud's views and those of a young challenger. The personalized accentuation of the differences of their theoretical and technical formulations with those of Freud strongly suggests that the young challengers had intense feelings about these differences. Much of the more subtle dynamics of the early group probably are no longer available for scrutiny, but what we can assess is the influence of cultural factors on the different viewpoints that evolved and the use of ideology to support and rationalize more personal struggles.

What was the influence of Freud's rigidity in asserting his viewpoints? In all fairness, the enormous scope of Freud's discoveries

and the continuous broadening of the world of unconscious conflicts and their consequences that he opened up would make it reasonable to think that it was difficult for the early group to absorb in
addition the theoretical and clinical breakthroughs stemming from
his disciples. When such contributions were asserted with an aggressive assertion of revolutionary "uniqueness" like that of Adler
and, eventually, Rank, an impatient rejection of their ideas seems
understandable. I believe, however, that what haunted the psychoanalytic movement, and continues to haunt organized psychoanalysis to this day, is that the clinical basis of psychoanalytic discoveries, the knowledge learned from psychoanalysis as an investigative
tool, is fraught with methodological difficulties. The mutual influences of analysts' theories and patients' regressive deployment
render decisions regarding alternative theoretical formulations
very difficult to make. The inevitable subjectivity and uncertainty of
the clinical process will be resolved (if ever) only after an entire
generation of analysts has approached the problem from different
viewpoints and sufficient knowledge has been accumulated for the
entire psychoanalytic movement to move on.

For example, Ferenczi's (1949) stress on the importance of the
mother/infant relationship and, with it, the emphasis on preoedipal
development, turned out to be an extremely important advance in
psychoanalytic understanding. It was elaborated later on by Melanie Klein, Winnicott, and Mahler, but it would take still another
generation to establish a synthetic view that would integrate the
preoedipal and oedipal stages of development in the concept of the
archaic oedipal constellation. Similarly, Adler's stress on the importance of competitiveness and aggression would only later be integrated into the psychoanalytic mainstream, under the influence
of newly accumulated information from the psychoanalytic treatment of severe psychopathologies, leading to Freud's discovery of
the importance of repetition compulsion and superego pathology.

It might be argued, of course, that psychoanalysis as an institution might have been more open to new ideas had the leadership
been more functional and less authoritarian. New ideas might then
have been welcomed, studied, elaborated, and integrated rather
than having to undergo periods of dissidence and reencounter. But
the enormous difference between Freud's creativity and the dependent attitude of his disciples probably constituted such a powerful
dynamic that a more relaxed search for consensus might have
slowed down the pace of Freud's own discoveries and contributions. Here the question of the extent to which it is functional that

the psychology of the institution adapts to the personality of the creative leader becomes relevant. In other words, some degree of authoritarianism on the part of an extremely creative leader may represent a reduction in an organization's optimal functioning but a price well worth paying for supporting such a leader. In all fairness, one also may grant the dangerous nature of experimenting with a new investigative tool—namely, psychoanalytic exploration—as causative in bringing about the inappropriate aspect of the behavior of those early disciples.

The Impact of Ideological Crosscurrents on the Development of Dissidence

Bergmann (M.S. Bergmann, "Rethinking the Problem of Dissidence and Change in the History of Psychoanalysis," unpublished manuscript, 2001) describes convincingly Jung's deep adherence to religion and mythology, with its linkage to German romanticism and ultimately to racist nationalism and anti-Semitism, and his irresponsible immersion in the Nazi culture. By the same token, Freud's profound identification with the rationalist and atheist culture of the nineteenth century may have contributed to Jung's rationalization of his departure from the psychoanalytic movement (McGuire 1974).

It is only in the last 30 years that various psychoanalytic contributors have reflected on the subtly militant atheism of psychoanalysis' ideological stance toward religion, expressed in the not infrequently heard statements in the 1950s and the 1960s that a well-analyzed person could no longer be a religious one. The concern over psychoanalysis becoming a "weltanschauung" was first expressed by Chasseguet-Smirgel (Chasseguet-Smirgel and Grunberger 1969) and has led in recent time to a meaningful reexploration of the relation between psychoanalysis and religion, for example, in the Mainz seminars in Germany in recent years (Kernberg 2000b).

Marxism became the ideological crosscurrent that influenced the dissidence of Wilhelm Reich, was already a factor in Alfred Adler's partisan political stance regarding the Social Democratic party in Austria, and reemerged in Erich Fromm's critique of capitalist societies. Perhaps the most extreme representatives of this

ideological development were Herbert Marcuse's utilization of
psychoanalytic thinking as part of what might be called a Marxist
theology of liberation and Althusser's utilization of the superego
concept, bringing together Lacan and Marx in analyzing the ideological superstructure of capitalism. The demise of Soviet Communism and the loss of popularity of Marxist ideology in general have
brought about a curious disappearance of the psychoanalytic communities' concern with the relation between psychoanalysis and
Marxism, but we must remember how it agitated the entire psychoanalytic generation in the 1960s and 1970s, leading, for example,
to the splitting off of Marxist groups from the psychoanalytic societies in Argentina. Those Marxist groups have, in the meantime,
disappeared entirely.

The most recent of these cross-cultural currents has been the
feminist critique of Freud, expressed along a broad spectrum, from
the thoughtful contributions of Melanie Klein and Edith Jacobson,
correcting Freud's assumptions about early superego development
in women, to the general critique of the primary nature of penis
envy in women, and to the dissidence of Karen Horney (Benjamin
1986; Blum 1976; Horney 1967). The marginalizing of Horney is especially to be regretted in the light of the later integration of new
understanding of early development in both genders, stemming
from both North American and European recent literature. Karen
Horney's departure from the New York Psychoanalytic Society was
probably determined less by the heretical nature of her ideas than
by the internal conflicts of the then monolithic institution to which
she belonged.

It is difficult to assess concurrently—rather than with hindsight—
to what extent ideological currents infiltrate psychoanalytic thinking and codetermine the differential characteristics of psychoanalytic institutions in different countries today. When a general
cultural agreement prevails in a certain region of the world, psychoanalytic institutions may not even be aware of those cultural influences on psychoanalytic development. For example, the strong
adaptational stress on the part of American ego psychology, the assumed normal adaptation to an "average expectable environment,"
the Hartmann era emphasis on the positive functions of the ego in
facilitating adaptation, and the tendency to reject the concept of a
primary aggressive drive (let alone the concept of a death drive) all
flourished in the optimistic cultural development of the United
States after the end of the Second World War (Bergmann 2000).
Meanwhile, predominance of concern over primitive aggression

was strongly developed in Great Britain during and immediately after the war years.

The spread of Lacanian psychoanalysis, with its stress on philosophy and rejection of Anglo-American empiricism, has had a strong impact on Latin American psychoanalytic societies living within a francophone cultural environment, while it has left only the merest traces in the humanities departments of American universities. It is interesting, furthermore, how the recent emphasis on genetics within the biological sciences and the revolution in neurosciences have prompted psychoanalysts to reexamine the relation between mind and brain, an interest totally absent from the psychoanalytic culture of only 20 years ago. It is significant, it seems to me, that the idolatrous attitude toward Freud of most of his followers during those years did not include recognition of his great interest in neurology and the relation of mind and brain.

My point is that during periods of rapid cultural shifts, when new ideological currents clash with traditional influences upon psychoanalytic thinking, that clash may contribute to the development of dissidence, eventually exaggerated as a system of rationalization for opposition that has deeper roots in psychoanalytic institutional dynamics.

Intrinsic Challenges of Psychoanalytic Theory and Technique to the Conventional Assumptions of Mass Culture

Here I enter a problematic area of argument. One often hears, particularly in conservative psychoanalytic circles, that the hard times psychoanalysis is presently undergoing are related to the enduring threat of Freud's findings to conventional assumptions of mankind. I believe that this argument tends to underestimate the serious problems that psychoanalysis has created for itself by accepting, indeed enacting its reputation as isolationist, elitist, and biased against empirical research. However, I believe the argument holds in terms of the persistence, within conventional culture, at least of the Western world, of the myths of the sexual innocence of childhood, the basic goodness of human beings, and the positive consequence of any human encounter in which at least one of the two parties is attempting to help the other. Max Gitelson put it in a simple sentence: "There are many people who believe in psychoanalysis, except sex, aggression, and transference."

These conventional assumptions are often called "resistance" to psychoanalytic concepts, an unfortunate misuse of a term whose specific meaning in psychoanalysis has to do with the manifestation of defensive operations in the psychoanalytic situation. This definition has particular implications for a contemporary theory of technique: more about this later.

The assumption of infantile sexuality, one of the most revolutionary discoveries of Freud, will probably be accepted in theory by every psychoanalyst. In practice, however, the ignorance or neglect of infantile sexuality shows up again and again, in the theorizing of dissidents as well as in various technical approaches within the psychoanalytic establishment. Thus, Jung's stress on the collective unconscious and archaic archetypes pointedly neglected infantile sexuality, and, as Bergmann pointed out, Jung accused Freud of having elevated sexuality to the equivalent of a religious commitment. Rank's stress on the fundamental importance of the relationship of the infant to mother likewise deemphasized infantile sexuality, and even Ferenczi, in accentuating the devastating effects of sexual abuse and traumatization of the child, implicitly turned back to that innocent view of childhood.

Melanie Klein's formulations, although they incorporated the concept of the premature oedipalization as a defense against preoedipal aggression, in practice stressed preoedipal conflicts almost to the exclusion of the erotic quality of the relationship between infant and mother. Only in the last 20 years, probably under the influence of contacts with French psychoanalysis, has the focus on oedipal conflicts again been accentuated in the work of Kleinian authors. Karen Horney, Kohut's self psychology, and the intersubjective and relational psychoanalytic schools evince an underemphasis of unconscious oedipal conflicts. It is as if the vicissitudes of infantile sexuality have to be rediscovered, again and again, against this cultural trend influencing psychoanalytic practice and theorizing.

The rejection of Freud's dual drive theory of libido and aggression and its replacement by an object relations approach also reflect the tendency to underestimate both infantile sexuality and aggression (Kernberg 2001). This shows clearly in the clinical illustrations of intersubjective, relational, and self psychological case material (Kernberg, in press 2011). Perhaps self psychology has been most outspoken in this regard, and Kohut's proposal that aggression derives from the traumatic fragmentation of the self may be the most specific formulation of that view. Erich Fromm's views imply that, in an optimally arranged society, the degree of aggression would decrease significantly (Fromm 1941). As Bergmann pointed out, Fromm was deeply critical of Freud because of his pessimistic stance in this regard.

The empirical research on attachment, of significant clinical as well as theoretical importance regarding early development, tends to focus primarily on the traumatic effects of mother's lack of normal responsiveness to the baby. Extrapolating from that research, the intersubjective and relational approaches have focused on the analyst's inevitable failures to understand as traumatic, requiring repair via appropriate interpretation before the analytic process can go on. In this regard, they follow a path not dissimilar from the techniques of self psychology. As in the theories of Fairbairn, the emphasis on the traumatic origin of neurosis and unconscious conflict implicitly denies the central importance of the disposition to aggression.

In the light of contemporary affect theory and the probability, as I have suggested, that the drives are supraordinate integrations, respectively, of positive and negative affects, one may question the primary nature of the drives but not the primary nature of both negative and positive affects and the disposition to rage, anger, hatred, disgust, as well as joyful contact and erotic pleasure. The primary nature of both intense positive and negative affect states and their influence on structure building supports, I believe, Freud's basic dual drive theory (Kernberg 1992a). It may be argued that only under pathological circumstances may aggression become so dominant that the effort to destroy all relationships—including the self—may become the dominant motivation, thus crystallizing as a death drive in some severely psychopathological conditions. That is a far cry, however, from the systematic underemphasis on the importance of the conflict between libido and aggression at all levels of psychological development implicit in many dissidents' objections to Freud's dual drive theory.

Regarding the transference, the painful reality that unconscious negative dispositions from many sources are an important aspect of the unconscious relationship of the patient with the analyst, of the defensive object relations in the transference that we call "resistance," and of the technical challenges for the analyst, is another culturally supported source of denial. The stress on the "real" relationship between patient and analyst, not as a consequence of transference interpretation but as a precondition for transference analysis, has led to an ever-reemerging tendency to induce the patient's cooperation seductively with supportive interventions. The problematic trend in earlier ego psychological approaches to stress the "overcoming" of resistances, and the misinterpretation of their functions only more recently corrected in the work of Paul Gray and Fred Busch, also serve as rationalization for an "antiauthoritarian," implicitly supportive technical approach (Kernberg 2001).

Here I cannot resist the temptation to explore somewhat further the issue of resistance and the culturally influenced questioning of the technical implications of this concept in the service of denial of the importance of the aggressive components of negative transference developments. Resistances should be analyzed in terms of the functions of the corresponding object relationship in the transference. Many years ago, Hanna Segal (1964) defined defensive operations, stating that resistances and the impulses against which they had been erected reflect, respectively, object relations activated defensively to deal with object relations activated by impulse. In this connection, I believe that the contemporary stress on a "two-person psychology," on the mutual influences of transference and countertransference, tends to undermine the more subtle aspects of transference analysis represented by a "three-person psychology," the analyst being split into one part responding in the countertransference to the patient's transference and into another part reflecting on that very development. The analyst's analysis of his or her countertransference as a preliminary step to analyze the transference-countertransference bind tends to be flattened by the premature utilization of countertransference by either adjusting to the patient's assumed reaction to an assumed stance of the analyst or communicating the countertransference to the patient. Under these conditions, the analytic dialogue shifts excessively into an analysis of the present interpersonal situation, to the detriment of the exploration of the deeper layers of the patient's unconscious conflicts around aggression and eroticism.

My point is that various dissidents, in their global reaction to psychoanalytic theory and technique, have incorporated an identification with conventional cultural assumptions and that this identification is not necessarily related to any "unanalyzed" personal psychopathology. Such cultural adaptation may contribute to the development of dissident theories into a broad replacement of psychoanalytic theory in toto.

Perhaps the strangest dissidence in this regard is Lacan's (Benvenuto and Kennedy 1986; Clement 1983). Leaving aside the problematic nature of his personality, his mystifying style of communication, and the question to what extent he distorted some basic Freudian concepts while assuming that he was providing the most faithful clarification and development of Freud's thoughts, his most significant dissident approach was his complete neglect of transference analysis and of the actual transference-countertransference relationship. This attitude was reflected in the arbitrary shortening of the analytic session according to the analyst's assessment whether meaningful communication was coming from the patient. The assumption that "empty talk" warranted ending the session meant brushing aside the analysis of unconscious defenses and, in the process, returning to a truly "one-person psychology" (or rather, a "one-person psychology" being enacted simultaneously by two persons in the same room…). To this day, one of the most problematic aspects of Lacanian psychoanalysis is the lack of presentation of clinical data that characterizes the entire Lacanian literature. There is no doubt that there are important theoretical contributions stemming from Lacan, particularly his proposals regarding archaic oedipal developments, the transformation of a dyadic relationship marked by the imaginary into a triadic one represented by the symbolic and its relation to the oedipal situation. So, returning once more to Gitelson's phrase, I believe it does summarize impressively the nature of the attitude of major dissenters and "paradissenters" toward basic psychoanalytic theory and technique.

The Influence of Institutional Dynamics on the Development of Dissidence

Returning to Bergmann's (M.S. Bergmann, "Rethinking the Problem of Dissidence and Change in the History of Psychoanalysis," unpublished manuscript, 2001) comments on the influence of the personal relationship with Freud on the thinking of the early dissidents, obviously, those who had no direct relationship with Freud still evinced an intense conflictual attachment to his basic ideas. I believe that this apparent focus on Freud's thoughts may mask major institutional dynamics of psychoanalysis, in addition to the other causal factors of dissidence mentioned so far. Psychoanalytic institutions developed strongly authoritarian tendencies, perhaps culminating at the time of maximum cultural prominence and popularity of psychoanalysis in its major centers in London, the United States, Buenos Aires, Argentina, and Paris, France.

I have referred to this issue in earlier contributions (Kernberg 1992b, 2000a) and only wish to summarize here my main proposal—namely, that the carrying out of psychoanalytic treatment within an institutional context led to institutional structures intended to protect candidates and training analysts from massive acting out of transference and countertransference, but these structures in fact had some unfortunate effects. While psychoanalytic treatment was considered as a combination of a science and an art, it was taught within an institutional structure that resembled a combination of a religious seminary and a technical professional school. The dominant administrative distortion was the development of the training psychoanalysis system, with the concentration of all authority regarding teaching, supervising, analyzing, and administrative leadership in the hands of the training analysts. This created a privileged class and an underclass (the candidates), with chronic institutional aggression acted out in the form of transference splitting, idealization of some subgroups, and paranoid developments regarding other subgroups and outsiders.

An atmosphere of submission and rebelliousness, of monolithic theorizing and indoctrination, while professing a flexible analytic understanding became major characteristics of psychoanalytic institutions, particularly when their social prestige and influence assured the stability and legitimacy of their educational enterprise. Within this atmosphere, I believe, dissidence became an expression of rebelliousness against the status quo, affecting to various degrees both early and particularly later dissidents. The case of Karen Horney illustrates this problem and so, more dramatically, does the fascinating summary of Rycoff's withdrawal from the psychoanalytic institution that Bergmann (M.S. Bergmann, "Rethinking the Problem of Dissidence and Change in the History of Psychoanalysis," unpublished manuscript, 2001) provided in the addendum to his paper. I believe that it is not a coincidence that Kleinian and Kohutian groups developed in the United States within the most conservative ego psychological institutions, and, at times, these same analysts then shifted from a Kleinian commitment to a self psychology or intersubjective one.

The "controversial discussions" in Great Britain (King and Steiner 1991) that prevented a split between the groups of Melanie

Klein and Anna Freud may have unwittingly permitted the enormous development of psychoanalytic contributions of the British
Psychoanalytic Society in the 1940s through the 1960s, by assuring
an institutionalized tolerance of alternative ideas and implicit con-
frontations of those ideas in the context of evaluation of clinical material over time. Yet the fact that candidates trained by Kleinian
psychoanalysts remained Kleinian and candidates trained by analysts of the middle group and of Anna Freud's group remained
within those respective groups points to the enormous pressure of
institutionalized psychoanalytic ideology in distorting the psychoanalytic process and in determining the position of the student body
regarding their respective training analyst's allegiances.

Authoritarian pressures in institutes may brand innovators as
dangerous rebels and force potential "modifiers" into an oppositional stance. Institutional splits or the development of dissidence
can be the result if one of the mutually split groups represents of-
ficialdom and the other is expelled and declared "nonpsychoana-
lytic." This is what happened in 1949 with the group of Schultz-
Henke in Germany, expelled from the International Psychoanalytic
Association, not because of what many years later was assumed to
be related to their past contamination by Nazi influences but because of the rejection of the concept of the death drive by Schultz-
Henke and the determination of the International Psychoanalytic
Association at that point that this position was incompatible with
psychoanalytic theory. Little did the psychoanalytic community expect that large segments of it would reject the concept of a death
drive, particularly in the United States, 50 years later.

Institutional dynamics typically show up as conflicts between
groups that appear, on the surface, as conflicts between charismatic
individuals in leadership positions of these groups. Charismatic leadership undoubtedly helps to crystallize groups around the leader, but
the institutional dynamics leading to such mutually split-off groups,
described by Bion as the basic group assumption of "fight-flight," lie in
institutional dynamics. Fortunately, the psychoanalytic community
has painfully learned that the expulsion of individuals and groups because of differences in theory leads to dissidence and a potential
weakening of the psychoanalytic movement and that the containment
of theoretical differences may have a beneficial effect on psychoanalysis as a whole. This principle operated already in the controversial
discussions and later on in the capacity of the American Psychoanalytical Association and the International Psychoanalytic Association to
contain Kohut's self psychology—in spite of its rejection of basic psy-

choanalytic theories that earlier would have led to a split. I have recently been able to observe the surprising development of a strong and articulate "intersubjectivity" group in the Chilean Psychoanalytic Association that used to be rigidly Kleinian, a counterpart to the developments in Argentina, where the traditionally rigidly Kleinian Argentinean Psychoanalytic Association has experienced the development of a powerful Lacanian group.

I believe that a variety of controversial issues regarding psychoanalytic technique are influenced by these same institutional dynamics. The confusion of the concept of resistance as the clinical manifestation of defensive operations in the transference with opposition to the psychoanalytic treatment "that has to be overcome" outside as well as inside the consulting room seems to me a typical manifestation of an authoritarian influence of the psychoanalytic institution on psychoanalytic technique. The questioning of the authority of the psychoanalyst on the part of self psychology, the intersubjectivity, and relational approaches seems to me equally an effort to react to institutional authoritarian pressures by injecting a political, democratic ideology into the analytic process. As another example, the transformation of the concept of technical neutrality into the "anonymity" of the psychoanalyst proposed by both ego psychological and Kleinian schools in the 1950s and 1960s seems to me a direct consequence of the efforts to protect the untouchable training analysts from contamination with the candidates' social body rather than the alleged effort to protect the "purity" of the transference.

Implications for the Future of the Psychoanalytic Enterprise

It seems to me that if the factors I have referred to are indeed fundamental contributors to the development of dissidence within psychoanalytic institutions, and if we are willing to learn from our history in considering the future development of psychoanalysis, we do have some major tasks at this time. First, the development of scientific research in the broadest sense is an urgent task. It will include both the gradual development of psychoanalytic expertise through the analysis of the effects of alternative approaches to the clinical situation over time and empirical research, in the sense of setting up experimental designs by which alternative theories can be tested and the field developed in this context.

It is obvious that there are enormous difficulties in the objective study of the psychoanalytic process, but we are gradually advancing in our capacity to carry out such studies. There are methods from other sciences that we may appropriate in addition to the use of the psychoanalytic situation per se as our major investigation of the unconscious. The dogmatic affirmation that only psychoanalytic treatment permits us to learn more about the dynamic unconscious and to resolve questions about alternative theories and techniques has been used to protect our institutions against the strengthening of psychoanalytic research in the broadest sense, in addition to isolating us from the surrounding world of science.

Second, we must tolerate the development of alternative approaches in our midst, both theories and methods, and see it as our task to evaluate them systematically, not in order to absorb and integrate eclectically everything that comes along but to develop our understanding in depth of what is essential about the psychoanalytic process and needs to be reaffirmed in the face of new developments. What has been called the "age of pluralism" only means that we have multiple theories and approaches and not that all of them have to be accepted or integrated. They have to be used as challenges, as tests of our science, and they cannot be avoided, because they confront us with the influence of cross-cultural, ideological, and fundamental scientific discoveries occurring in fields at the boundary of psychoanalysis. The temptation to use neurobiological findings merely to affirm that "Freud was right all along" can be as destructive as the systematic ignorance of such findings. We have to be prepared to modify our theories and techniques in the light of controversies and not as an effort to politically accept a bland pluralistic eclecticism.

Strengthening our scientific enterprise implies fundamental changes in psychoanalytic education, the development of an authentically scientific atmosphere where faculty and students jointly study our field, openly recognize and articulate areas of uncertainty and ignorance, and discuss how we can proceed to obtain new knowledge. I am aware that every time this challenge is formulated, there is an immediate response of "We are doing all of this anyhow": and it usually takes a long time to show that this may not be so at all.

If the proposed dynamics regarding ideological crosscurrents and consistent conventional cultural assumptions are true, there may be some battles that have to be fought again and again: the pendulum switch between genetic and intrapsychic versus environmental and traumatic determinants of unconscious psychic conflicts also may have to be elaborated again and again. In earlier work (Kernberg 2001), I pointed to the present development of a mainstream of psychoanalytic technique that combines fundamental contributions from ego psychology, Kleinian psychoanalysis, the British Independents, and the French mainstream, while an alternative development has been the consolidation of a relational/intersubjective/self psychological approach. These developments may illustrate the extent to which Freud's basic discoveries regarding aggression, sexuality, and transference have to be worked through, again and again, in the process of the development of psychoanalytic knowledge.

Finally, one of the most astonishing blind spots in the development of psychoanalysis has been the neglect of the development of psychoanalytic psychotherapy for a broad spectrum of patients whose psychopathology does not respond to standard psychoanalytic treatment. The denial of this issue, on the one hand, and the development of significant breakthroughs in psychoanalytic psychotherapies, on the other, often outside the context of psychoanalytic institutions, is a major paradox. Veikko Tähkä's book *Mind and Its Treatment* (1993) provides a helpful overview of these new developments. This paradox reflects, I believe, the ongoing insecurity of psychoanalysis regarding the survival of its science and, therefore, the need to protect the mythical "identity" of psychoanalysis, on the one hand, and a self-destructive avoidance of full integration of some of the most important contributions of psychoanalysis to the field of psychotherapy, on the other. We may be at the beginning of the breakdown of this denial, and of the awareness that a broad spectrum of psychoanalytically derived techniques can be explored, applied, and scientifically evaluated, strengthening the contributions of psychoanalysis to society. The development of independent societies of psychoanalytic psychotherapy functioning in parallel and even in competition with psychoanalytic societies is one form of unrecognized institutional dissidence that has been very damaging to psychoanalysis and needs to be overcome. This is the subject of future work.

References

Benjamin J: The alienation of desire: women's masochism and ideal love, in Psychoanalysis and Women: Contemporary Reappraisals. Edited by Alpert JL. Hillsdale, NJ, Erlbaum, 1986, pp 113–138

Benvenuto B, Kennedy R: The Works of Jacques Lacan: An Introduction. London, Free Association Books, 1986

Bergmann MS: The Hartmann Era. New York, Other Press, 2000

Blum HP: Masochism, the ego ideal, and the psychology of women. J Am Psychoanal Assoc 24:157–191, 1976

Chasseguet-Smirgel J, Grunberger B: L'Univers contestationnaire. Paris, Petite Bibliothèque Payot, 1969

Clement C: The Lives and Legends of Jacques Lacan. New York, Columbia University Press, 1983

Ferenczi S: Confusion of tongues between adult and child. Int J Psychoanal 30:225–230, 1949

Fromm E: Escape From Freedom. New York, Farrar & Rinehart, 1941

Horney K: Feminine Psychology. London, Routledge & Kegan Paul, 1967

Kernberg OF: Aggression in Personality Disorders and Perversions. New Haven, CT, Yale University Press, 1992a

Kernberg OF: Authoritarianism, culture, and personality in psychoanalytic education. Journal of the International Association for the History of Psychoanalysis 5:341–354, 1992b

Kernberg OF: A concerned critique of psychoanalytic education. Int J Psychoanal 81:97–120, 2000a

Kernberg OF: Psychoanalytic perspectives on the religious experience. Am J Psychother 54:452–476, 2000b

Kernberg OF: Recent developments in the technical approaches of English-language psychoanalytic schools. Psychoanal Q 70:519–547, 2001

Kernberg OF: Divergent contemporary trends in psychoanalytic theory. Psychoanal Rev (in press, 2011)

King P, Steiner R (eds): The Freud-Klein Controversies, 1941–1945. London, Tavistock/Routledge, 1991

McGuire W (ed): The Freud/Jung Letters: The Correspondence Between Sigmund Freud and C.G. Jung. Bollingen Series XCIV. Translated by Manheim R and Hull RFC. Princeton, NJ, Princeton University Press, 1974

Segal H: Introduction to the Work of Melanie Klein. New York, Basic Books, 1964

Tähkä V: Mind and Its Treatment: A Psychoanalytic Approach. Madison, CT, International Universities Press, 1993

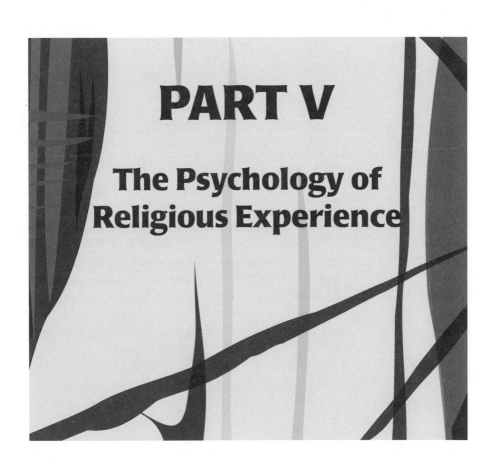

PART V

The Psychology of Religious Experience

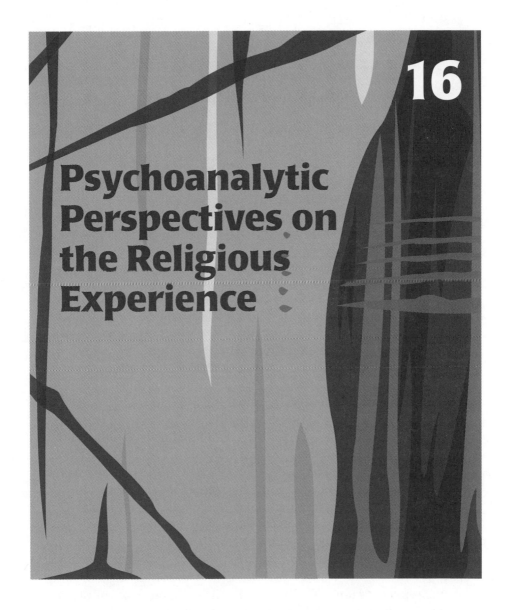

Psychoanalytic Perspectives on the Religious Experience

Presented at a conference on "Psychoanalysis and Religion," of the Main-zen Psychoanalytische Arbeitsgemeinschaft, Mainz, Germany, July 11, 1998. This chapter was reprinted from Kernberg OF: "Psychoanalytic Per-spectives on the Religious Experience." *American Journal of Psychother-apy* 54:452–476, 2000. Used with permission.

In this chapter, I explore the origins of the drive toward the establishment and security of an integrated system of ethical values as an essential aspect of the personality and its relation to the religious experience. This moves the focus of this volume from the individual pathology of nonintegrated love and hate to the expression of this antinomy at the level of social and cultural expression of the relevant conflicts and explores the crucial function of the religious experience to deal with them. In the process, I review the significant changes that psychoanalytic theory has undergone in its relation to religion.

A Critical Review of Freud's Position

Historically, psychoanalysis has been widely perceived as implicitly questioning religious values and organized religious systems, primarily because of Freud's (1927/1961) critical writing about religion. In spite of the contributions of a distinguished group of psychoanalysts (Chasseguet-Smirgel [1973], Meissner [1984], Ostow [1982], Rizzuto [1979], Zilboorg [1958], and others) whose writings pointed to the compatibility of religious convictions and the psychoanalytic identity, I believe it is fair to state that a tendency toward an atheistic philosophical position has prevailed among many leading psychoanalysts and that this cultural tradition has only recently changed. In what follows, I shall summarize my own views regarding this issue, basing myself upon strictly psychoanalytic considerations regarding individual development and psychopathology, and the application of psychoanalytic understanding to mass psychology and the formation of ideologies.

In "The Future of an Illusion" (1927/1961), Freud spelled out his critical view of religion and his expectation that, in the long run, a rational system of moral convictions and rationally based ethics would replace organized religions. He drew a picture of cultural requirements and expectations characteristic of humankind, centered on the need to understand and control nature, with the related gratification of human needs. He also suggested that a major challenge of culture was the regulation of interpersonal relationships and the distribution of the produce of human labor. Freud considered that these cultural aspirations were challenged by the animosity toward culture derived, within the individual, from the drives—both sexuality and the destructive aspects of aggression, from mass psychology, and from the limitations of the educability of the human being.

He proposed that culture relies on the obligation to work and to renounce acting upon the derivatives of the drives, particularly in the
form of incest, cannibalism, and violence.

Freud proposed that the superego reflects the internalization of
the external demands posed by culture, controlling by means of its
prohibitions the discontent of disadvantaged social classes and providing narcissistic and substitute gratifications through the positive
influence of ideals and artistic creativity. He proposed that religious
imagination contributed to achieving the overall cultural objective
of civilizing interpersonal relationships by reinforcing prohibitions
against drive-derived behavior and interpersonal aggression, while
providing consolation regarding the uncertainties of human destiny
and explaining the apparent indifference of nature by humanizing
it. Animism as a primitive religion reflected that humanization,
while infantile dependency on the parents and longings for their
protection were projected into the longing for the protection by an
all-powerful God. Thus, the functions of polytheism and, later,
monotheism, Freud went on, were to control the frightening aspects of nature, to control the cruelty of human destiny and death,
and to enforce cultural restrictions.

Freud suggested that insofar as science has reduced the sense
of impotence in the face of the uncontrollable cruelty of nature,
destiny, and death, religious beliefs have focused more and more
on the imposition of cultural demands. In essence, God dominates
nature, even death; God will reward what is good, punish evil, and
control destiny; God determines the fundamental laws of culture.
Freud proposed that the unitary character of God reflects the paternal principle, protects against the dominating power of nature,
and legitimizes the limitations imposed by culture.

Freud traced the history of religion to totemism as the beginning of belief in a protective deity, embodied in a sacred animal that
could not be hunted as ordinary prey. The ritual killing and eating
of the totem symbolically reflected the murder of the father and the
appropriation of his power. The transformation of animal gods into
multiple human-faced gods evolved toward the monotheistic concept, while the unique God reflected the ultimate protection of the
helpless child against nature and the fulfillment of his or her longing for an omnipotent, protective father. The ambivalence toward
father, Freud proposed, was reflected in the combination of idealization and fear of God.

Freud referred to the demands of religious dogma of faith that
cannot be justified scientifically, faith based in the tradition of the

fathers, the proofs of tradition, and the prohibitions against doubt. Religious dogmas, he proposed, are illusions in the sense of not being open to demonstration or to refutation. They correspond to childlike wishes, the projection of infantile demands and prohibitions. Yet Freud conceded, all universal concepts (Weltanschauungen) are illusions. Furthermore, without religion, the human being confronted with death and required to submit to cultural demands would be overwhelmed by his or her own helplessness and frustration. Freud suggested that science reduces the territory of religion but that the likelihood persists that culture can only be protected by the strict suppression and threats of punishment that organized religion provides. But religion had to tolerate "sin" in order to be tolerable.

Freud believed that the commandment "not to kill" is a rational prohibition. It should be possible to abandon the idea of God, he felt, and put culture on a rational basis of expectations and prohibitions. Yet, he went on, passion is stronger than reason, and inasmuch as murder of the father was the origin of all prohibitions, cultural prohibitions are thus derived from the original Father and his Godliness. Only through the affectively imposed superego prohibitions can the drives be suppressed, and, in this regard, religion is analogous to an obsessive neurosis.

Freud stated that intelligence offers an alternative to religion as a means to control the expression of instinctual demands. He granted that many people are not able to achieve that but believed that science will help us. It is at this point that Freud made his famous statement "the voice of intellect is soft, but it doesn't rest until it has been listened to." He believed that intelligence fosters the love of other human beings and that science, developing constantly through trial and error, actualizes the sublimated wish to reduce suffering, and science is no illusion.

In summary, Freud saw the historical development of religion as beginning in the original conflicts around the murder of the father of the primitive horde, with totemism as the precursor of polytheism and monotheism as the highest form of religion. He saw the embrace of religions as a human disposition resulting from infantile helplessness, longing for the father, and the projection of the infantile superego. Freud acknowledged that rationality is undermined by sexual and aggressive drives, by the dangers derived from mass psychology, and by the challenges from suppressed social classes. And he granted that organized religion has had a powerful influence upon the flourishing of learning and artistic expression.

What seems to me most striking in this analysis, reexamined in the light of the experience of the twentieth century, is Freud's expression of faith in the triumph of rationality and his conviction that a universal system of morality can develop out of rational considerations and in the light of our rapidly developing scientific knowledge. This is striking, because Freud himself, in his work on religion (Freud 1927/1961) as well as throughout the entire body of his developing formulations, stressed the unavoidable infiltration of consciousness and rationality by unconscious motivation, particularly the primitive aspects of unconscious aggression. He himself, throughout the late developments of his theoretical formulations, was forced to conceptualize the death drive—the profound destructiveness and self-destructiveness of human beings—as an instinctual force as powerful as libido (Freud 1920/1955).

In addition, his acknowledging the unavoidable nature of the conflict between suppressed or disadvantaged social groups and those in power, and the dangers derived from mass psychology that he himself had so dramatically formulated, is in direct contradiction to his—one might almost say, irrational—faith in the assured final triumph of rationality. Also, what he describes as the psychological origin and development of religiosity as a fundamental human tendency speaks to the profound nature of religious convictions as an essential part of human beings, but it does not deal with the objective nature of the existence of God or the validity of religious systems in general. Here, I believe, psychoanalysis touches its boundaries with philosophy and enters the danger zone of becoming a weltanschauung in itself, running counter to the scientific spirit of psychoanalytic exploration.

Freud's assumption of the possibility of creating a universal system of ethical values on the basis of rational considerations would seem questionable not only on the basis of his own convincing findings regarding the unavoidable infiltration of rational thinking by unconscious motivation but also, on a vast social, political, and cultural level, on the basis of the experience of the twentieth century. As François Furet (1999) has convincingly pointed out, this century has been under the shadow of two major competing ideological systems that pretended to develop a rational, universal basis of morality rooted in the "scientific" analysis of historical developments in modern Western society. Nationalistic fascism and Marxist communism developed systematic and universal ethical systems supposedly based on a rational analysis of contemporary society. Both, in their purest and unrestricted forms dominating modern nations, led to the most horrendous crimes and mass murder in the history of humanity. The "rational moralities" of Naziism and communism co-opted science, without which the scope of their depredations would have been seriously curtailed.

The Holocaust in Nazi Germany, the Reign of Terror in the Gulag in the Soviet Union, and the Cultural Revolution in China illustrate the practical failure of "scientific" rationality, reconfirming sadly, in contemporary history, Freud's cautionary statements regarding the universality of the death drive and the dangers of mass psychology. Freud, almost as an aside, granted the autonomous existence of art and artistic values as values that were independent from rationality and science. In what follows, I will argue for the need to grant an equally independent existence to the potentiality of a universal system of values not subordinated to reason and science.

The Nature of Evil and the Psychology of Religiosity: Some Psychoanalytic Contributions

Freud (1920/1955) reached the conclusion that basic human motivation was constituted by libido or the life drive and thanatos or the death drive. He reached this conclusion on the basis of his systematic exploration of unconscious motivation in his experiences with patients, the growing database of psychoanalytic exploration in general, and also his application of psychoanalytic theory to the study of social and cultural phenomena. The overwhelming evidence pointing to destructive tendencies not only as part of psychopathology but also as a potential in all human beings and, at the same time, a potential for activation in mass movements and mass psychology in general lent conviction to these fundamental assumptions in Freud's formulations.

One dramatic source of evidence is the prevalence of social violence; that is, the emergence of violent behavior as a mass phenomenon under certain socioeconomic, political, or ideological conditions. I am explicitly excluding here "ordinary" belligerent behaviors as an expression of warfare, in which the combination of nationally mandated participation in the armed forces; the actual presence of armed, belligerent opponents; and a nationalistic ideological superstructure foster and tolerate violence on a large scale.

I am suggesting that social sanction of the massive killings of civilians and of the torture and persecution of minorities reflects the operation of the death drive as currently formulated by André Green (1993), that is, a fundamentally destructive and self-destructive drive directed against the establishment and maintenance of object relations. I propose that this fundamental destructiveness operates in groups, institutions, and social and national conflicts and that, without ignoring the specific historical, political, economic, social, and cultural origins of intergroup violence, psychoanalysis may contribute to the response to the basic question: What explains the sudden shift of massive human behavior from ordinary civilized interaction and respect for human life to massively expressed and sanctioned social violence? I have already referred to the dramatic and frightening evidence of social violence as a major fact of the past century. From the Gulag, the mass starvation of peasants, and the terror in the former Soviet Union to the extermination of the Jews by Nazi Germany; from the terror of the Cultural Revolution in Communist China to the mass killings of the Pol Pot regime; and from the murderous oppression of minorities in the Middle East and Africa to military dictatorships in South America and the savage fighting in the Balkans at the end of the last century, there is more than ample evidence of the universality of the phenomenon, although one could argue that the most extreme manifestations of it are reserved for ideologically totalitarian regimes in contrast to the more restricted violence of ordinary military dictatorships (Furet 1999).

Some focused sociological observations and experiments provide more direct evidence of the sudden shift in behavior of ordinary human beings when mass psychology is activated. Bette Bao Lord (1990) describes how, reflecting back on the Cultural Revolution, a history professor confessed to her his own regressive violence during that time. He had been a young student of a professor who had been branded as counterrevolutionary by the Red Guards and was subjected to public humiliation and beating by the entire group of his former students. He described how, standing in the circle surrounding his former professor, he realized that his fellow students could identify him with the counterrevolutionary behavior of his formerly admired and beloved teacher and found himself participating in the savage beating of his professor, in a frenzy that he was unable to reflect on until many years later.

Henry Dicks's (1972) study of 28 German SS concentration camp guards, serving prison terms in Great Britain for torturing and killing concentration camp inmates, revealed ordinary, severe, but not violent narcissistic personalities in most of them and a common background of ideological indoctrination and training "on the job." These criminals had reverted to rather bland and nonaggressive behavior, once in British jails. Victor Klemperer's (1995a, 1995b) diaries are perhaps the most lucid documentation we have of the massive social regression toward a tolerant indifference to, if not active engagement in, the gradual dehumanization of Jews in Germany as preliminary to their mass murder; and Wolfgang Sofsky (1993) has described the machinery of the concentration camps involving tens of thousands of functionaries fully aware of the nature of that terror. Zinoviev (1984), in his sociological analysis of mass corruption as an essential consequence of the socialist ideology and dictatorial system of the Soviet Union, has described the essential logic and overwhelming dominance of socially sanctioned dishonesty as a culturally accepted principle of coexistence. The Milgram (1974) experiments showed how intelligent, culturally privileged university students could be induced to participate in experiments of slow torture under the guise of scientific objectivity.

There are specific developments in the psychoanalytic research on mass psychology and group psychology that point to the universal tendency to react with an upsurge of generally shared intense rage and hatred in certain regressive group situations.

Freud, in his study of "Group Psychology and the Analysis of the Ego" (1921/1955), described the mutual identification of all the members of the mass movement in their idealization of the leader, the shared projection of their superego onto the leader, and the resulting sense of freedom, power, and lust for destructive aggression that characterizes the mass movement or the mob. This activation of unbridled aggression when a mob or a mass movement has crystallized has been studied further in the analysis of small unstructured groups carried out by Wilfred Bion (1961). He demonstrated that when the task orientation of a group breaks down, there is an immediate regression into one of three "basic assumption groups," namely, the assumption of "dependency," "fight-flight," or "pairing."

In the basic assumption group of "dependency," the group tends to idealize a grandiose, self-assured leader, the dependency on whom gives them a sense of security and gratification, while all the members feel incompetent and unskilled without the protection of such an idealized leader. Not surprisingly, individuals with strong narcissistic features tend to be induced to assume the leadership role by such groups. When, conversely, the group regresses to the fight-flight basic assumption, mutual distrust, suspiciousness, competition for power, and dominance emerge. The group may either unite in a fighting spirit against an out-group or subdivide into an in-group and an out-group. Leadership falls on the most paranoid individual of the group, well disposed to lead them in a fight against real or assumed enemies. Finally, in the basic assumption group of "pairing," there is a tendency of the small group to turn to a couple, heterosexual or homosexual, in the hope that their developing relationship will infuse the group with a sense of meaning and excitement and thus assure its future.

The psychoanalytic understanding of these group developments is that the "choice" of a basic assumption is based on the depth of the group's regression, which in turn is likely determined by the severity of the trauma involved in the initial loss of the group's functioning as a task group. Thus, the pairing group, with its emphasis on sexuality and relatedness, represents a defense against the more primitive dependent and fight-flight groups, in which the idealization of the narcissistic leader of the dependency group is a defense against the still more threatening regression into the fight-flight group led by a paranoid leader. The general implication is that a potential exists in all individuals functioning within a small group to regress in one of these ways if and when ordinary task structures or work orientedness breaks down.

Pierre Turquet (1975) studied the behavior of unstructured large groups of 50–150 individuals. He demonstrated that such a large group, when it has no task other than to observe its own behavior, generates extreme anxiety and rapidly regresses into a state of diffuse fear of aggression, in which nobody listens to anybody else, efforts to form subgroups to defend against the fear of imminent outbreak of aggression are ineffectual, and aggression readily breaks out among the subgroups. "Innocent bystanders" develop within the large majority, and there is a general, resolute rejection of any rational leadership that might start to emerge. The large group only tolerates the leadership of a narcissistic individual—who, *au fond,* is despised by everybody although his or her cliché-ridden conventionality has a soothing effect on the group— or else they select a paranoid leader who transforms the chaotic large group into Freud's mob.

I have suggested in earlier work (Kernberg 1998) that the large group constitutes, in effect, the basic situation against which the development of mob and mass psychology, on the one hand, as well as small group psychology, on the other, are defensive operations. In other words, in unstructured group situations, in which ordinary status-role relationships become inoperant, there is an immediate upsurge of fear of aggression that reflects the massive projection of aggressive tendencies on the part of all involved and against which the development of a narcissistic or a paranoid orientation is a defensive structure. The ultimate explanation of these developments is that under such "groupish" situations, the ordinary disposition to relate to dyadic and triadic family and social situations breaks down. The individual now experiences himself or herself as surrounded by multiple others with whom he or she is related in an uncertain way, a situation that reproduces the intrapsychic condition before the development of what ego psychology refers to as object constancy. The multiplicity of external objects reproduces the multiplicity of primitive, split part-object representations and the need to sort them out into "all good" and "all bad" internal objects. This immediate reproduction under regressive social situations of a very early developmental stage of individual development leads us to the contributions of psychoanalytic object relations theory. In Kleinian psychoanalytic psychology, this state is described as the "paranoid-schizoid" position. Because Kleinian object relations theory offers an explanation of both the evolution of the capacity for love and affiliation and the proclivity to regress to suspiciousness, hatred, and violence under certain conditions, I shall lay out the basic principles of object relations theory.

Psychoanalytic object relations theory accounts, in effect, for the origin of love and hate, the core emotions, respectively, of libido and the death drive. Psychoanalytic object relations theory assumes that the earliest relationship of the infant to his or her mother consists of moments when affects are rather low key and ordinary learning takes place and other moments when affects are intense or extreme and hence result in the internalization of affective memory structures, constituted by the representation of self relating to the representation of mother under the dominance of the peak affect. In short, peak affects are structured into internalized object relations, which constitute the "building blocks" of the psychic structures that culminate in the ego, superego, and id in Freud's formulations.

A fundamental contribution of Melanie Klein (1940, 1946) was her proposal that in infancy a split is maintained between the internalized object relations that are under the affective dominance of aggression and frustration and those that are dominated by elation and sensual stimulation, in order to preserve the illusory purity of ideal relationships between infant and mother, and to protect the infant from the terror of the paranoid fantasies connected with internalized object relations controlled by rage and hate. These splitting operations and their related defense mechanisms determine for the infant, Melanie Klein suggested, an unconscious world of multiple ideal self-representations interacting with ideal object representations, sharply split off from the multiple "bad" self-representations interacting with their "bad" objects. This state of internal affairs characterizes what Melanie Klein called the paranoid-schizoid position. Throughout the first year of life, the overcoming of that splitting under the influence of predominantly benign, pleasurable, and loving interactions together with ongoing cognitive development leads to the integration of idealized and persecutory aspects of the self and its objects, an integration that significantly strengthens and is strengthened by the cognitive potential for self-reflection and for realistic perception of external reality. This internal integration is what Melanie Klein referred to as the depressive position.

The depressive position, with its appreciation of the mother who frustrates as identical with the one who gives pleasure, permits the infant to internalize those aspects of the parents that imply demands and prohibitions. The acceptance of frustration in the realization that it is a price to pay for love and security thus originates the early superego. Under conditions of severe traumatization and sadistic and persecutory parental demands, a pathological superego may be constituted, with sadistic demands for perfection. Such a superego may turn a significant part of aggression against the self, leading to depreciation and impoverishment of the self that resonate with impoverishment of the self-experience in the face of subsequent separation and object loss. An intolerable, excessively sadistic primitive superego mostly reprojected onto the environment may lead to weakness or absence of superego functions, paranoid suspiciousness and hypersensitivity, and uninhibited expressions of aggression. Under favorable conditions, however, the superego evolves into an organization of internalized ethical and moral values, with aggressive responses mitigated by the sophisticated affects of guilt and concern.

What interests us here is that in these early processes of integration of affect dispositions and internalized object relations, profoundly significant developments occur that will constitute both the origin of religiosity and the manifestations of what under a worst-case scenario will constitute the most severe disposition to hatred, destruction, and self-destruction. When intensely frustrating, rageful interactions prevail in the life of the infant and young child, the corresponding internalized object relations tend to fixate the disposition of the individual toward rageful destruction of perceived enemies. Hatred develops as a structured object relation under the dominance of chronic rage and the resultant wishes to destroy, control, and make suffer a potentially threatening object. Both a constitutional disposition to excessive rage reactions and severe traumatization in early childhood contribute to the dominance of such a disposition to hatred.

When frustration and hatred are dominant, splitting between idealized and persecutory relations tends to persist, with the typical manifestations of either a protective self-aggrandizement and devaluation of others—narcissistic defenses—or a tendency to project aggression with a suspicious, fearful, and controlling attitude to the environment—paranoid defenses. When sufficiently severe, these tendencies give rise to the corresponding narcissistic and paranoid personality disorders.

In contrast, when the integration between the idealized and persecutory self- and object representations is successful, a tolerance for both good and bad aspects of self and others evolves, with a corresponding deepening of the relationship to the parental figures and a capacity for more realistic self-evaluation and for concern and guilt over one's own aggression. Now emerge wishes for reparation and, along with tolerance for ambivalence, the desire to restore an ideal relationship that leads to the wish to live up to internalized demands and prohibitions, to obtain a sense of security and well-being by being at peace with one's own superego and ego ideal.

To the extent that the early relationship with mother is primarily infused with euphoria and joyous sensuality, the associated feelings of love and a wish for fusion with mother give rise to dispositions to empathy, dependency, and a sense of union, even at a distance, that facilitate the experience of oneness with the world, a sense of transcendence.

Gratitude for love received, as well as the capacity for guilt feelings over one's own aggression, and the wish to repair damage done constitute the origins of sublimation, of the emotional experience of sinfulness and desire for expiation, and mourning as a capacity to miss and long for a lost good object. This constellation defines Klein's depressive position. While contemporary psychoan-

alytic thinking no longer assumes an early symbiotic stage of development in which self and objects are consistently fused or not
yet differentiated, there do apparently exist states of early fusion
under the impact of peak affect states (both of love and of hatred).
The peak affect state of love gives rise to a profound capacity for
empathy, compassion, and mercifulness and also, as Rayner (1994)
has proposed, to a fundamental sense of justice in terms of the expectation of reciprocity of love and fairness in mutual treatment.

In contrast, lack of achievement of the depressive position and
the predominance of object relations infused with rage and hatred
establish the potential for severe distortions and destructiveness in
all object relations. In the antisocial personality proper, this takes
the form of a tendency to destroy all relationships with significant
others. In narcissistic personalities, one can observe chronic sadistic pleasure in making others suffer, along with inordinate envy.
Such envy may lead to the unconscious destruction not only of what
is experienced as bad or dangerous but also of what is experienced
as good and desirable in other persons, so that the extremely envious person has to destroy what he or she so desperately longs for
(Klein 1957). Clinically, we call "perversity" a clinical syndrome in
which the afflicted patient tries to extract love from others in order
to destroy that love and the person who gives it.

Winnicott (1965), who first described the capacity for concern
as a consequence of the achievement of the depressive position,
also described how, at an early stage of development, the infant
tends to find a "transitional object"; that is, a belonging such as a
blanket or a toy that is felt to be both part of the self and not part of
the self. The transitional object represents the significant other and
yet is totally under the control of the infant, an object that can be
cuddled and attacked and that survives, that is always there, part
of reality and part of fantasy. It expresses the infant's capacity for
object investment and, at the same time, for building up a world
of fantasy reflecting the internalization of that good object. This
illusional transitional world, Winnicott proposed, is the origin of
creative fantasy, of culture, art, and religion as a combination of
fantasy structures and objectively created external reality. Winnicott thus traces the very origin of the drive for the production of cultural values, in the areas of both art and religion, to a basic human
tendency active since infancy.

Edith Jacobson (1964), who has developed the most elaborate
theory of the organization of the superego, has described successive layers of the superego from a most primitive, negative, fantas-

tically forbidding, and punishing layer; to a later idealized layer of demands reflecting those of the idealized parental images; to the more realistic superego of the oedipal period, in which the first two layers merge and thus reduce the extreme nature of primitive internalized morality. These developments open up the child to the internalization of more realistic demands and prohibitions throughout childhood, eventually leading to processes of deperson-ification, abstraction, and individuation of the mature superego, that integrates the ethical value systems of the individual reaching from deep unconscious levels to preconscious and conscious guide-lines of moral behavior.

The understanding of the psychopathology of the superego when normal development fails has facilitated our understanding of the frightening psychopathology of the antisocial personality dis-order, an extreme form of psychopathology in which there is no ca-pacity for feelings of guilt and concern and no capacity for the "milk of human kindness," and unmitigated hatred reigns in the form of aggressive or exploitive destructiveness.

Bion (1970) enriched our understanding of the basic structures of the normal superego by pointing to three mutually incompatible "vertices" that express libido and orient human behavior and rela-tionship to reality: they are 1) the epistemological vertex, leading to knowledge and to defining and acquiring truth; 2) the aesthetic vertex, leading to the search for beauty; and 3) the ethical vertex, the drive toward what is good and toward ethical value systems. He pointed to the mutually irreducible nature of these vertices, in the sense that none of them can be subsumed under the other two. The vertex of ethics, in turn, is linked to the search for love and intimate relations with others, opposed to the destructive nature of primitive hatred, the expression of thanatos, that constitutes the counterpart of all three of these vertices. The death drive operates against lov-ing relationships, against the recognition and acceptance of truth, and against the acquisition of knowledge in general and, of course, against normal morality reflecting ethical systems.

In this connection, Bion described three types of basic object re-lationships: "symbiotic," "commensal," and "parasitic." Symbiotic relationships are geared to produce growth and development of something new in the relationship and expressed by creativity; commensal relationships are simply surface contacts without any deeper development of anything new; and parasitic relationships are geared to bring about mutual destruction. Donald Meltzer (1988), in exploring related issues, described the "aesthetic conflict" as the conflict between, on the one hand, loving and implicitly erotic impulses of the baby toward mother, expressed in the idealization of the surface of mother's body and leading to the capacity for a sense of beauty; and on the other, the projection of aggression into the interior of mother's body, leading to the fear of the interior of her body and derived hypochondriacal fears of bodily destruction. The predominance of love in the mother-infant relationship fosters the development of the depressive position, with its consequences for superego development referred to before, in contrast to the predominance of hatred, which may corrupt and destroy love, as in the syndrome of perversity already mentioned.

From a different perspective, Ronald Fairbairn (1954) described the "moral defense" as a basic psychological tendency to transform aggressive demands and punishment from the parents into acceptable internalized demands, out of the profound need to make sense of the world and to develop an internalized guidance system to deal with it. He explained the excessive severity of the superego in patients subjected to extremely traumatic experiences as the internalization of sadistic parental behavior into the superego because "it is preferable to live in a world of a cruel God than in the world of the unpredictable devil."

In my own research on the unconscious relationship of the couple in love (Kernberg 1995), I have suggested the simultaneous development of three levels of relationship of the couple: the sexual, the object relational, and the ego ideal levels. I have proposed that the projection of the mature aspects of the ego ideal onto the beloved other transforms an internal value system into an external, embodied, ideal other, thus transforming external reality into the realization of an intrapsychic longing, as an important aspect of the experience of transcendence. Love thus includes both an "illusion" and a "reality." My considerations were based on the systematic studies of the ego ideal by Chasseguet-Smirgel (1973, 1984), who has contributed, perhaps more than anybody else, to reexamining the relationship between psychoanalysis and religion. She pointed to the real existence of evil and the function of religion to control evil by the establishment of boundaries and the law.

Chasseguet-Smirgel, in her fundamental book *Creativity and Perversion* (1984), described the "perverse solution" to experiences in infancy and childhood that greatly intensify the traumatic effects of the crucial challenges faced by all children. Starting from the oedipal situation as a universal human conflict, she pointed first to the narcissistic trauma of the exclusion of the infant and child from the intimate relations of the parents and the humiliation of being unable to compete with the parent of the same gender for the parent of the other gender. This trauma is reinforced by the universal seductiveness derived from the unconscious erotic currents linking the infant to the parent of the opposite gender and by castration anxiety as the most primitive form of unconsciously feared punishment for the oedipal wishes involving incest and murder. The inordinate intensification of these traumas in cases of severe pathological development lead, Chasseguet-Smirgel suggested, to the "perverse solution," which takes the form of defensive denial of the differences between the genders in order to deny castration anxiety, denial of differences of age in order to make incest permissible, and denial of the privileged functions of the genitalia. These defensive distortions render all aspects of the body equal: there are no differences of age, gender, and organs. This universal equivalence destroys all law and order, facilitates the dominance of aggression in condensation with sexuality, and initiates the "anal" transformation of object relations—in the sense that the relations with an object acquire a completely undifferentiated, devalued, and expulsive characteristic.

Chasseguet-Smirgel describes the world of de Sade as characteristic of this state of affairs: the dominance of polymorphous perverse infantile sexuality suffused by aggression and coinciding with the denial of law and order as well as of God and religion. Religious and sexual ecstasies are condensed under the dominant affect of aggression, with idealization of the destructive rupture of all boundaries. Perversion, Chasseguet-Smirgel concludes, is a re-creation of a primitive chaos, within which anal relationships of dominance, expulsion, and soiling replace normal relations. These patients who have found the "perverse solution" to childhood trauma present a denial of reality and an idealization of anality in terms of a pseudoaesthetic attitude that hides a profound tendency to treat all relationships as excrement.

Chasseguet-Smirgel points to the reality of the existence of evil as represented by this perverse tendency to re-create a primitive chaos; religious commands and prohibitions constitute a universal, intuitive reaction against, and protection from, such chaos. She analyzes the Ten Commandments in terms of their underlying structure that requires respect for the authority of God, demands respect for older generations, and forbids incest, murder, and the destructive invasion of other people's rights and property. The Ten Commandments and related and derived commands and prohibitions, such as those made explicit in Leviticus 18–20, represent a fundamental moral law directed against the dominance and triumph of evil. Chasseguet-Smirgel concludes that religion constitutes a fundamental recognition of, and radical opposition to, the nature of evil and perversion as its psychopathological representation.

André Green (1990, 1993) has expanded upon Chasseguet-Smirgel's contributions on the nature of evil, pointing to the profound influence of the death drive on psychic functioning at all levels. On the basis of the exploration of the most severe forms of destructiveness and self-destructiveness in individual patients, and in society and culture, he proposes that the essential characteristic of the death drive is that of "deobjectification"; that is, a radical destruction of all object relations, in contrast to the "objectifying" function of libido, reflected in the drive to establish, maintain, and deepen object relations; to give and receive love; and to express creativity in the context of gratifying object relations. Green (1993) described the thrust of evil as the expression of the death drive, as implying that everything that exists is without meaning; evil obeys no order or law, has no objective, and seeks only to achieve one's will and obtain one's object of appetite by the exertion of power. Evil has no reason. In a fundamental development of our contemporary understanding of the death drive, Green, in his book *Le travail du négatif* (1993), described radical destruction of the need for significant relationships with others as a manifestation of the death drive. This is much more severe than sadomasochistic relationships with objects that indicate at least some fusion between libidinal and aggressive strivings.

In summary, recent psychoanalytic studies have contributed significantly to our understanding of religiosity with all its components of compassion, concern, guilt, reparation, a solid system of ethical principles as an indication of normal superego development, and the dominance of love and commitment, in contrast to the characteristics of evil reflecting the most severe manifestations and derivatives of the death drive. The fact that evil operates as a basic component of group regression and mass psychology as well as an aspect of individual psychopathology points to the unavoidable, overarching nature of the threat of evil as part of human destiny. One particularly severe manifestation of evil is the interlocking quality of the manifestations of severe psychopathology in leadership, on the one hand, and the regression of group processes and mass movements under the influence of sociopolitical conditions, on the other.

The Relationship Between Individual Psychopathology, Group Regression, and Sociocultural Developments

The two paradigmatic personality disorders that reflect, respectively, the idealizing and the persecutory "all good" and "all bad" aspects of earliest experience are the narcissistic and the paranoid personality disorders. In the narcissistic personality disorder, as a defense against threatening activation of the split-off paranoid experience, a defensive self-idealization takes place, in which a pathological grandiose self "absorbs" the characteristics of the idealized objects and thus wards off the threat of dependency and need of others. This self-idealization shows in the patients' grandiosity, self-centeredness, overdependence on admiration, devaluation and greedy exploitation of others, lack of empathy, and difficulties in commitment. Conscious and unconscious envy reflect the underlying unconscious hatred against which narcissistic grandiosity, aloofness, and exploitiveness are defenses as well as being their indirect expression. These patients need to be admired in order to protect their self-esteem, and they are powerfully motivated to occupy positions of power and potential admiration. We have already found them as the natural leaders of the small group assumption of "dependency" and the large group attempting to protect itself against the upsurge of aggression.

The paranoid personality disorder, rather than being a defense against the nonintegrated early paranoid experience, may be considered its prototype. These patients' intense hostility tends to be projected onto others, determining intense suspiciousness, distrust, hyperalertness, and "righteous indignation" when some rationale can be found to justify the attack on assumed or real enemies. This is the typical leader of the "fight-flight" group and of the mass movement or mob as an alternative organization to the large group. Paranoid personalities—similarly to narcissistic personalities—thus also emerge as natural leaders in certain regressive group situations.

In addition, a particularly severe personality disorder is constituted by the syndrome of malignant narcissism, in which narcissistic and paranoid features are combined and condensed (Kernberg 1992). Here the patients' grandiose self is infiltrated with aggression, and these patients obtain their sense of security and grandiosity by exercising power and threats, inspiring terror, and exerting sadistic control. These patients, in short, present a combination of narcissistic and paranoid features, with absence of superego functions manifested by antisocial behavior and ego-syntonic aggression directed against self or others. As an illustration, from all we know, both Hitler and Stalin clearly presented these features of malignant narcissism. Participants in mass movements dominated by such leaders are expected not only to submit to them but also to admire or love the leader, who is feared. The projection of the individual superegos of members of the mass movement onto such a leader may lead to the unbridled development of massive antisocial behavior. The totalitarian regimes of Nazi Germany and the Soviet Union illustrate these developments on a large social scale.

The implications of this relation between group regression, on the one hand, and certain features of leadership, on the other, are made more complex by the fact that even normal, functional leadership of institutions requires from the leader not only high intelligence, moral integrity, and understanding of others in depth but also small doses of narcissism and paranoia: narcissistic features in order to protect his or her internal security in the face of the ambivalence to which leaders are exposed and paranoid features as opposed to naïveté, that is, a motivated innocence that protects them from diagnosing accurately the negative currents that may limit or threaten leadership functions in an organization.

Regressive group processes and psychopathology of leaders that emerge under such regressive conditions reinforce each other. The situation is made even more dangerous by two social mechanisms that, on the one hand, may control group regression and protect the functional quality of institutions but, on the other, also may be infiltrated by destructiveness, thus worsening even further the institutional regression into violence.

These two social mechanisms are bureaucratization and ideology formation (Kernberg 1998). Bureaucratization refers to the organization of procedures, rules, and regulations that control the functioning of a group, or of groups within institutions, or institutions relating to one another. It controls group regression precisely by transforming an unstructured group situation into a structured one. *Robert's Rules of Order* are the simplest example of maintaining the structure of an assembly; the indispensable rules and regulations that control the relationships among staff and between supervisors and subordinates in organizations are another example of this structuring.

The problem is that, while such bureaucratic structures are indispensable for the functioning of social organizations, bureaucracies themselves tend to evolve into privileged groups with their own interests. In its interactions with those outside its boundaries, such an entrenched bureaucracy may express the same "fight-flight" characteristics that regressed groups display in their interior. In other words, aggression controlled within the bureaucratic organization may be displaced to its periphery and be reflected in the proverbial sadism of the lowly members of the bureaucracy toward outsiders and of the "guardians of the gates" of all institutions. At the same time, in large social institutions, such as state governments, an efficiently functioning bureaucracy may amplify and exaggerate the negative effects of the regressive leadership of a narcissistic, paranoid, or malignantly narcissistic leader. The immediate totalitarian transformation of Germany upon the assumption of Hitler was a testimony to the highly effective German bureaucracy. In a somewhat similar process, the Russian communist regime's bureaucracy was able to extend its powers throughout the entire Soviet Empire.

The second social mechanism for controlling group regression is the development of an ideology that cements relationships within a group and, when humanitarian in nature, may counteract the tendency to regressive activation of violence. The psychoanalytic study of ideologies illustrates that they, in turn, may vary along a broad spectrum, the polarities of which are characterized, on the one extreme, by what might be called narcissistic trivialization, and, on the other extreme, by a violent, paranoid fundamentalism. The middle region of ideologies usually is characterized by humanistic value systems.

Thus, for example, the lip service to communist ideals during the last two decades of the Soviet regime, an indispensable requirement to ascend the social and political ladder of the "Nomenclature," was cynically regarded by the large majority of the Soviet Union's population, a typical example of narcissistic trivialization. In contrast, the fundamentalist Marxism of terrorist groups, such as the Shining Path in Peru, the RAF in Germany, and the gangster regime of Pol Pot, illustrates the paranoid-fundamentalist polarity of Marxism where socially sanctioned violence dominates. The humanitarianism of western European Marxist movements in the 1970s and 1980s may be considered the humanist center of the ideology. As Green (1969) has pointed out, humanist or mature ideologies typically include respect for the individual, respect for autonomy and differences of viewpoints, and tolerance and protection of the privacy of the sexual couple and of family structure, as opposed to the efforts of fundamentalist ideologies to assert the social community's total control of individual life in all its aspects. Whether an individual enters a totalitarian ideological system, as Green also pointed out, depends on the maturity of the superego and of the ethical value systems of the individual: there is a complementary relationship between socially dominant ideologies and individual psychopathology.

There also exists an intimate connection between ideology formation and historical traumas. Vamik Volkan (1999) has pointed to how national identity is built into early ego identity by means of language, art, customs, food, and the intergenerational transmission of narratives of historical triumphs and traumas as part of this commonality of culture. The multiplicity of other individuals surrounding the infant, child, and young adult, all connected by common cultural traditions, contributes to the consolidation of ego identity in establishing common features of multiple self-representations in relating to multiple objects that have to be integrated in the shift from the paranoid-schizoid into the depressive position. By the same token, during severe group regression, such sociocultural commonalities become fundamental in linking the members of a social group with one another, cementing a common ideology, and compensating for the loss of individual identity with a group identity based upon both identification with a leader and a heightened sense of cultural identity embedded in a common historical background.

A number of factors, singly or in combination, can promote a shift of a dominant social or political ideology in the paranoid-fundamentalist direction, particularly in a culture with strong trends toward racism and religious warfare. These include severe social traumas, such as the loss of a war or territory, economic crisis, the threat of internal foreign groups or external enemies, or belonging to socially disadvantaged or suppressed social classes. Any of these conditions can foster group regression into a violent mob or mass movement.

To summarize: the various conditions that may determine the massive regression of a population and foster socially sanctioned violence and breakdown of ordinary morality and civilized human interaction are various combinations of unmetabolized social traumas; fundamentalist ideologies; primitive, particularly malignant narcissistic leadership; an effective, rigid bureaucracy; and the dissolution, by financial crisis or social revolution, of ordinary social structures and the task systems linked to them.

As Bracher (1982) pointed out, the ascent of a totalitarian leadership is fostered, in addition, by state control of the economy, the armed forces, and, particularly, the media. Moscovici (1981) has expanded Freud's analysis of mass psychology in pointing to how, historically, the printed word, the newspaper, radio, and television have successively increased the simultaneity of information for large masses, creating, in the process, an instant mass psychology with its inevitable regressive potential. This process continues with the growth of electronic communication. When watching television, we automatically tend to react in a more passive-narcissistic and/or paranoid way than would be the case when reading, for example, as a way of absorbing and metabolizing information in an individualized, autonomous manner.

Thus, regressive features of modern society emerge as a powerful counterpart to the increased opportunity for information sharing and education provided by the development of contemporary media. Media and mass psychology tend to move socially accepted systems of ideas regarding the meaning and history of the social structure in regressive directions, fostering a narcissistic superficiality or a paranoid sharpening of socially dominant ideology systems. Efficient bureaucracies and powerful control by the state apparatus may indirectly contribute to the activation of violence under conditions of social breakdown, if a fundamentalist party achieves control. In areas of poverty and extreme density of population, when such density and poverty are accompanied by destruction of family structure and traditional values, including, of course, those of religion, the activation of large group processes may induce random violence even within a society with stable social structures, a democratic system of government, and control of violence throughout society at large.

The characteristics of the massive regression of social groups include the lust for cruelty, dehumanization of out-groups, primitive self-idealization, conventionality and thoughtlessness, envy, and destructiveness: in short, both the characteristics of patients with severe personality disorders, particularly malignant narcissism, and the characteristics of regressive large group psychology. These, in essence, are the manifestations of evil not only at the level of the individual but at the level of group processes and political movements that may affect an entire society or nation.

Obviously, the description of the mutual reinforcement of individual, social, political, and cultural factors that determine the activation of unbridled aggression and social violence also implies potentially corrective factors, the urgency of which has become more evident, given the disastrous developments within the century that has just concluded.

In this chapter I cannot explore potentially preventive and controlling measures in detail, although it may be stated without exaggerating that we do know some corrective features, some preventive measures, and some means of control, although we have not achieved the ability on a social level to implement measures that could counteract the potential for malignant regression in communities or nations. Our present knowledge, stemming to quite an extent from psychoanalytic studies of individuals, indicates the importance of prevention of severe psychopathology from infancy and early childhood on; the protection of democratic systems of government; the importance of well-functioning social organizations as opposed to breakdown of task systems; and the need to achieve systems of distribution of the products of human labor that mitigate and control the effects of poverty, population density, and family disorganization.

The importance of the protection of the humanistic center of ideologies at the social and political level is the counterpart to the assurance of the development of healthy systems of moral values and ethical commitments on the part of the individual. Healthy superego structures of the individual are permanent structures, but socially dominant ideologies may shift rapidly toward regression, causing deterioration at the level of groups and social masses, of the effectiveness of individual ethical systems. The value of universally valid ethical systems such as those provided by organized religion has emerged as a major counterforce to the threats of massive group regression. Organized religion, of course, may also be infiltrated by socially sanctioned aggression in its shift into fundamentalist polarities, or lose its humanizing power through regressive trivialization at the narcissistic polarity, or become a corrupt and self-serving bureaucracy in opposition to the legitimate needs of society. This brings us back to the antinomy of evil and religiosity as basic characteristics of the human being.

Mature Religiosity: The Characteristics of the Deity and of Mature Religions

In what follows, I am carrying out a restricted analysis on the basis of psychoanalytic findings and concepts rather than attempting a philosophical and theological approach to religion. With regard to the individual superego, its characteristics include an integrated system of personal ethical values, a universal set of rules of behavior and rights, and a universal value system that transcends the individual.

More in detail, mature religiosity includes an integrated value system that transcends the individual's interest and has truly universal validity that applies to all human beings. It is a comprehensive and harmonious system, and its fundamental principles are love and respect of others and of the self. It includes a sense of responsibility for this value system that transcends all concrete laws, and expects such a sense of responsibility also on the part of other human beings, but with understanding, compassion, and concern in combination with a sense of universal justice. Such a mature religiosity includes the capacity for reconciliation, forgiveness, and reparation on the basis of understanding the unavoidable ambivalence of all human relationships. This value system includes prohibitions against murder and incest and the regulation of sexual relationships. Such regulation implies tolerance and protection of the loving couple and of the marital couple and of the privacy of their sexual freedom. Such a mature religiosity also includes tolerance, hope, confidence in goodness without denial of evil, and a sense of responsibility toward a higher moral instance that corresponds to the common ideal of humanity. Mature religiosity includes the investment of work and creativity as a contribution to the creation of what is good and the struggle against destructiveness. Mature religiosity, finally, includes respect for the rights of others and tolerance for unavoidable envy and greediness without letting them control one's own behavior.

It should be obvious that such characteristics, directly opposing the manifestations of evil within the individual, also may act as a powerful countercurrent against the temptation of seduction into a regressive mob, with its paranoid-schizoid ideology of dividing all humanity into good and bad, self-idealization and dehumanization of the enemy, rationalized cruelty and destructiveness, and blind obedience to a leader's autocratic rules of morality.

It is of interest to compare these characteristics of mature religiosity as an essential aspect of normal psychology with the nature of God as described in the religious systems of Western culture. In the Judeo-Christian tradition, God is described as sovereign of nature, the creator of the world; He maintains lawfulness of nature; He is kind, compassionate, forgiving yet punishing. He is transcendent, and His wisdom is the source of human understanding. Through revelation, He relates himself to humankind, and through redemption, He sanctifies all existence.

The correspondence between the characteristics of mature religiosity, derived from the various sources of development of the ego ideal and the superego and reflecting a dominance of love over hatred, of libido over the death drive as an aspect of psychological health and maturity, on the one hand, and the characteristics of the Deity in Judeo-Christian religions is striking. The emergent desire and necessity of a transcendent system of ethical values is one crucial *vertex*—to use Bion's term—of psychic functioning that evolves in parallel to the search for knowledge and truth and the search for, and creation of, beauty.

Returning once more to Freud's views of religion: his idealization of rationality missed, I think, the irreducible nature of the aspiration for a universal ethical system that transcends the rational needs of the individual, although it certainly considers them. His equalizing the psychological origins of religiosity with the illusional character of religion preempted unnecessarily a philosophical and theological approach. In all fairness, it obviously preceded the discovery of the creative and transcendent quality of the transitional aspect of psychological functioning in Winnicott's work.

Psychoanalysis may be considered one of the basic psychological sciences, together with the neurobiology of the central nervous system, but the understanding of human functioning cannot leave out the corresponding social psychological and cultural anthropological sciences in general. In the same way that psychoanalysis cannot provide a comprehensive analysis of artistic creation (although it certainly has much to say about the unconscious origins, motivations, and inhibitions of aesthetic creativity), I believe this also is true for the reality of a transpersonal, supraordinate system of ethical values as a basic precondition of human survival. Freud himself contributed to our understanding of the psychological origins and unavoidable reality of evil, in discovering the overshadowing influence of the dynamic unconscious on human existence.

Organized systems of religion are undoubtedly not free from such unconscious influences and from the regression toward the polarity of ideological systems referred to before. Our experience with patients illustrates how religion may be used as a rationalization for personal cruelty and destructiveness, how it may be transformed into obsessive-compulsive systems, and how the psychopathological deterioration and destruction of superego functions may lead to destructive and self-destructive antisocial behavior. But psychoanalysis cannot provide the answers for the truth value as opposed to the origins of universal ethical systems: it cannot become a weltanschauung. The psychological and social functions of religion as a hierarchically supraordinate, universal system of values, and the conception of God as the guarantor, or abstract principle, or unifying concept of a religious system may have its intuitive origin in the development of the psychic apparatus but cannot be contained, I believe, within the "scientific vertex" of psychoanalytic theory.

In contrast to Freud, I would conclude that science and reason cannot replace religion, that religiosity as a fundamental human capability and function has to be integrated in our understanding of normality and pathology, and that a universal system of morality is an unavoidable precondition for the survival of humanity. Psychoanalysis has given us fundamental information regarding the origin of religiosity but not a world conception or an arbitration of the philosophical and theological discussion regarding God.

At a clinical level, one of the functions of the psychoanalyst is to explore the extent to which religiosity as a mature desire for a transpersonal system of morality and ethical values as outlined is available to our patients. The function of the psychoanalyst is not that of a pastoral counselor or a guide to such a universal system of values; rather, the psychoanalyst's function is to free the patient from unconscious conflicts that limit this capability, including the systematic confrontation, exploration, and resolution of unconscious conflicts that preclude the development of concern, guilt, reparation, forgiveness, responsibility, and justice as basic aspirations of the individual. Psychoanalysis also has to help certain patients to free themselves from the use of formal religious commitments as a rationalization of hatred and destructiveness directed against self or others. Perhaps one might add, to Freud's suggestion that love and work are the two main purposes of life, that the commitment to morality and the appreciation of art are two further, major tasks and sources of meaning for the human being.

References

Bion WR: Experiences in Groups. New York, Basic Books, 1961
Bion WR: Attention and Interpretation. New York, Basic Books, 1970
Bracher KD: Demokratie und Ideologie im 20. Jahrhundert. Bonn, Germany, Bouvier-Verlag, 1982
Chasseguet-Smirgel J: Essai sur l'idéal du moi. Paris, Presses Universitaires de France, 1973

Chasseguet-Smirgel J: Creativity and Perversion. New York, WW Norton, 1984

Dicks HV: Licensed Mass Murder. New York, Basic Books, 1972

Fairbairn WRD: An Object Relations Theory of the Personality. New York, Basic Books, 1954

Freud S: Beyond the pleasure principle (1920), in The Standard Edition of the Complete Psychological Works of Sigmund Freud, Vol 18. Translated and edited by Strachey J. London, Hogarth Press, 1955, pp 1–64

Freud S: Group psychology and the analysis of the ego (1921), in The Standard Edition of the Complete Psychological Works of Sigmund Freud, Vol 18. Translated and edited by Strachey J. London, Hogarth Press, 1955, pp 65–143

Freud S: The future of an illusion (1927), in The Standard Edition of the Complete Psychological Works of Sigmund Freud, Vol 21. Translated and edited by Strachey J. London, Hogarth Press, 1961, pp 5–56

Furet F: The Passing of an Illusion. Chicago, IL, University of Chicago Press, 1999

Green A: Sexualité et idéologie chez Marx et Freud, Paris, Etudes Freudiennes, 1969, pp 187–217

Green A: Pourquoi le mal? in La folie privée (Recueil d'Articles 1971–1988). Paris, Gallimard, 1990, pp 370–401

Green A: Le travail du négatif. Paris, Les Editions de Minuit, 1993

Jacobson E: The Self and the Object World. New York, International Universities Press, 1964

Kernberg OF: Aggression in Personality Disorders and Perversions. New Haven, CT, Yale University Press, 1992

Kernberg OF: Love Relations: Normality and Pathology. New Haven, CT, Yale University Press, 1995

Kernberg O: Ideology, Conflict, and Leadership in Groups and Organizations. New Haven, CT, Yale University Press, 1998

Klein M: Mourning and its relation to manic-depressive states, in Contributions to Psycho-Analysis, 1921–1945. London, Hogarth Press, 1940, pp 311–338

Klein M: Notes on some schizoid mechanisms. Int J Psychoanal 27:99–110, 1946

Klein M: Envy and Gratitude. New York, Basic Books, 1957

Klemperer V: Ich will Zeugnis ablegen bis zum Letzten: Tagebücher 1933–1941. Berlin, Aufbau-Verlag, 1995a

Klemperer V: Ich will Zeugnis ablegen bis zum Letzten: Tagebücher 1942–1945. Berlin, Aufbau-Verlag, 1995b

Lord BB: Legacies: A Chinese Mosaic. New York, Knopf, 1990

Meissner W: Psychoanalysis and Religious Experience. New Haven, CT, Yale University Press, 1984

Meltzer D, Williams MD: The Apprehension of Beauty: The Role of Aesthetic Conflict in Development, Art, and Violence. Perthshire, Scotland, Clunie Press, 1988

Milgram S: Obedience to Authority. New York, Harper & Row, 1974

Moscovici S: L'âge des foules. Paris, Librairie Arthème Fayard, 1981

Ostow M (ed): Judaism and Psychoanalysis. New York, KTAV, 1982

Rayner E: What determines interpretation? The intuition of justice as a factor in interpretation. Revista Chilena de Psicoanálisis 11(2):31–41, 1994

Rizzuto A-M: The Birth of the Living God: A Psychoanalytic Study. Chicago, IL, University of Chicago Press, 1979

Sofsky W: The Order of Terror: The Concentration Camp. Princeton, NJ, Princeton University Press, 1993

Turquet P: Threats to identity in the large group, in The Large Group: Dynamics and Therapy. Edited by Kreeger L. London, Constable, 1975, pp 87–114

Volkan V: Das Versagen der Diplomatie. Gieen, Germany, Psychosozial-Verlag, 1999

Winnicott D: The development of the capacity for concern, in The Maturational Processes and the Facilitating Environment. New York, International Universities Press, 1965, pp 73–82

Zilboorg G: Freud and Religion. London, Geoffrey Chapman, 1958

Zinoviev A: The Reality of Communism. New York, Schocken Books, 1984

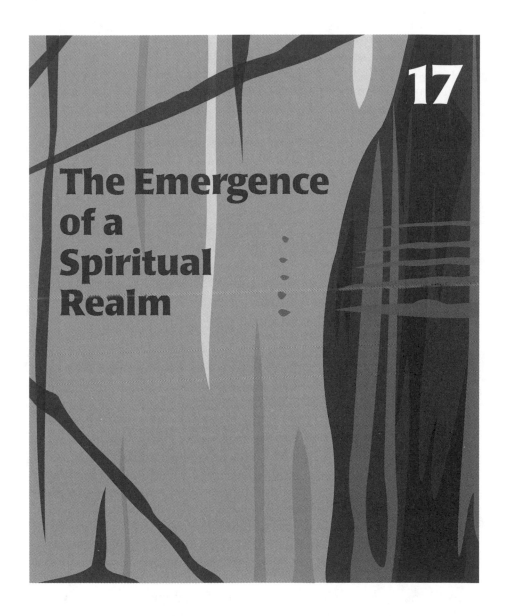

17

The Emergence of a Spiritual Realm

Presented at the Delphi International Psychoanalytic Symposium, Delphi, Greece, October 24–30, 2008.

Continuing the exploration of the experience of religiosity as a fundamental human potential, in this chapter I explore the functions of the spiritual dimension of human psychology. I describe the development, from internalized object relations, toward the creation of values in a world of spiritual aspirations, and relate this development to the establishment of formal religious belief systems.

The relationship between psychoanalysis and religion illustrates the general problem of the influence of ideological currents on scientific thinking. In recent years, we have been able to observe how, when the focus is on the conceptualization and classification of psychological illness, the closer the manifestations of psychopathology come to issues in the realm of cultural conflicts, the more supposedly scientific decisions are influenced by conventional morality and political ideology. I believe that psychoanalysis is not free from such influences. The controversy, for example, regarding the conceptualization of homosexuality, as well as the psychology of women, illustrates this point. Freud's analysis of the origin of religious beliefs in "The Future of an Illusion" (1927/1961) spelled out his critical view of religion and his expectations that, in the long run, a rational system of moral convictions and ethics would replace religion. He laid the foundation for our contemporary understanding of the infantile roots of religiosity and its fundamental function in dealing with the drives, particularly the relation between oedipal conflicts and childhood representations of God. However, Freud's faith (pun intended) in the replacement of religion by reason and, in a more general sense, by science stands in contrast to his theory of the profound influence of unconscious motivation over human life and of the correspondent limitations of reason. Freud assumed, as Lütz (2007) pointed out, that the belief in God was an illusion, and thus he started from an implicit, but clear, atheistic philosophical viewpoint. Several authors have criticized Freud's philosophical approach and the related implication that psychoanalysis be considered a weltanschauung. This critique was formulated, among others, by Chasseguet-Smirgel (1973), Meissner (1984, 1987), Ostow (1995), Rizzuto (1979, 1988), and Zilboorg (1958), whose writings pointed to the compatibility of religious convictions and a psychoanalytic identity. More recently, an excellent collection of essays on the relation of psychoanalysis to religion, edited by Black (2006), reveals a positive, open-minded exploration of the psychology of religious belief, its psychodynamic origin, and the philosophical questions raised by its relation to the truth hypothesis of religious convictions.

I believe that although an atheistic philosophical position prevailed among many leading psychoanalysts of an earlier generation, this may no longer be the case (Parsons 2006; Symington 2006). In what follows, I shall try to separate a psychoanalytic perspective from a strictly philosophical one, leaving open the philosophical question of the existence of God. I shall focus on the origin of religiosity as a dimension of spirituality derived from the internalized world of object relations but transcending it into a realm of experience no longer to be subsumed within that internal world.

Edith Jacobson (1964) described the gradual consolidation of the mature superego as the integration of successive layers of sadistic superego precursors, idealized superego precursors—reflecting, in turn, idealized representation of self and objects and, finally, the later oedipal phase of superego development. In this later phase, moral demands and prohibitions integrate with an earlier matrix in which sadistic/persecutory and idealized superego precursors are integrated. Overall, this process establishes a sense of morality that, while initially repressing infantile sexuality linked to oedipal conflicts, is eventually reworked in adolescence, leading to acceptance of mature love relationships, achieving the capacity for a commitment to a relationship in depth, and the integrations of erotic and tender emotions. Simultaneously, the superego's control of the transformation of aggressive impulses into adaptive autonomy and self-assertion contributes to the capacity to integrate libidinal and aggressive strivings at the service of developing generalized ethical systems and general laws of morality that involve the search for fairness and justice.

The optimal adult superego includes such an integrated system of personal ethical values and a universal set of rules of behavior and of rights and responsibilities. What characterizes this value system, beyond the reparative tendencies of the depressive position, and the derivatives of the resolution of oedipal conflicts, is its transcendence beyond the individual's instrumental interests; that is, the search for a truly universal validity that may apply to all human beings. Optimally, it is a comprehensive and harmonious system, and its fundamental principles are love and respect for others as well as the self. Responsibility for this value system transcends conventional laws, assumes a shared social and human contract with other human beings, and incorporates understanding, compassion, and concern for others in combination with a sense of universal justice.

I believe that these are the characteristics of a mature religiosity as a psychological function that includes the capacity for reconciliation, forgiveness, and reparation on the basis of understanding of the unavoidable ambivalence of all human relationships. This value system includes prohibitions against murder and incest and principles of regulation of sexual relationships. Such regulations imply sexual tolerance and the protection of a loving couple within the privacy of their sexual freedom. A mature religiosity also includes tolerance, hope, confidence in goodness without denial of evil, and a sense of responsibility toward moral principles that correspond to a common ideal of humanity. Mature religiosity includes the recognition of the need for investment in work and creativity as a contribution to what is good and to struggle against destructiveness. Finally, mature religiosity includes respect for the rights of others and tolerance for unavoidable envy and greed without letting them control one's own behavior.

Superego development reveals its origin in the struggle between love and hatred, in the reparative and sublimatory aspects of drives; and in this regard, it is clearly rooted in the developmental history of internalized object relations. This development includes the achievement and working through of the depressive position, the transformation of early transitional objects into the integration of cultural values, the transformation of the illusory nature of the transitional object into symbolic expression, and identification with cultural and ethical values. And, of course, the aspiration for love and justice incorporates the superego working through of the oedipal situation.

Bion (1970) has pointed to the mutual irreducibility of the "vertices" of truth, the scientific dimension; of beauty, the aesthetic dimension; and of goodness, the religious dimension. From a psychoanalytic viewpoint, the aesthetic sensibility and pleasure with our relationship with the arts; the ethical experience involved in conflicts around justice, punishment, reparation, and forgiveness; the complex structure of the experience of love; and the exciting search for scientific evidence seem, indeed, very different ways to approach human reality, but they do, ultimately, have common roots in the early internalization of object relations that constitute the matrix of the psychic apparatus. I believe that the evidence for the gradual transformation of the predominance of paranoid schizoid mechanisms into the depressive position, regardless of the timetable involved, has been amply confirmed by the study of early normal development as well as in severe psychopathologies and has relevance for the origin of all three "vertices" of experience.

The integration of love and hatred—of idealized and persecutory early object relations—is crucial for the establishment of the archaic superego, the tolerance of feelings of guilt and reparative impulses as normal aspects of the mourning process. An early acceptance of responsibility for one's actions, an early notion of justice, punishment, redemption, and forgiveness, is derived from such integrative processes.

Meltzer's (Meltzer and Williams 1988) hypothesis of the idealization of the surface of mother's body as the counterpart of the projection of aggression into the interior of her body and of the origin of the experience of beauty in this idealization of the surface of mother's body is, I believe, a reasonable hypothesis that may be linked to the idealization of the transitional object and transitional phenomena, so that the idealization of the breast, of mother, and of beautiful objects have a common origin. As Chasseguet-Smirgel (1984) has pointed out, artistic creativity also involves the sublimatory and defensive transformation of anal impulses in the aspiration and sense for beauty.

By the same token, efforts to understand and control nature and the material world, in order to influence and transform it, are linked to the sublimatory expression of aggressive impulses with reparatory trends, the motivation involved in instrumental and scientific creativity.

But the later developments in the realm of beauty, truth, and ethical values evolve into independent spheres of human experience and activity. Scientific evidence, ethical value systems, and artistic creativity evolve, indeed, into independent "vertices" in the approach to reality. But the autonomous development of these different realms of human experience implies a process of transformation that adds an element of transcendence to the individual's discovery of the values of his or her particular culture. This transcendence is expressed in the nature of the moral system that protects and elevates the entire social community, the exploration of the boundaries of our knowledge of space and time, the experience of the universal quality of great art, and the spiritual quality of a union in love. It is a world of values that point to the construction of meaning in the conscious life of human beings and constitute a higher level of cognition and experience in relation to the material world, the spiritual realm of experience. The content of this spiritual world of values is explored by philosophy, but the capacity of the individual to enter and develop within such a world of values, and deal with its limitations, belongs in the realm of psychoanalysis. It is this intermediary space, the individual's capacity to sense a spiritual reality, that applies to the relation between psychoanalysis and religion.

The major thesis of my presentation is that there exists a point at which experiences, judgments, and values derived from the internal world of object relations acquire a sense of universality that takes them out of the discrete world of internalized object relations and provides them with a sense of transcendence, of universal value within their respective domain. This development evolves into a spiritual realm. At the same time, that transcendental quality appears as rooted in external reality in a correspondence between internal experience and general laws affecting the human community and nature; that is, the world at large.

This raises the question to what extent, in that development, there exists an intuitive generalization of personal experience that corresponds to the perception of an objective reality independent of this development of human values. Does our development of spiritual values evolve into a global projection of such values, or does it correspond to the intuitive perception of a new realm of reality independent of human experience?

Psychoanalysis does not have the answer to this question, but it points to the universality of the psychological developments that make posing this question unavoidable. The transcendental nature of human spirituality leads to the quest for a realm of reality beyond material human limitation, in the realms of love relationships, in the discovery of beauty through the arts, and in the realm of moral law—a transcendental sense of justice. In a parallel development, in the search for truth in the scientific realm, there is equally a sense that scientific discoveries at the boundaries of human knowledge acquire a transcendental quality: here intellectual knowledge transcends into questions regarding the overall nature, origin, and sense of matter, space and energy, and time.

Simultaneously, there evolves a significant function of the spiritual realm to provide the basis for a humanistic ideology as the counterpart of the emergence of primitive aggression in the context of regressive group processes, particularly of large, unstructured groups (Kernberg 1998; Volkan 2004). One might say that religious ideologies play a potentially crucial role in the protection of social structures against such a regression, although, of course, religious ideology itself may be penetrated by regressive aggression. And not only mature superego functions, but also infantile prohibition against sexuality influence religious ideologies.

In the realm of love relationships, there is a significant difference between the search for fusion and primitive idealization in the infant-mother and child-parental relationship in general and that implied in falling in love in adolescence and adulthood. Adult love implies a broader knowledge of reality and a sense of nature, history, and art that provides the intimate relationship of the couple with a commonality of experience that infuses the love relationship with a sensitivity that constitutes an entirely new experience of universal values. To jointly experience art, enjoy nature, and examine the history of one's own past bring about the possibility of a dimension of love as a window of existence that opens a new and shared world of values that can be experienced together.

Here, then, the concrete implication of love as a maturational development of internalized object relations acquires a spiritual value—that is, a sense of a new, jointly created capacity to capture the intensity of beauty, the dramatic nature of the surrounding world, and the universal value of art that is difficult to achieve by an individual's isolated approach to those realities. The corresponding emotional experience may be rooted in the original "oceanic experience" linked to the emotional fusion of infant and mother, but its content has a general, transcendental value: a spiritual realm of the new encounter of love that cannot be equalized to its origin in early infancy and childhood. And, of course, adult love implies the overcoming of oedipal prohibitions and conflicts involving sexual intimacy.

Examining more closely the individual's relation to art, a similar development may be traced. From the admiration of mother—particularly, the idealization of her body surface—as the initial impulse to the experience of beauty, and the construction of a transitional object and its later substitutes (Winnicott 1953/1971), to the gradual capacity for the experience of the beauty of art is a long way. The capacity to symbolically express deep emotional contents of the mind gradually evolves in children's capacity to express themselves in painting and playful constructions and in their emotional reactions to and participation in music, theater, stories, and visual material. Gradually, when children and adolescents are provided with a facilitating social environment and the opportunity to acquire knowledge of the language of artistic expression, this capacity evolves into their sensitivity for the transcendental aspects of the message of art and its relation to universal human experience of the mysteries of beauty and nature, of love, and of the religious experience itself. The objective, material aspect of the artistic creation requires a corresponding sensitivity of the individual confronting it and opens a world of meanings that transcend the concrete world of individual experience. Just to use one example, Breugel's painting "The War Between Life and Death," in the Prado Museum, represents the human struggle between love and aggression, the collision of unmitigated destructiveness with the sublime qualities of music and love, all in the presentation of an objective world that veers from a condensed space of intense intimacy in love to the frightening infinity of the space of the legions of death.

And again, in the realm of superego development, from the primitive persecutory superego precursors and the idealizing structures of the ego ideal and the integrating features of the oedipal superego to the individualization, personalization, and abstraction of ethical values of the mature superego, a point is reached where the identification with the oedipal couple and its demands and prohibitions, rules, and expectations are transformed into a personal sense of moral values that include a sense of justice, generosity, forgiveness, and autonomy. This development transcends the instrumental aspects of daily life and the practicalities of life in an ordinary social environment and includes the aspiration for the triumph of those universal values that give sense and meaning to human existence. Obviously, such values and judgments are influenced by social and cultural environments and structures and, particularly, by religious commitments and ideology.

Here, in the realm of moral values and ethical systems, there exists both a protection of meaningful human existence and the threat of the infiltration of this realm by aggression itself, particularly in the implications of paranoid, fundamentalist ideologies and the regressive, narcissistic devaluation of ethical value systems.

This process of transformation of the world of internalized object relations into spiritual values also may be observed closely in the process of normal mourning, perhaps particularly in the case of the mourning over the loss of a beloved person with whom one has lived for many years. That mourning process frequently includes a painful sense of not having made use fully of all the opportunities that such a long life together would have provided. It is, as Rabbi Moshe Berger observed (personal communication, June 2006), as if only at a point of infinite absence were it possible to fully recognize the full value of the time of finite presence in love. That recognition is painful and reinforces the grief and longing for the object that has been lost. At the same time, this development stimulates an intense impulse to correct, compensate, and repair the experience that has been missed while the loved person was alive. Such repair is not possible in reality, there can be no forgiveness after death, and the solution that gradually emerges stems from the very persistence of the internal object relation with the lost object.

In the context of that permanent internal object relation, the unfulfilled life project of the person who has departed emerges as an internal mandate, an aspiration to be fulfilled by the mourner. This mandate, in turn, originates the search for experiences and actions that will fulfill the spirit of the desires, hopes, and expectations of the lost person, and these aspirations and actions acquire a spiritual meaning that transcends the concrete relationship in the context of which they are activated. This development becomes an ongoing source of pressure toward actions inspired by corresponding ideal value systems.

One general conclusion I draw from this development, from internalized object relations toward the creation of values in a world of spiritual aspirations, is that there exists a commonality of pressures in this direction in the various realms of human experience involving beauty, truth, justice, and love. These aspirations have their roots in the infantile experience of idealization of mother and the oedipal couple, the transitional world, and the developments of the depressive position. They operate in the direction of the actualization of transcendental values that jointly define religiosity as the aspiration for a general principle of the search for truth and knowledge, overall goodness and love, overall power committed to justice and protection against evil, and overall protection and creation of beauty.

Religiosity as a general function of the human psyche finds an expression in formalized religious convictions, whether a highly individualized commitment to a vaguely formulated but integrated system of values, or the adherence to one of the major religions of the Eastern or Western world, or some variation of them. Such religious systems provide order and integration and in their objectivity as cultural values, the reassurance for the power and the permanence of such values.

This brings us to the psychological aspects of the concept of God as the ultimate objective cause of reality and of the origin and mandate of the religious system of values. From the viewpoint of historical development, religious systems have been a universal characteristic of human societies, evolving from totemism to polytheism, and finally, to the monotheism of present-day mature religious systems. Throughout history, the attributes of God have increasingly reflected transcendental value systems that correspond to those emerging in the conscious and unconscious development of the ethical value systems of the human mind.

From a psychoanalytic viewpoint, the search for a personalized God, modeled, as Freud suggested, upon the idealized experience of the oedipal father, may explain an important source of religiosity but cannot, I believe, be considered to reflect an objective assessment of the existence of God. In fact, as mentioned before, Freud started from an atheistic philosophical position to analyze religion or, rather, religiosity. He assumed that the idea of God was an illusion. It is an open question, however, that transcends psychoanalytic exploration, to what extent religiosity as a human function corresponds to a development of a psychic apparatus that allows us to perceive and understand aspects of the objective reality of the universe, or whether the human mind is using psychic operations to project a spiritual reality onto the universe that really derives from a strictly human psychological experience. Is God a creation of the human being, or are we coming to understand aspects of reality that can best be subsumed in the concept of God as an ultimate omniscient, omnipotent, benign, and generous entity dominating the world? This is a question for philosophy and science, and I believe that psychoanalysis needs to avoid the temptation of becoming a weltanschauung.

Psychoanalysis has made essential contributions to the understanding of the origin of the capacity for religious experience, aspirations, and convictions, their roots in the unconscious life of the struggle between libido and aggression, in the context of the internalization of object relations, and in the vicissitudes of intrapsychic conflicts derived from the corresponding structural developments. Furthermore, in analyzing severe pathologies, we have expanded our knowledge about the limitations and distortions in the development of the superego and the evolution of the normal ego ideal. Severe deficits in the establishment and functioning of ethical values, as intrapsychic guidance and control systems, lead to and are part of severe psychopathology with antisocial features. A true capacity for full development of the religious experience, regardless of the system of religious convictions this applies to, is an important part of normal psychological functioning. And, correspondingly, mature religious systems should be centered on corresponding ideologies of love and tolerance, appreciation of goodness, protection against aggression, affirmation of the sanctity of human life, and respect for every individual's rights and autonomy.

The functions of a spiritual dimension of human psychology, whether embedded in a formal religious belief system or an idiosyncratic, searching spirituality, include the participation in a transcendental world of values that enriches personal life, creates a new level of human relationships, and deepens the capacity for love, the responsibility to moral values, and the resistance to the dangers of aggressive regression in group processes and ideological systems. Religious convictions, faith in God's existence, undoubtedly strengthen all these functions, regardless of whether or not they correspond to an ultimate truth that religiosity equips the individual to be able to perceive.

This brings us to the problem of significant distortions of religious experience derived from the aggressive infiltration of narcissistic and paranoid phenomena typical of culturally determined large group regression and the development of paranoid ideological systems. I referred in an earlier work (Kernberg 1998) to the humanistic center of contemporary religious systems, which may be contrasted to their potential regression into a paranoid polarity in the form of religious fundamentalism, on the one hand, and, on the other, into a narcissistic conformist conventionalism that preserves the religious tenets but deprives them of their profound meaning. This is particularly true under conditions of societal regression into cultural stagnation in dominant but decadent, frail social structures. Applying a psychoanalytic analysis of large group processes, religious systems may be examined in terms of the extent to which form and content, basic principles, and the reality of social behavior are harmonious and consistent with correspondent universal norms of justice, respect, and protection of individual and society against the dominance of aggression.

From the viewpoint of the psychoanalyst's focus on the religious experience of individual patients, the view expressed in this chapter implies the need for profoundly respecting religious convictions of our patients if they are part of a harmonious, integrated system of ethical convictions and do not serve the purpose of rationalized regressive superego pressures on self and on others. Sadistic superego features are frequently rationalized and masked as enactments of religious commands and prohibitions, and carefully sorting out the misuse of religion from such a sadistic motivation should permit the transformation of the sadistic attitude in the patient's religious system, confronting the rationalizations of aggression. By the same token, severe splitting operations, by which the nonconflictual adherence to a religious system with a reasonable, integrated morality coexists with an unmitigated dishonesty and unethical behavior, require the analysis of these defensive operations and exposure of the hypocritical and dishonest use of ideological convictions as a denial of immoral and antisocial behavior.

The role of the psychoanalyst, as Ernst Ticho (1972) pointed out many years ago, is not to be moralistic but to operate from a moral viewpoint. And this, I believe, holds true also for psychoanalysis as an institution, where authoritarian pressures may cause immoral institutional behavior running counter to the general ethical system commonly agreed upon as part of the governance of psychoanalytic institutions. Freud believed that, at the end, reason would replace religion: but this belief, as we have seen, was contrary to Freud's deep conviction that the forces of the unconscious would always overshadow human behavior, and his profound pessimism regarding a morally ordered world seems more realistic today than ever. The efforts in the twentieth century of fundamentalist ideologies to replace religion by "scientific" systems of ethical principles led to the rationalized murder of millions of people by Marxist communism and Fascist nationalism (Furet 1999).

From a psychoanalytic viewpoint, we have to be alert to the possibility that all ideological systems, including religious ones, may be infiltrated by primitive aggression, but this does not deny the importance of these very ethical principles to provide social and cultural assurances against socially tolerated aggression. The struggle within the individual to transform the superego into a normal guidance system against distorted regressive ideological influences repeats itself in the social realm.

In conclusion, psychoanalysis has important contributions to make to the understanding of the origin, development, and functions of religiosity as a fundamental human principle, and to the ideological distortions of religious systems, but not in regard to the objective truth of the ideological assumptions of religious convictions. From a viewpoint of open system theory, the development of intrapsychic structures into a spiritual world of value systems may be considered as parallel to the development of neurobiological structures, particularly perception, cognition, affects, and memory, into a realm of psychological structures: the intrapsychic structures and their development explored by psychoanalysis. These structures are the basis of the humanistic core of religious systems, parallel at a social and cultural level to the functions of the mature superego for the individual.

References

Bion WR: Attention and Interpretation. New York, Basic Books, 1970

Black DM (ed): Psychoanalysis and Religion in the 21st Century: Competitors or Collaborators? New York, Routledge, 2006

Chasseguet-Smirgel J: Essai sur l'idéal du moi. Paris, Presses Universitaires de France, 1973

Chasseguet-Smirgel J: Creativity and Perversion. New York, WW Norton, 1984

Freud S: The future of an illusion (1927), in The Standard Edition of the Complete Psychological Works of Sigmund Freud, Vol 21. Translated and edited by Strachey J. London, Hogarth Press, 1961, pp 5–56

Furet F: The Passing of an Illusion. Chicago, IL, University of Chicago Press, 1999

Jacobson E: The Self and the Object World. New York, International Universities Press, 1964

Kernberg O: Ideology, Conflict, and Leadership in Groups and Organizations. New Haven, CT, Yale University Press, 1998

Lütz M: GOTT. Munich, Germany, Pattloch Verlag, 2007

Meissner W: Psychoanalysis and Religious Experience. New Haven, CT, Yale University Press, 1984

Meissner WW: Life and Faith: Psychological Perspectives on Religious Experience. Washington, DC, Georgetown University Press, 1987

Meltzer D, Williams MD: The Apprehension of Beauty: The Role of Aesthetic Conflict in Development, Art, and Violence. Perthshire, Scotland, Clunie Press, 1988

Ostow M: Ultimate Intimacy: The Psychodynamics of Jewish Mysticism. Madison, CT, International Universities Press, 1995

Parsons M: Ways of transformation, in Psychoanalysis and Religion in the 21st Century: Competitors or Collaborators? Edited by Black DM. New York, Routledge, 2006, pp 117–131

Rizzuto A-M: The Birth of the Living God: A Psychoanalytic Study. Chicago, IL, University of Chicago Press, 1979

Rizzuto A-M: Why Did Freud Reject God? A Psychodynamic Interpretation. New Haven, CT, Yale University Press, 1998

Symington N: Religion: the guarantor of civilization, in Psychoanalysis and Religion in the 21st Century: Competitors or Collaborators? Edited by Black DM. New York, Routledge, 2006, pp 191–201

Ticho EA: Termination of psychoanalysis: treatment goals, life goals. Psychoanal Q 41:315–333, 1972

Volkan V: Blind Trust: Large Groups and Their Leaders in Times of Crisis and Terror. Charlottesville, VA, Pitchstone, 2004

Winnicott DW: Transitional objects and transitional phenomena (1953), in Playing and Reality. New York, Basic Books, 1971, pp 1–25

Zilboorg G: Freud and Religion. London, Geoffrey Chapman, 1958

Index